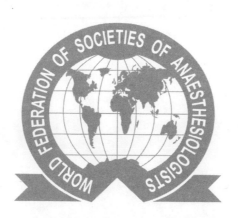

"to make available the highest
standards of anaesthesia
to all peoples of the world"

*(The Netherlands Official Gazette
of Friday, August 17ᵗʰ, 1956)*

Springer
Milan
Berlin
Heidelberg
New York
Hong Kong
London
Paris
Tokyo

A. Gullo - J. Rupreht (Eds)

World Federation of Societies of Anaesthesiologists
50 Years

Contributors
D.R. Bacon • T.C.K. Brown • M. Chobli • E.A. Damir • M. Dobson
R. Eltringham • C.H. Hoskins • M. Mauve • O. Mayrhofer • A.E.E. Meursing
E.M. Papper† • N. Parbhoo • C. Parsloe • J. Robins • M. Rosen • K. Shimoji
P. Sim • M. Vickers • D.J. Wilkinson • J.S.M. Zorab

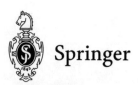 Springer

ANTONINO GULLO
Department of Perioperative Medicine,
Intensive Care and Emergency
Trieste University School of Medicine
Trieste, Italy

JOSEPH RUPREHT
Department of Anesthesiology
Erasmus University, Rotterdam, The Netherlands
and University of Ljubljana, Slovenia

Springer-Verlag is a part of Springer Science+Business Media

springeronline.com

© Springer-Verlag Italia, Milano 2004

ISBN 88-470-0252-4

Library of Congress Cataloging-in-Publication Data:
World Federation of Societies of Anaesthesiologists: 50th anniversary book / A. Gullo, J.
  Rupreth, eds. ; foreword by P. Scherpereel.
     p. ; cm.
  Includes bibliographical references and index.
  ISBN 8847002524 (alk. paper)
     1. World Federation of Societies of Anaesthesiologists--History. 2.
  Anestesiology--Societies, etc.--History. I. Title: 50th anniversary book. II. Gullo, A. III.
  Rupreth, Joseph, 1946- IV. World Federation of Societies of Anaesthesiologists.
  [DNLM: 1. World Federation of Societies of Anaesthesiologists. 2.
  Anesthesiology--history. 3. Societies, Medical--history. WO 11.1 W927 2004]
  RD82.W676 2004
  617.9'6'0601--dc22

                                                                    2004042741

Typesetting and cover design: Graficando (Milan, Italy)
Printing and binding: Grafiche Erredue (Cirimido, Italy)

Printed in Italy

SPIN: 10988855

*Sponsored by
an unrestricted educational grant
from Organon, a leader
in the research and development
of neuromuscular blocking agents
since 1964*

Congratulations to the WFSA
on the occasion
of its **50ᵗʰ anniversary**
celebrated at the
WCA Congress 2004

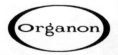

FOREWORD FROM THE PRESIDENT OF THE 13ᵀᴴ WORLD CONGRESS OF ANAESTHESIOLOGISTS

Ph. Scherpereel

The World Federation of Societies of Anaesthesiologists (WFSA) will celebrate this year the 50th anniversary of its creation. WFSA was formally constituted at the World Congress of Anaesthesiologists (WCA) in Scheveningen, the Netherlands, in 1955. The French Society of Anaesthesiologists (SFAR) is proud to host the 13th WCA and to open a new chapter of the history of this venerable institution. During this half century, the WFSA has grown and developed many activities. From 28 initial founder member societies, the WFSA now has over 100 member societies grouped in regional sections.

WFSA is mainly involved in education through educational programmes in many developing countries worldwide, in intensive courses and training centres. Its publications of books and regular issues of *Update in Anaesthesia* in five languages (French, Spanish, Russian, Mandarin, and English) constitute a substantial contribution to the development of anaesthesia in the developing world. Not less important than education is the major role that WFSA plays in the development of solidarity and friendship among anaesthesiologists of all nations.

Today, when fast means of transportation shorten distances and electronic mailing greatly reduces the time for communication, the world is becoming a large village and people need to meet, to share knowledge, and to avoid conflicts.

The history of WFSA has been punctuated with superb congresses, which were all successful and marked by prestigious anaesthesiologists who have contributed to the tremendous progress of the specialty during these first 50 glorious years.

To celebrate this golden jubilee the WFSA has produced a commemorative book. Antonino Gullo and Joseph Rupreht have collected chapters from many contributors to tell the story of the first half-century of the WFSA. It was a huge and difficult job, but the result is brilliant and I am convinced that many colleagues will be delighted to have this exciting book, dedicated to the memory of the World Federation of Societies of Anaesthesiologists.

Foreword from the WFSA Honorary Secretary and from the President

A.E.E. Meursing, T.C.K. Brown

The path along which anaesthesia has developed in the quest for expanding knowledge, skills, and experience was trodden at first by but a few, then by many. In the last 50 years, the scope of anaesthesiology has widened and many aspects of our specialty have formed due to the enormous growth in scientific and medical discoveries. Thus, national anaesthesia societies - already present in some countries - were formed and came to flourish.

The World Federation of Societies of Anaesthesiologists was founded in September 1955 after informal meetings had commenced in 1951 to explore the possibilities of a world body in anaesthesia. Their aim was and is:

to make available the highest standards of anaesthesia, pain treatment, and resuscitation to all peoples of the world

Appreciative that some of the founders were around, able, and willing, the WFSA executive committee (1998) agreed to commission this 50-year commemorative book to be presented to the national member societies on the occasion of the World Congress of Anaesthesiologists in Paris, France, in 2004.

The editors Professor A. Gullo and Professor J. Rupreht are to be warmly congratulated on a task excellently completed. The contributing authors, in particular Maarten Mauve, and John Zorab, deserve our appreciation. We owe thanks to Organon International that this book could be printed and disseminated at this time.

May the contents of this book provide insight and knowledge of the history of anaesthesia, not from a professional but from an organisational aspect. Without this organisation many patients in the world would still be suffering. After all, we do not know where we are going if we do not know where we come from.

TABLE OF CONTENTS

APPENDIX

1 WFSA 50 YEARS EDITORIAL REMARKS

J. Rupreht, A. Gullo

Writing history of anaesthesia

The World Federation of Societies of Anaesthesiologists (WFSA) was established much later than the most-famous national societies of anaesthesia but much earlier than most of its constituent members. This is why the organisation saw a fivefold increase of its membership within 50 years.

Half a century is long enough a period to estimate the value of an organisation to society, its viability, and prospects for the future. Changes in society may strengthen any organisation or make it dissolve. The WFSA is very mature being 50 next year, but is not old. The organisation has adapted to the ever-changing world by remaining youthful, enabling it to readjust its course to the ever-elusive goal of better anaesthesia for all people of the world.

A historical record of the WFSA is a sign of organisational and professional maturity. The decision to produce the commemorative book was not an isolated one but was a part of the very popular writing of the history of anaesthesia. The catalyst for a history of professional anaesthesia was the First International Symposium on the History of Anaesthesia at Rotterdam in 1982. This was regarded as a historical event by the famed historian Gwenifer Wilson, and has been repeated at 4-yearly intervals ever since, with ever increasing success. Each time a valued book of proceedings is produced. Several national societies of anaesthesiologists have produced commemorative books to celebrate and document either 40 or 50 years of existence. Without trying to be exhaustive, such books have been published in Australia, South Africa, Great Britain, The Netherlands, Scandinavia, Switzerland, and Germany. The latest 2003 addition to this remarkable body of medical and cultural history is the *Origins of Anaesthesia*, which was published in Spain.

To commemorate WFSA-50 years

It was during the WFSA-sponsored East Africa anaesthesia meeting in Harare, Zimbabwe, 1977, that a decision was taken to produce a commemorative book - WFSA-50 years. It was de facto Anneke Meursing's idea based on knowledge of very successful national anaesthesia history books. The WFSA officers wished the book to appear at the time of the 13th World Congress of Anaesthesiologists in Paris in 2004. There seemed to be a wealth of time and opportunity to produce the book.

Anneke Meursing, the Honorary Secretary of the WFSA, approached the past WFSA President John Zorab with the request to produce a commemorative book and an offer to be a member of the editorial board. The other two proposed members were Professor Maarten Mauve and Joseph Rupreht. M. Mauve had been the secretary to the World Congress of Anaesthesia in 1955 when the WFSA was established. For participants of the 10th World Congress, also in The Hague, he wrote a remarkable early WFSA history, in 1992. Joseph Rupreht had experience with editing historical essays on anaesthesia (*Essays*, 1985) and with helping to co-edit the 40 years' history of the Dutch Association of Anaesthesiologists. John Zorab was asked to chair the editorial board or committee, "with his capable skills and enthusiasm".

Dr. Meursing's letter of 28 August 1977 was promptly answered and John Zorab wondered whether it was time to say yes or no. He wanted it to be established who would take over as editor-in-chief should someone fall by the wayside. Furthermore, Zorab envisaged a large editorial board to aid the chief and the two assistant editors. Furthermore, financial help would be required. The initial office and mail expenditure would become much larger as, in the course of time, the book neared production. At that time no one knew what a book would cost and where the money would come from. Zorab wanted to clarify many issues about the enterprise before saying yes. This letter raised so many questions and gave no answer. It was sent to A. Meursing, M.D. Vickers, M. Rosen, T.C.K. Brown, and R. Eltringham, but not to the two assistant editors. The early idea was to describe the WFSA history decade by decade.

Early problems with the book

No straightforward answers to many of Zorab's questions were forthcoming by the end of 1997. An expense of U.S. $ 40,000 was envisaged, for which approval of the WFSA Executive Committee officers was sought but was not obtained. Such matters, it was thought, could only be settled during the meetings in connection with the 4-yearly World Congresses. John Zorab suspended editorial activities and so did M. Mauve. There was a brainstorming meeting of A. Meursing and J. Rupreht on 1 May 1998, at Rotterdam. It was thought that preparations for the book should continue while all efforts were made to secure finances. The idea to produce only a very limited number of copies was discarded so that every delegate to the Paris 2004 congress would get a copy. After many attempts to secure money, A. Meursing successfully negotiated sponsorship of the book by the Organon Company. This solution also ensured that the book would be printed in thousands, allowing some extra copies for public relations purposes.

Before the end of 1998, J. Zorab and M. Mauve resigned from the project. This caused problems on two fronts because they stopped writing their contributions and all negotiations with publishers were discontinued.

The *deus ex machina* solution to all troubles evidently was the energetic and encouraging promise to J. Rupreht by A. Gullo from Trieste to join A. Meursing's WFSA book project. Not only had Professor Gullo edited dozens of books, he also was the best negotiator with the new publishers, Springer-Verlag Italia. Gullo's role as co-editor made it largely unnecessary to depend further on external editorial advice. The prospect of producing the book seemed very promising in 1999 and there seemed to be time enough to do so before the Paris congress.

Final choice of contents

It became obvious that a repetitive presentation of the WFSA history would do no justice to a myriad of interesting topics. Instead of writing decade by decade only, many contributions relate to the WFSA connections with different regions of the world, to educational and financial aspects, to World Congresses, and to future challenges, along with hopes for the WFSA of the future. The proposal for the new contents and for the co-authors was presented at the Montreal meeting of the Executive Committee. With minor changes, all the suggestions of Rupreht/Gullo were accepted and, at long last, A. Gullo officially became a co-editor. Thankfully, the previous editors Zorab and Mauve were among the co-authors once more.

As the period from 2000 to 2003 passed, there were several factors causing delay, one of which was a problem with the sponsorship. The deadline was moved repeatedly forward and our working partners at Springer-Verlag, Dr. Hofmann and Dr. Rizza, deserve many thanks for their patient understanding.

Several transcontinental joint sessions have taken place to prepare the WFSA-50 years for publication. The editors met in Trieste, Brussels, Lille, Rotterdam, Montreal, and Milan. In the end, it has taken the joint effort of many individuals to produce the first history of the WFSA. The Departments of Anaesthesiology at Rotterdam and Trieste merit the sincerest appreciation for playing the decisive background role, yet again re-establishing their international place in education.

2 THE LONG WAY TOWARDS THE ESTABLISHMENT OF THE WFSA

M. Mauve

Introduction

Although not a historian, I have nevertheless assumed the task of writing a chapter on the history of the establishment of the WFSA. So I am a historian now! E.H. Carr [1], in his reflections on history and on the role of the historian, compares the course of history with a moving procession winding along the past. "The metaphor", he writes, "is fair enough, provided it does not tempt the historian to think himself as an eagle surveying the scene from a lonely crag or as a V.I.P. at the saluting base. Nothing of the kind! The historian is just another dim figure trudging along in another part of the procession." And he concludes: "The historian is part of history. The point in the procession at which he finds himself determines his angle of vision over the past."

These words have prompted me to write a few lines about myself. After 8 years as a general practitioner, which included World War II, I decided to become an anaesthesiologist. From 1947 I was trained for that specialty, which at the time did not exist in my country. From 1953, in my capacity as President of the newly founded Netherlands' Society of Anaesthesists, I was concerned with the organisation of a World Congress of Anaesthesiologists, to be held in 1955 in my country, with the object of establishing the World Federation of Societies of Anaesthesiologists (WFSA). So my vision is limited to those years and this determines my perspective. The rest of my knowledge is derived from archives in The Netherlands, in London, and in Paris, and from literature and letters from or discussions with anaesthesiologists active at the time.

With regard to the text of this article the following remarks are made. For historical reasons all countries are named as they were at the time of the foundation of the WFSA. The term "anaesthesiologist" is used, even when at the time or currently other terms are used, the original terms and spelling ("e" versus "ae") are followed. Finally the author wishes to stress that much of this record, both text and illustration, is derived from his study published at the 10th World Congress of the WFSA in 1992 in The Hague, The Netherlands, [2] by courtesy of its publisher.

The beginning

The WFSA, established 9 September 1955 at the World Congress of Anaesthesiologists held at Scheveningen, The Netherlands, owes its origins to several events in a variety of countries spread over a period of decades. The question arises: which circumstances facilitated the eventual birth? For the success of any organisation to be set up, the time has to be ripe for its purposes and, vise versa, the purposes have to fit into the time. Considering this view, in this record of the birth of the WFSA attention is paid to the desire for international relations, which emerged strongly after World War II, to the state of anaesthesiology at the time, to early and later relevant events, to the wisdom of the concerning parties to steer the enterprise into the right channels, to the many anaesthesiologists from countries all over the world who have contributed to the creation of the WFSA and, last but not least, to the most-welcome material and financial assistance from outside.

The post-war desire for international relations and the state of anaesthesia at the time

The desire for cordial international relations after World War II is well documented and understandable. In the field of medicine this desire led to the establishment of international contacts and, above all, to travelling. Many specialists went abroad, mainly to Great Britain and the United States, in order to increase their knowledge and skills to international levels. It is noteworthy that many specialists, again mainly from Great Britain and the United States, visited other countries in which medicine was less well developed, to lecture on the development of their specialties. In addition, this travelling in itself stimulated the trend for international relations.

In this climate, the setting up of international projects in anaesthesia seemed logical. One of the first was the foundation of the Confederacion Latinoamericana de Sociedades de Anestesiologia (CLASA) [3, 4], which was announced at the Argentine Congress in 1949, although established de facto some years after. Other examples are the Scandinavian Society of Anaesthesiology, founded in 1949 [5] and the series of combined congresses of the Austrian, German, and Swiss Societies of Anaesthesiologists, which started in 1951. On a much smaller scale were the combined meetings of the Belgian and Dutch societies, started in 1948. Apart from their shared scientific interests, these organisations also had in common linguistic and geographical aspects. Their actual influence on the foundation of the WFSA may have been negligible but they certainly helped to set the stage.

In this context the establishment of the Anaesthesiology Centre in Copenhagen occupies a special place. It was set up in 1950 by a joint venture of the World Health Organisation, the National Health Service of Denmark, and the Medical Faculty of the University of Copenhagen, with the object to provide basic training in anaesthesia to medical personnel from countries all over the world. The relatively short courses were conducted until 1973 and had a total of 650 trainees from 65 different countries [6]. In the beginning many of the leading teachers were from Great Britain and the United States and several were later involved in the setting up of the WFSA.

Great Britain and the United States were far ahead of other countries in the field of anaesthesiology after World War II. There were only a limited number of other countries where the practice of anaesthesia was based on sound physiological and pharmacological principles.

During World War II with its attendant isolation of large parts of the world, the possibilities for the development of anaesthesiology were very limited. A great deal had to be made up and great was the assistance rendered by anaesthesiologists from Great Britain and the United States. It was a very lively period during which the basic views on anaesthesia, which today are common knowledge, were absorbed by the trainees.

The realisation that anaesthesia not only had to keep up with progress in surgery but also that anaesthesia, in itself, made certain surgical procedures possible was very stimulating, as was also the participation in pre- and post-operative patient care. Concurrent with the efforts to fill the post-war anaesthetic vacuum, many societies of anaesthesiologists were founded and several new journals of anaesthesia were published.

To summarise, the rapidly progressing state of anaesthesia in conjunction with the strong trend towards internationalism made the time ripe for a worldwide organisation of anaesthesiologists.

Early relevant events

For the early events, one has to go back to the well-known American anaesthesiologist Francis Hoeffer McMechan (Fig. 1) (1879-1939), the intrepid advocate for the progress and the co-ordination of anaesthesia, first in the United States and Canada, and subsequently also in other parts of the world, including Latin America, Europe, and Australia. In 1919 he established the National Anesthesia Research Society from which in 1925, by amalgamation of several regional societies, the International Anesthesia Research Society (IARS) was born [7]. This society operated and still operates extensively in the United States and Canada and in a smaller way in other countries. In 1934 McMechan, hearing the news of the establishment of the French Society for the Study of Anaesthesia and Analge-

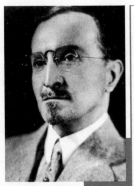

Fig. 1.
Francis Hoeffer McMechan (photograph courtesy of the Wood Library/Museum of Anesthesiology, Park Ridge, Illinois, USA)

sia sent a letter to Paris in which he urged mutual co-operation. Two years after, the French surgeon Desmarest attended the IARS congress in Philadelphia [8]. McMechan then suggested the French organise an anaesthesia congress in Europe. This suggestion bore fruit and the decision was taken by the surgeon Robert Monod (1884-1970) (Fig. 2). To organise the First French Anaesthesiology Congress in Paris in July 1940. Although this congress would not attain international status, it was expected that a large number of different countries would be represented [9]. However, due to world events this congress had to be cancelled.

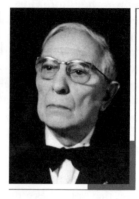

Fig. 2.
*Robert Monod
(1884-1970)*

Later events and the spark that set things on fire

After the war the plan to organise an anaesthesiology congress in Paris was revived by Monod and this eventually led to the International Anaesthesiology Congress in Paris from 20 to 22 September 1951 [10]. (Note the change in its title from "French" to "International"). One of the topics on the scientific programme was the "Creation of an International Movement for the Study of Anaesthesiology", to be introduced by the surgeon Marcel Thalheimer.

For a better understanding of what follows a short intermezzo is inserted. The French Society differed in essential respects from the IARS. Whilst the purpose of both societies was to promote research and to publish a journal, the French society was founded by surgeons and it was not planned to develop into an association of anaesthesiologists [11]. It was open to all physicians and scientists interested in anaesthesia, whereas the IARS, like the British Association, was founded by anaesthesiologists and its membership restricted to that category.

It was evident that the Société Française, which in 1950 consisted of only 16 anaesthesiologists among its 108 ordinary members [12] and which was, moreover, run by surgeons, would require the co-operation of other anaesthesiologists. The obvious choice for this purpose was the large and well-organised Association of Anaesthetists of Great Britain and Ireland. The contact was made by letter from the French Embassy in London, dated 1 February 1951 [13] and on 2 March an unofficial meeting took place in that city [14]. Present were Alexander Low, President of the association, John Gillies (Fig. 3) Ronald Jarman, Ivan Magill, and Geoffrey Organe (Fig. 4) and, from France, the surgeon Marcel Thalheimer. The latter expounded his plan for the founding of an international society with the French ideas as a guideline for its membership. To this author's mind the British must have been surprised by these ideas as well as to be confronted with an anaesthetic society run by surgeons. The discussions led to the conclusion to hold a further exploratory meeting in Paris in May.

The Paris meeting, on 5 May 1951, was presided over by R. Monod [15]. Amongst the 14 present were also representatives from Belgium, Denmark (also for Norway and Sweden), Italy, The Netherlands, and Switzerland who were invited by a letter circulated from the French society. Thalheimer again expounded his concept for an international society. Very soon a serious difference in opinion developed between those wishing to gather together specialised anaesthesiologists only and those who wanted to include all physicians and scientists interested in anaesthesia. In view of these contradictory ideas, the British anaesthesiologists suggested that there should not be too great a hurry to form an international society, but this was reject-

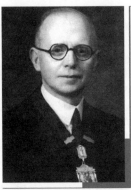

Fig. 3.
John Gillies

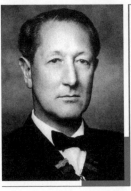

Fig. 4.
Geoffrey Organe

ed by Thalheimer. In a letter to Thalheimer [16] dated July 1951, Low emphasised the strong British sentiments concerning the admission of any members other than anaesthesiologists. He suggested contacting the anaesthesiologists in the United States, but to no avail.

In the meantime Organe had sounded out the opinion of anaesthesiologists from a number of English-speaking countries [17]. It was unanimously agreed that there must be an international society, but including only anaesthesiologists and certainly not surgeons. Opinions were, however, divided as to whether an entirely new society should be set up, some thinking that an adaptation of the existing International Anesthesia Research Society would be sufficient.

With a view to the further developments, it should be noted that 2 weeks prior to the French congress in Paris from 20 to 22 September 1951, another congress of anaesthesiologists was held in London, namely the combined congress of the International Anesthesia Research Society USA and the Association of Anaesthetists of Great Britain and Ireland from 3 to 7 September 1951. As this congress also attracted members from other countries, it provided a natural opportunity to discuss Thalheimer's projects. On 6 September an informal meeting of representatives from 15 different countries took place with H.R. Griffith (Canada) in the chair. The report by John Gillies of this meeting

has been preserved [18]. Besides Grif-
fith (who also represented the Inter-
national Anesthesia Research Society),
the British representatives John Gillies,
R. Jarman, K. Lloyd Williams, I.W.
Magill, and G.W.S. Organe and the
French surgeon Marcel Thalheimer.
The following anaesthesiologists were
present: O. Felder-Argentine, E. Lopes
Soares-Portugal, F. Leventhal-Australia,
D. Monton-Spain, A. Goldblat-Bel-
gium, G.F.V. Anson-New Zealand,
O.V. Ribiero-Brazil, T. Gordh-Sweden,

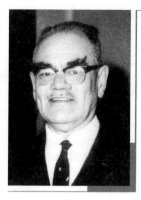

Fig. 5.
*C.R. Ritsema
van Eck*

G. Cousineau-Canada, A.W. Friend-USA, E. Ciocatto-Italy (Section of Anesthetics AMA), V.O. McCormick-Ireland, W. Metz-USA, C.R. Ritsema van Eck
(Fig. 5) The Netherlands.

During the general discussion on the steps so far taken by the French to
initiate an international organisation of anaesthesiologists, most participants
were of the opinion that the whole matter should proceed carefully and
slowly. The representatives of a few European societies, however, felt that
action should be taken soon and thus followed the French lead. With regard
to the creation of an international anaesthesia society open to non-anaesthesiologists as strongly proposed by Thalheimer, a considerable majority
was against this form of membership.

It was even feared that this might have the unfortunate effect of splitting
the anaesthesiologists into two groups, for and against, with each group having their own society. In fact, voices were heard to that effect. The proposal to found a second international anaesthesia organisation also caused some
hostility. It was considered that the International Anesthesia Research Society (USA) had done reasonably well in the international field for many years.
In reaction to this the opinion was advanced that its objectives were limited
and that its influence in Europe was negligible. To summarise, strongly conflicting views about the setting up of a world organisation of anaesthesiologists, desired by all parties, manifested themselves in rather a sharp way.

In a letter of 17 September [19] Organe warned Thalheimer not to proceed too hurriedly, as the resistance to his plans was really very great. He suggested that a small committee be formed to draw up the rules for an international society and to adapt them until they were acceptable to all national societies, "a formidable task". Nevertheless, on 22 September 1951, at the
final session of the international congress in Paris under the chairmanship of
Monod, Thalheimer put forward his proposals for an international society in
the form of a federation of national societies, open to all medical personnel
interested in anaesthesia. Its members would be divided into different sections
for anaesthesiologists, surgeons, physicians, chemists, pharmacologists, phys-
iologists, and veterinary surgeons [20].

To cut a long story short, after fierce discussions the representatives of 32 national societies participating at the congress, in accordance with Organe's advice, unanimously came to the resolution to form an "Interim Committee" that would take all further decisions for the setting up of an international association in the form of a federation of national societies of anaesthesiologists [21].

To this committee were elected Pierre Huguenard, temporarily replacing Jacques Boureau, France, John Gillies, Great Britain and Ireland, Alexandre Goldblat, Belgium, Torsten Gordh, Sweden, and Harold Griffith, Canada. As advisor to the committee Jean Francisque Delafresnaye, representative of the Council of International Organisation of Medical Sciences (CIOMS), a joint organisation of WHO and UNESCO, was co-opted.

In the context of the above it seems appropriate to quote the originator of the French project, Robert Monod, the founder of the French Society for the Study of Anaesthesia and Analgesia. In his opening speech to the congress he explained himself clearly [22] Translated it reads: "I will probably be the last surgeon ever asked to chair a congress in anaesthesiology. I will therefore take this opportunity to assert what I always have asserted: anaesthesia must be freed from tutelage. But, in so doing - the necessity that this specialty be recognised officially - must one go so far as to ban those who do not exclusively practise anaesthesia from societies and congresses in anaesthesia? We believe not. Anaesthesiologists will be making a great mistake if they consider their specialty purely as a technique. If anaesthesia cuts itself from all the medical sciences it will function in a vacuum", and he continued: "Anaesthesiology has only succeeded in advancing and will only continue to progress with the help of collective efforts. It seems to me essential that not only anaesthesiologists engage in these efforts but also all those concerned with anaesthesia or who contribute to its aims and promote its efficiency".

So much for "the spark that set things on fire", that is to say the turbulence of the year 1951, caused by the French conception and tenacity. But then, from sharp contrasts and open discussions good results may emerge.

The Interim Committee

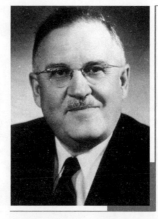

Fig. 6.
Harold Griffith

The choice of the members of the Interim Committee was a happy one; all documents reveal the harmony in which they worked. From the very onset Harold Griffith (Fig. 6) was chairman. No details are available concerning his election. Torsten Gordh stated briefly: "Harold was appointed by nature" [23] and most probably he hit the nail on the head. Harold Griffith was a kind and wise man with a natural gift of leading discussions, patiently listening to everyone but at the same time to the point. He held a variety of important offices, amongst others President of the IARS in 1948 and chairman of its board of trustees from 1949 to 1952. His professional merits are great; he is well known for the introduction of the use of curare in anaesthesia.

Alexandre Goldblat (Fig. 7) was secretary to the Interim Committee, a function for which he was well suited. He combined a quiet manner with great dynamism, was highly intelligent, and could swiftly reach the heart of the matter. Moreover, he was able to express himself clearly in several languages. In 1942, during World War II, he succeeded in crossing over from occupied Belgium to England and joining the Belgian and British forces. From 1945 he became a pupil of Ivan W. Magill at the Westminster Hospital where he also came to know Geoffrey Organe. Back in Belgium he belonged to the small group of pioneers who established in that country the specialty of anaesthesiology.

John Gillies was the leading Scottish anaesthesiologist of his day. He was well known through the textbook which he wrote together with R.J. Minitt and also through his work with H.W.C. Griffiths (mind the s, he is not the same as Harold Griffith) about the - in those days - revolutionary method of controlled hypotension. Gillies held many important functions, amongst others President of the Association of Anaesthetists of Great Britain and Ireland and President of the Anaesthetic Section of the Royal Society of Medicine. John Gillies was devoid of any ostentation, he was a personal friend of Harold Griffith.

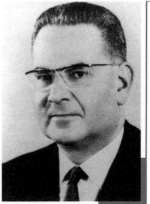

Fig. 7.
Alexandre Goldblat

Torsten Gordh (Fig. 8) is one of the anaesthesiologists who originally wanted to become a surgeon. Being the youngest of the surgical trainees, he was delegated to handle anaesthesia not know-

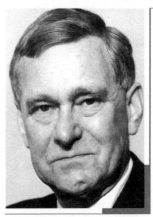

Fig. 8.
Torsten Gordh

ing much about it [24]. Dissatisfied with the result, he underwent training in anaesthesiology in the United States under Ralph Waters from 1938 to 1940. Back in his country, Sweden, Gordh became the pioneer in the development of anaesthesiology throughout the whole of Scandinavia. In 1950, together with Henning Poulsen of Denmark, Eero Turpeinen of Finland, and Otto Molestad of Norway, he established the influential Scandinavian Society of Anaesthesiologists.

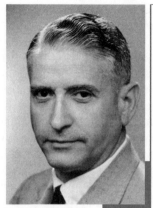

Fig. 9.
Jacques Boureau

Jacques Boureau (Fig. 9) was one of the champions in France for the official recognition of anaesthesiology as an independent medical specialty. In 1946 he was one of the founders of the Syndicate of French Anaesthetists of which, until 1953, he was President. In 1951, Boureau became the first anaesthesiologist to be chosen as General Secretary of

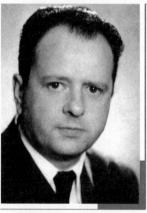

Fig. 10.
Jean Francisque Delafresnaye

the French Society for the Study of Anaesthesia and Analgesia, the committee of which had, hitherto, been entirely in the hands of surgeons. In 1958, Boureau was elected President; meanwhile the name of the society had been changed to Society of Anaesthesia, Analgesia and Resuscitation.

This section on the members of the Interim Committee would not be complete without paying due attention to its advisor Jean Francisque Delafresnaye (Fig. 10) who guided the work from the beginning to the end. Ritsema van Eck, who later was co-opted to the committee, states: "Invaluable help was received from the CIOMS in the person of its secretary Dr. J.F. Delefresnaye, Paris, France. He was always willing to aid in constructing a society that would receive the approbation of all, that remained within the boundary put by custom and law and in developing statutes and by-laws acceptable to us. His knowledge in judicial matters, but above all his linguistic proficiency and his friendliness made him an estimable man in this constructive period. He became a "good friend of us all" [25].

The wise men who steered the initiative into the right channels

The Interim Committee was set up in order to make suggestions concerning the form, objectives, and membership of the international society of anaesthesiologists, which would be acceptable to all the national societies. Most probably the members of the committee had already exchanged ideas in Paris, but no written account has been preserved. Griffith, in his *History of the WFSA* [26] simply states: "We went to our homes and got to work. We had no definite plans, no funds and not much idea about what kind of organisation we should form. Our first task seemed to be to gather information regarding anesthesiology and the status of anesthesiologists from every country in which there was any existing organisation. So Goldblat and I divided up the world between us, and gradually accumulated a great deal of information regarding national societies of anesthesiology, the status of anesthesiologists and their numbers."

A questionnaire containing nine items was sent to all known national societies for return to Griffith [2]. The questions were related to the name of the society, to composition of the board, to the number of its members, and to the publication of a bulletin. There was also a question about the existence in the same country of other scientific bodies concerned with anaesthesia. The last questions concerned the approval of the eventual establishment of an international society set up as a federation of national societies, about its purpose and organisation and, finally, about the time and place for a World Congress of Anaesthesiologists to establish such a society. In addition, Goldblat sent out a letter containing a draft constitution for an international federative society, no doubt made up in conjunction with Delafresnaye but, unfortunately, no copy of the letter has been discovered. By the beginning of 1953 it became clear that there should be a meeting of the Interim Committee. At the invitation of Goldblat the meeting took place in Brussels.

The first meeting of the Interim Committee, Brussels, 18-20 June 1953

From the agenda and the extensive minutes, which both are preserved [27], the following is a compilation. With the intention to widen the horizons of the Interim Committee, leading anaesthesiologists from several countries were also invited to this meeting. In all were present: Canada, Harold Griffith, chairman of the Interim Committee, member of the board of IARS, Wesley Bourne, advisor in anaesthesiology to the University of Paris (WHO); Belgium, Alexandre Goldblat, Honorary Secretary to the Interim Committee, secrétaire Section d'Anesthésie de la Société Belge de Chirurgie, J. de Walle, président Association Professionelle des Spécialistes en Anesthésiologie, Henri Reinhold, vice-président Association Professionelle des Spécialistes en Anesthésiologie; Great Britain and Ireland, W.A. Low, President of the Association of Anaesthetists of Great Britain and Ireland, John Gillies, vice-president Association of Anaesthetists of Great Britain and Ireland, member Interim Committee, G.S.W. Organe vice-president Association of Anaesthetists of Great Britain and Ireland, R.W. Shackleton, Honorary Secretary Association of Anaesthetists of Great Britain and Ireland; Sweden, Torsten Gordh, member Interim Committee; France, Jacques Boureau, président du Syndicat Anesthésistes Français, vice-président de la Société Française d'Anesthésie et d'Analgésie, member Interim Committee; United States A.W. Friend, member of the board of the International Anesthesia Research Society, unofficial observer Society of American Anesthesiologists, T.H. Seldon, member of the board of the International Anesthesia Research Society, unofficial observer Society of American Anesthesiologists, R.J.Whitacre, member of the board of the International Anesthesia Research Society, unofficial observer Society of American Anesthesiologists; Italy, E. Ciocatto, secretary of the Società Italiana di Anestesiologia; The Netherlands C.R. Ritsema van Eck, past President Nederlandse Anaesthesisten Vereniging; Australia J.E. Gillespie, member of the committee of the Australian Society of Anaesthetists, CIOMS J.F. Delafresnaye, advisor to the Interim Committee, secretary to the Council for International Organizations of Medical Science.

According to the letter paper used later, it appears that the representatives, W.A. Low, G.W.S. Organe, R.P. Shackleton, C.R. Ritsema van Eck, E. Ciocatto, W. Bourne, R.J. Whitacre, A.W. Friend, and T.H. Seldon were co-opted as associate members of the Interim Committee. Together with the original members, they formed the "Committee for the Organization of the World Federation of Societies of Anaesthesiologists".

After the summing up of delegates, Griffith cleared up any confusion about the two American societies existing together next to each other, namely the International Anesthesia Research Society (IARS) and the American Society of Anesthesiologists (ASA). "There is not any friction between the two", he said, "most members intermingle. The IARS had sent delegates to this meeting as it takes an interest in all matters pertaining to anesthesiology in the world, but it should be understood that, if a federation of national societies should come into being, the anaesthesiologists of USA should be represented by ASA. In view of the large number of members of ASA it was not possible to consult them in time, hence no official representatives of ASA were present but only unofficial observers."

On Griffith's questionnaire, responses were received from 22 national societies of anaesthesiologists, representing approximately, 7,000 members (e.g., 888 from Great Britain and about 4,000 from the USA) [28]. Organe's archives contain only 17 of these responses, namely from Australia, Belgium, Brazil, Canada, France, Germany, Great Britain, Italy, The Netherlands, Norway, the Philippines, Portugal, South Africa, Spain, Sweden, and Switzerland. Their answers contained the following information.

The committees of these 17 societies, with the exception of France and

Italy, consisted entirely of anaesthesiologists. Five societies published a journal, namely Belgium, Brazil, France, Italy, and Great Britain; Australia and Canada sent regular newsletters. All were of the opinion that their society would agree to an international society set up as a federation of national societies. The question about the purpose of an international society was left unanswered by 4 societies, the responders made suggestions concerning friendship, exchange, and congresses (by 5 societies), organisation, committees, and membership (by 4 societies), anaesthesia apparatus etc. (by 4 societies), training of anaesthesia (by 3 societies), and research and teaching (by 2 societies).

In a letter dated 18 February 1953 from Delafresnaye to the members of the Interim Committee, the following suggestions for the aims of the future international society were also made: to promote the creation of national societies, to promote exchange of information, to lay down minimum requirements for training all over the world, to standardise pieces of equipment, to lay down safety rules, to compile lists of fellowships granted by existing bodies, and to give advice to national and international bodies.

The two enumerations seem to reflect the practical way of thinking of the representatives of the - in most cases - relative young specialty of anaesthesiology. In reaction to this, Dr. A.W. Friend (USA) conveyed Dr. Morris Nicholson's opinion[1] that the primary aim of the society should not be a better position for the anaesthesiologists, but better anaesthesia for more patients throughout the world. This suggestion was seconded by Gillies and unanimously accepted as the base for the exact wording of the aim of the international society, a decision reflecting the idealism of the time.

The draft constitution had been sent out in 1952 by Goldblat. Unfortunately, no copy of this draft or of the replies have been found. As the minutes of the meeting refer to the draft by numbers of the subjects only, the discussions are not easy to follow, hence I confine myself to general remarks. As to the statutes of the future society, Delafresnay suggested that the meeting had better limit itself to general guidelines, a more-precise formulation could be best left to CIOMS experts[1]. On the proposal of Gillies, a draft committee was set up which later was called the Committee on Statutes and By-laws. It consisted of: H.R. Griffith, A.Goldblat, G.S.W. Organe, and J.F. Delafresnaye.

On the proposal of Organe, who played an important role throughout the meeting, the following basic resolutions were definitely accepted:
- the establishment of an international society of anaesthesiologists,
- that this society be formed as a federation of national societies,
- that only one society would represent each country,
- that it should bear the name of "World Federation of Societies of Anaesthesiologists."

---

[1] Dr Morris J. Nicholson was a member of the Board of Trustees of the IARS and a proficient author in the Current Researches of Anesthesia and Analgesia

Furthermore on Organe's proposal, the voting rights in the federation were laid down. Since the societies with few members were afraid of being outvoted by the large societies, it was decided that at the General Assembly each society should be entitled to one delegate if the number of its members was 250 or less, to two delegates if its membership numbered 250-500; to three delegates if it numbered from 500 to 1,000, and to one extra delegate per 1,000 members over 1000.

It was decided that the Executive Committee should carry out the decisions of the General Assembly and take, within the limits of those decisions, all measures that would further the purposes of the Federation. The Executive Committee would consist of nine members of whom at least one must be from Europe, the United States and Canada, Latin America, and Asia and Australia. The Executive Committee would have the power to co-opt up to three additional members who would serve until the next period of election.

The problem of financing the Federation was not solved. At Organe's suggestion it was decided that the national societies should contribute in proportion to their number of delegates to the General Assembly and that the scale of the annual contributions would be decided by the General Assembly. However, such contributions could not be expected until the World Federation had been established. Until then the committee for the organisation of the World Federation depended on help from outside. In this connection Griffith recorded: "Throughout the period of the organization of the World Federation it was the financial assistance, more than any other factor, which made possible the whole "development"[26].

To this statement it may be added that the assistance came from CIOMS and, particularly, from the IARS who acted as a guarantee for all deficits [29]. There was also a gift of U. S. $ 1.000 from Messrs. Becton and Dickinson.

The last item to decide was where, in 1955, the congress was to be held, at which congress the official establishment of the World Federation should take place. In the post-war years, that was not a simple question, not only because of the existing sentiments but, above all, because of financial and travelling constraints. Torsten Gordh proposed Amsterdam, as in those days The Netherlands was comparatively cheap and for most European countries not too far away. This proposal was agreed to and the target date for the congress was set for June 1955.

The second meeting of the Interim Committee was planned to take place in June 1954, also in Amsterdam. Because of the venue of the congress C.R. Ritsema van Eck, past-president of The Netherlands' Society, was co-opted to the Interim Committee.

Later the plans had to be changed. Because of the relatively short time for the preparation of the congress, the target date was shifted from June to September 1955. As in that month Amsterdam could not guarantee sufficient hotel accommodation, preference was now given to Scheveningen, the seaside resort of The Hague, where in September the busy season is over. It was also decided to hold the second meeting of the Interim Committee there.

During the interval between the first and second meeting of the Interim Committee contacts between the members, as well as with the national societies of anaesthesiologists known at the time, were maintained by correspondence only, due to luck of finances to cover travelling expenses.

A circular letter dated 13 February 1954 from the secretary Alexandre Goldblat was sent to the national societies [30]. "I have the pleasure", he wrote, "to bring officially to the notice of your society the project of creation of a World Federation of Societies of Anaesthesiologists based upon a resolution passed at the time of the Paris Congress of Anaesthesiology in 1951". The societies were informed about the activities of the Interim Committee to date. Their attention was drawn to the rapidly increasing interest in anaesthesiology world-wide, to the increasing number of anaesthetic societies under exclusive control of anaesthesiologists, and to the general need for an international organisation of anaesthesiologists. The societies were asked to discuss the enclosed draft constitution proposed at the Brussels meeting. Finally, Goldblat brought to their notice the organisation of the congress of anaesthesiologists to be held in The Netherlands in 1955. Comments on the draft constitution, together with precise information on the name and address of the society concerned, on its constitution, board, and members (are non-anaesthesiologists admitted as ordinary members?) were to reach the Interim Committee before 1 June 1954, in good time for the meeting of the committee at Scheveningen. No other written accounts of the activities during the interval have been found.

The second meeting of the Interim Committee, Scheveningen, 24-27 June 1954

Unfortunately only a few documents of the meeting are available. From this author's reminiscence and from accounts of other participants the following reconstruction transpires. Present were the members of the Interim Committee: H.R. Griffith, chairman, Goldblat, secretary, J. Boureau, J. Gillies, T. Gordh, C.R. Ritsema van Eck, President of the future congress, and J.F. Delafresnaye, advisor to the committee. From Great Britain were present: G.S.W. Organe, T.C. Gray, and R.W.P. Shackleton; from the United States L.J. Durshordwee, representing the IARS [26], probably A.W. Friend and T.H. Seldon, and an unofficial representative of ASA as well; from West Germany R. Frey; from Israel F.F.Foldes; from The Netherlands M. Mauve President of The Netherlands' Society of Anaesthetists, Honorary Secretary of the World Congress, and L. Boeré, honorary treasurer of the World Congress.

The agenda has been recovered [30] and is reproduced in full, as it gives a good impression of the course of the meeting. It consists of three main subjects:

1. New developments in the WFSA,
   a) Summary of the proceedings of the first meeting (June 1953)
   b) Exchange of letters with the various national societies
   c) Comments received regarding the draft constitution
   d) Applications for membership from various societies
   e) Progress of the idea of a World Federation.

2. World Congress-September 1955
   a) Material preparations from the Dutch representatives, finance, provisional organisation, setting up of various committees
   b) Scientific preparation, free subjects or various themes, symposia ?

3. Technical preparation for the installation of the WFSA
   a) The General Assembly: convocations, designation, etc.
   b) Preparation of the election of the Executive Committee, etc.

With regard to the first item, the new developments of the WFSA, valuable information was gained from the answers to the circular letter of 13 February 1954 from Goldblat to the national societies. Alas, no original replies from the societies are found. According to Griffith there had been enthusiasm for membership of the proposed Federation from almost all national societies and approval of the general principles of the constitution [26].

With reference to the second and third main subjects of the agenda, i.e., the World Congress 1955 and the preparation for the installation of the WFSA, the following information was given. In order to become a corporate body and to be able to arrange all financial matters, a foundation entitled "World Congress of Anaesthesiologists 1955" was set up by means of a legal deed, dated 20 February 1954. The board of this foundation consisted of C.R. Ritsema van Eck, President, M. Mauve (Fig. 11), secretary, L.A. Boeré, treasurer and A.M. Laterveer, J. van 't Oever, D.W. Swijgman, and B. de Vries Robles, members. Their task was, under the auspices of The Netherlands' Society, to prepare for the Congress in 1955. For this reason they are referred to as the "Organising Committee".

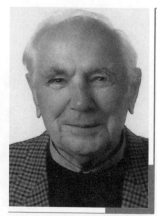

Fig. 11.
M. Mauve

A balanced budget for the congress had been determined. The expenses were kept low because the members of the Organizing Committee, with the help of only a few professionals, undertook the organisation of the congress themselves. The first outgoing costs were covered by loans from the, at the time, about 55 members of The Netherlands Anaesthetists Society and with the guarantee of a certain sum of money from the Dutch Ministry of Education, Art, and Sciences.

The Interim Committee was unable to give definite information on attendance, but it was estimated that some 350 anaesthesiologists would participate in the congress. The hotel facilities at Scheveningen were considered to be adequate. The Kurhaus Hotel at Scheveningen (Fig. 12) had three rooms with sufficient seating and spacious accommodation for the other congress functions. The congress languages were to be English, French, and German, simultaneous interpretation was to be provided.

As the main subjects for the congress were those that at the time were attracting the most attention, namely respiratory and circulatory physiology, hypothermia, and controlled hypotension. Panel discussions were planned to follow the papers on these subjects. Other subjects were muscle relaxants (the advent of succinylcholine was very recent), the teaching of anaesthesia and, of course, free papers. All suggestions were accepted by the Interim Committee, the exact date of the congress in September 1955 was left to the Organising Committee.

The name for the congress provoked a vigorous discussion. The Organising Committee suggested "World Congress of Anaesthesiologists 1955", but the members of the Interim Committee found that inadequate. They wanted the establishment of the WFSA to be announced in the title and they also wanted to proclaim it as the "First International Congress". The French found the latter unacceptable, their objection being that the first international congress had been held in Paris. The members of the Interim Committee considered a name such as "Second International Congress" equally unacceptable and so the original suggestion of "World Congress of Anaesthesiologists 1955" was retained.

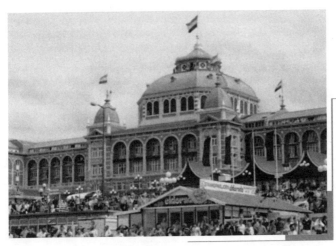

Fig. 12.
The Kurhaus Hotel at Scheveningen where the establishment of the WFSA took place

The draft constitution as revised June 1954

A copy of this draft constitution has been found [31] without a covering letter. Considering the date and the contents of the draft the supposition seems logical that it reflects the final outcome of the discussions at the meetings of the Interim Committee in 1953 and 1954, the views at these meetings are clearly recognisable. If so, this document must have been the basis for discussions with the candidate members of the WFSA before and during the World Congress 1955. The following is a general view of the draft.

IN SECTION I THE NAME OF THE FEDERATION AND ITS HEADQUARTERS ARE DEALT WITH

IN SECTION II THE PURPOSES AND THE FUNCTIONS OF THE WFSA ARE DETERMINED

Article 3
The object of the Federation is to make available the highest standard of anaesthesia to all peoples throughout the world.
In pursuit of this aim, the functions of the Federation shall in particular include the following:
To assist and encourage the formation of national societies of anaesthesiologists
To promote the dissemination of scientific information
To recommend desirable standards of training for anaesthesiologists
To provide information regarding opportunities for post-graduate training and research
To encourage research into all aspects of anaesthesiology
To encourage the establishment of safety measures including the standardisation of equipment
To advise upon request national and international organisations

SECTION III DEALS WITH MEMBERSHIP

Article 4
The members of the Federation shall be the national societies known to and certified by the Interim Committee for the establishment of this Federation including the national societies of Argentine, Austria, Australia, Belgium, Brazil, Canada, Chile, Colombia, Cuba, Denmark, Finland, France, West Germany, Great Britain and Ireland, Israel, Italy, the Netherlands, New Zealand, Norway, the Philippines, South Africa, Sweden, Switzerland, Spain, the United States of America, and Uruguay, together with such organisations as shall be approved by a vote of a majority of the aforesaid members present at the first General Assembly of the Federation which shall be held without notice immediately following the adoption of these articles.

It is worth noting the difference between the national societies mentioned in this section and those approving the definite statutes at the establishment of the WFSA in 1955 by their signature. In the draft no mention is made of India who signed the statutes, whereas New Zealand, the Philippines, and the United States are mentioned who did not. Supposedly, the societies mentioned in the draft are the responders to the circular letter of Goldblat of 13 February 1954.

Section IV is concerned with the General Assembly

Article 10
The Federation shall be governed by a General Assembly of delegates from member organisations.
In this article the number of delegates and the voting rights are regulated exactly as proposed by Organe and accepted by the Interim Committee at the Brussels meeting.

Article 13
The General Assembly shall meet in ordinary session on the occasion of each international congress.

Article 14
The General Assembly shall be the supreme body of the council and shall be entitled to take cognisance of all matters not explicitly precluded by these articles.
The principle functions of the Assembly shall be:
to determine the policy of the Federation
to elect the Executive Committee and the secretary/treasurer in accordance with these articles
to receive and approve the reports of the Executive Committee
to fix the scale of subscriptions, etc

Article 15
The Executive Committee shall prepare the agenda of the assembly, etc

Article 16
The General Assembly shall elect a President at the beginning of each session with three vice-presidents, etc

SECTION V DEALS WITH THE EXECUTIVE COMMITTEE

Article 19
The Executive Committee shall execute the decisions of the General Assembly and take within the limits of those decisions all measures designed to further the purposes of the Federation.
The Executive Committee shall consist of 12 members of whom at least 1 must be from (a) Europe, (b) the United States and Canada, (c) Latin America, (d) Asia and Australia, and 1 other member from each of the two largest member organisations.

Article 20
The chairman and his deputies will be appointed by the Executive Committee from among its members.
The Executive Committee shall nominate the secretary/treasurer 3 months in advance of the General Assembly.

Article 22
The secretary/treasurer may request the Executive Committee to take decisions by postal ballot.

SECTION VI, VII, AND VIII DEAL WITH THE FINANCE, THE DISSOLUTION, AND LIQUIDATION OF THE FEDERATION AND THE ENTRY INTO FORCE OF THE STATUTES

Article 27
These statutes shall become effective when ten of the organisations participating in the first General Assembly shall have accepted them.

Article 28
The English text of the statutes and by-laws shall be considered as authoritative.

World Congress of Anaesthesiologists 1955, Scheveningen, 5-10 September: final preparation for the WFSA

The preliminary notice of the congress and the application forms were sent out in December 1954 to the national societies known, and announcements were sent to the anaesthetic journals to be inserted. The preliminary programme followed 2 months later (Fig. 13).

The number of anaesthesiologists wanting to attend the congress exceeded greatly the estimated number; it leapt from 350 to over 800 from 44 countries, plus 400 partners [32]. Since such numbers could no longer be accommodated at Scheveningen and in The Hague, it became necessary to use hotels at Noordwijk, a seaside resort 25 km away and to organise a shuttle bus service to the congress.

The congress was held under the patronage of H.M. Queen Juliana of The Netherlands. Robert Monod, the French surgeon who, stimulated by Francis Hoeffer McMechan, took the initiative for the organisation of an international association of anaesthesiologists, was invited as an honorary member of the congress.

For the simultaneous translation the interpreters had to be familiarised with the terminology of the, at that time on the continent of Europe, new specialty. The technical facilities were by modern standards somewhat primitive. Everything was transmitted by cables, which ran over the floor. The apparatus was operated by student volunteers from the Technical University of Delft under the guidance of Jacques Boerée, son of the treasurer of the congress. A comical note is that all cables, headphones, apparatus, and interpreter boxes in the main hall of the Kurhaus had to be removed by 1800 hours so that the ticket holders could attend the concerts that had to take place despite the congress. During the night everything had to be replaced.

With regard to the organisation of the WFSA and its establishment at the closing session of the congress, the members of the Interim Committee held their conclusive meetings before and during the congress, as did the members of the subcommittees that had meanwhile come into being [33].

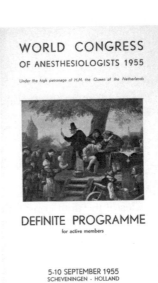

Fig. 13.
Programme of the congress at which the WFSA was established

On the 4 September 1955 the preliminary meeting of the delegates representing the national societies was held for the purpose of the election of the members of the Committee on Nominations. Elected were O. Mayrhofer, Austria, A. Goldblat, Belgium, O. Bastos, Brazil, R.A.Gordon, Canada, M.M. Curbelo, Cuba, E.O. Turpeinen, Finland, W.A. Low, Great Britain and Ireland, and E. Ciocatto, Italy.

On 6 September the Committee on Credentials met to examine the credentials of the delegates representing the national societies. The committee consisted of M. Bantz de Olega, Argentine, O. Secher, Denmark, P. Jacquenoud, France, chairman, R. Frey, West Germany, and R.P.W. Shackleton, Great Britain and Ireland. The committee was to report to the Interim Committee.

Also on 6 September the preliminary meeting of the delegates and observers took place [34]. Present were: H.R. Griffith, chairman Interim Committee, member Committee on Statutes and By-laws; A. Goldblat, Honorary Secretary Interim Committee, member Committee on Statutes and By-laws; J. Gillies, member Interim Committee; T. Gordh, member Interim Committee; J. Boureau, member Interim Committee; C.R. Ritsema van Eck, member Interim Committee; G.W.S. Organe, member Committee on Statutes and By-laws; J.F. Delafresnaye, advisor Interim Committee, member Committee on Statutes and By-laws.

The delegates included M. Bantz de Olega, Argentine; O. Bastos, Brazil; L. Cabrera, Chile; S. Campbell, Canada; E. Ciocatto, Italy; R.B. Curbelo, Cuba; G. Delgado, Columbia; R. Frey, West Germany; A. Gonzalez Varela, Argentine; C. Hoyer, Venezuela; P. Jacquenoud, France; N.R. James, Australia; E. Lopes Soares, Portugal; W.A. Low, Great Britain and Ireland; I. Lund, Norway; O. Mayrhofer, Austria; F. Roberts, South Africa; O. Secher, Denmark; R.P.W. Shackleton, Great Britain and Ireland; S. Talwalkar, India. The observers included L. Wright, the United States and A. Longhino, Yugoslavia.

The draft constitution was subjected to an extensive revision. It was proposed to register the WFSA officially in The Netherlands. The Dutch text of the statutes, requisite for registration, would then be binding for the WFSA. Ritsema van Eck would set the procedure in motion.

Dr. L. Wright, who was present as the official observer for the American Society of Anesthesiologists, took the opportunity to explain why the ASA did not wish to join the WFSA at that time. The only reason, he said, was the lack of sufficient liaison in the former days between the composing societies. In his opinion it was only a matter of time before the ASA joined the World Federation.

On 7 September the Committee on Nominations met [35]. With regard to the relevant articles of the draft constitution and the by-laws, the committee selected and proposed the nominations for the members of the board of the General Assembly as well as of the Executive Committee. The names of the candidates are mentioned below in connection with the closing session of the congress.

The closing session of the congress, Friday, 9 September 1955

Of this session, at which the WFSA was to be established (Fig. 14) a verbatim report by A. Goldblat has been preserved [36]. What follows is derived from this report and from what I remember.

At the middle of the large table is Harold Griffith with the members and advisers of the Interim Committee, on both sides are the delegates of the founding countries of the WFSA. At the right side are the sound technicians. The main hall of the Kurhaus Hotel is completely filled. A large table occupies the dais behind which Harold Griffith is sitting together with the members of the Interim Committee, Geoffrey Organe, and the delegates from 26 national societies who are about to establish the World Federation. Facing the table the students are sitting to operate the sound apparatus.

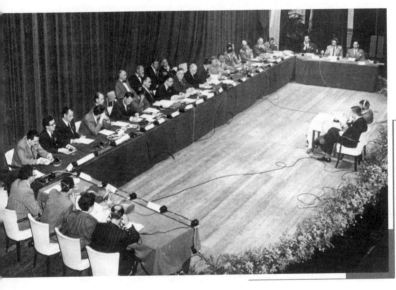

Fig. 14.
The meeting at which the WFSA was established during the closing session of the congress

Present were the delegates from:

Associacion Argentina de Anestesiologia; *M. Bantz de Olega, A.Gonzalez Varela*

Oesterreichische Gesellschaft für Anaesthesiologie; *O. Mayrhofer*

Australian Society of Anaesthetists; *N.R. James*

Association Professionelle des Spécialistes en Anesthésiologie (Belgium); *A. Goldblat*

Sociedade Brasileira de Anestesiologia; *O. Bastos (deputising for Z. Vieira)*

Canadian Anaesthetists' Society; *H. R. Griffith, R.A. Gordon, S. Campbell*

Sociedad de Anestesiología de Chile; *L. Cabrera*

Sociedad Colombiana de Anestesiología; *G. Delgado*

Sociedad Nacional de Anestesiología (Cuba); *R.R. de Curbelo*

Dansk Anestesiologisk Selskap (Denmark); *O. Secher*

Suomen Anestesiologiyhdistys (Finland); *E.O. Turpeinen*

Société Française d'Anesthésie et d'Analgésie; *J. Boureau, P. Jacquenoud*

Deutsche Gesellschaft für Anaesthesie (West Germany); *R. Frey*

Association of Anaesthetists of Great Britain and Ireland; *W.A. Low, G.W.S. Organe, J. Gillies, R.P.W. Shackleton*

Indian Society of Anaesthetists; *S. Talwalkar*

Israel Society of Anaesthetists; *F.F. Foldes*

Società Italiana di Anestesiologia; *E. Ciocatto*

Nederlandse Anaesthesisten Vereniging (The Netherlands); *C.R. Ritsema van Eck*

Norsk Anestesilegeforening (Norway); *I. Lund*

Sociedade Portuguesa de Anestesiologia; *E. Lopes Soares*

South African Society of Anaesthetists; *F. Roberts*

Associacion Española de Anestesiología; *D. Monton*

Svensk Anestesiologisk Förening (Sweden); *T. Gordh*

Schweizerische Gesellschaft für Anaesthesiol/Société Suisse d'Anesthésiologie; *K. Zimmermann*

Sociedad de Anestesiología del Uruguay; *A. Canellas*

Sociedad Venezolana de Anestesiología; *C. Hoyer*

Also present were official observers from the Societies of:
Czechoslovakia - H. Kessler
Egypt - El Gohari
Greece - S. Couremenos
Hungary - J. Pastarova
Jamaica - V. Keating
New Zealand - A. Slater
Poland - S. Pokrzywnicki
Rumania - N. Hortolomei
Turkey - Sadi Sun
USA (ASA) - L. Wright
USSR - J. Zaitsev
Yugoslavia - A. Longhino

The various reports differ according to the countries from which observers were present.
In the Proceedings of the Congress [36] are also mentioned:
Hawaii - E. You
Kenya - J. Mackenzie
Mexico - R. Rodriguez
Nigeria - P. Edwards

The annual report of WFSA for 1955-1956 by Goldblat and Organe [37] does not refer to these countries, nor is Hungary mentioned. However, according to the list of participants [31], all mentioned anaesthesiologists were present at the congress.

The establishment of the World Federation of Societies of Anaesthesiologists

On the 9 September 1955 at 1615 hours Griffith, by virtue of his position as chairman of the Interim Committee called the meeting to order. The first order of the meeting was the report of the Committee on the Credentials of the delegates. Goldblat, spokesman of the committee, informed the chairman that the credentials of the 33 delegates showed them to be the accredited representatives of their national societies. These delegates then were entitled to vote.

The next order of business was the adoption of the constitution and by-laws. Goldblat reported that in the preliminary meetings of the concerning committee the articles of the constitution and by-laws had been discussed until approved by all delegates. Subsequently the text was translated into Dutch, requisite for registration under the Dutch law.

Ritsema van Eck added that the Dutch text was under discussion in the Department of Justice. He suggested that after adoption of the constitution the delegates signed their names to that effect on a separate sheet to be added to the translated text (Fig. 15). The constitution and by-laws were put to the vote, the delegates were unanimously in favour of the adoption and signed their names as desired. Thereupon Griffith addressed the audience:

"Ladies and Gentlemen, the baby is now born. The confinement has been prolonged, but nevertheless, I think has been accomplished without serious complications."

The last duty of Griffith as chairman of the Interim Committee was to call upon the spokesman of the Committee on Nominations for the nominations for the positions of President of the General Assembly and of the vice-presidents. Dr. Gordon announced the names of the nominees: President H.R. Griffith; vice-presidents C.R. Ritsema van Eck, A. Goldblat, R. Frey, and R.R. Curbelo. All were elected amidst loud applause.

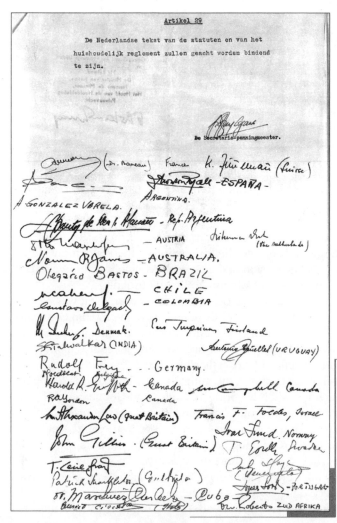

Fig. 15.
Signatures of delegates approving the Statutes of the WFSA

The next duty of Griffith, but this time as President of the WFSA, concerned the election of the secretary/treasurer of the newly founded Federation. Since only one nomination was received, namely of Geoffrey Organe, he was appointed to that office. Griffith said: "If we had looked through the world for one who is admirably qualified to fulfil such an "important post in the field of world anaesthesiology, no-one could have found anyone who is "better suited to that post". Time has shown how right he was.

The following order of business was the election of the Executive Committee, responsible for the affairs of the Federation in between meetings of the General Assembly. In accordance with the proposals of the nominating committee, the following were appointed: J. Boureau, France; E. Ciocatto, Italy; J. Gillies, Great Britain and Ireland; A. Goldblat, Belgium; T. Gordh, Sweden; H.R. Griffith, Canada; N.R. James, Australia; O. Mayrhofer, Austria; R.P.W. Shackleton, Great Britain and Ireland; A. Gonzalez Varela, Argentina; Z. Vieira, Brazil. A. Goldblat was elected unanimously as chairman.

There was still one item, which had to be discussed and to be decided, namely the matter of finances. According to the constitution, the WFSA is supported by contributions from member societies. In this context Organe proposed that the contributions be related to voting power, the larger the society the more delegates and the more subscription. He proposed a basic subscription of the equivalent of U.S. $ 0.75, per annum per delegate. In case of societies with fewer than 75 members, he suggested U.S. $ 1 per annum per delegate. All delegates were in favour of these proposals. The last subject for consideration was when and where the next World Congress would be held. On Griffith's proposal this was referred to the Executive Committee.

At the meeting the business was interspersed with speeches of thanks by Griffith, Goldblat, and Organe. Foldes proposed a vote of thanks to the members of the Interim Committee for the "tremendous amount of work and enthusiasm that they have put into the foundation of the Federation." Finally, Griffith declared this first session of the General Assembly of the World Federation of Societies of Anaesthesiologists to be adjourned.

Thus the Congress of Anaesthesiologists 1955 at Scheveningen was brought to a conclusion. Thanks to the efforts of the members of the Interim Committee and of many others, in particular of Geoffrey Organe, the dreams of Francis Hoeffer McMechan and Robert Monod had become a reality, namely the World Federation of Societies of Anaesthesiologists.

At the dinner after the congress the author of this chapter made the following speech which ran, slightly abridged. Ladies and Gentlemen, We have met already in my capacity of Honorary Secretary to the congress but now I have the pleasure to address you as President of The Netherlands Society of Anaesthesists, your host. In a young and small society like ours some members need to hold more than one function. It is a young society indeed, set up 7 years ago by half a dozen members. Nevertheless, when seed is sown into fertile soil, the plants, or let us say the tree, will grow prosperously. Thus it did, with branches and flowers and it was my duty to look after it.

Some 4 years later I discovered a new bud on our tree. It was a bud like a cuckoo, growing with ever-increasing speed and the branch bent heavily under its weight. Feeling my responsibility I chose for the care of the tree the best head-gardener I could provide Dr. Cornelis Ritsema van Eck. As things often go, if you give something, you will receive more in return and I was appointed to a sort of sub-boss of the garden, thereby assisted by other members of our society. Meanwhile the bud grew bigger and bigger and the branch bent lower and lower, so we had to look for more experienced help[1]. Miss De Beaufort and Mr. Fentener van Vlissingen came into the picture, but still the team was hardly strong enough to support branch and bud, and a disaster it would be if that bud were spoiled.

Fortunately great assistance was provided by many fellow anaesthetists from abroad as well as by their associations, and also by the Council for International Organization of Medical Sciences (CIOMS). In addition material help came from our Government and from the Municipality of The Hague.

With feelings of gratitude I mention the patronage of the Congress by Her Majesty Queen Juliana of the Netherlands. Thus, backed up from numerous sides, we succeeded to keep the bud alive.

Today, the 9 September 1955 at 4.15 p.m. it burst open and out came the most beautiful flower ever seen in the world of anaesthesia. All its petals were of a different size, shape and colour, forming together a magnificent combination.

Dr. Harold Griffith, you and your members of the Interim Committee, Dr. Jacques Boureau, Dr. John Gillies, Dr. Alexandre Goldblat, and Dr. Torsten Gordh have inoculated that bud on our tree, thereby trusting in our hands the care of your beloved flower: the Congress to establish the World Federation of Societies of Anaesthesiologists. On behalf of The Netherlands Society of Anaesthetists we thank you with all our hearts for that evidence of faith. We hope that the work has been done in accordance with your views. We also congratulate you on your rightly deserved election as the first President of the World Federation.

We owe a great debt of gratitude to our friends from all parts of the world for their liberal assistance; they are too numerous to mention all their names. You will agree that I should make one exception Dr. Geoffrey Organe.

At this moment the congress is in the past already. The petals of the flower are falling and will be spread all over the world, over the seas and through the air. It is our sincere wish that they will induce our fellows to inoculate many more buds, not only to the glory of our Federation but also to promote the fulfilment of its high ideals.

I invite you to drink with me on its prosperous future. Good luck to all!

---

[1] At that time professional congress organisations did not exist in our country, congresses were organised mainly by the doctors themselves with secretarial help.

The post-congress activities

The next day, the Executive Committee under the chairmanship of Alexandre Goldblat held its first meeting. Among other items it was decided (1) to co-opt to the committee C.R. Ritsema van Eck, The Netherlands, and S.G. Tawalkar, India; (2) the headquarters of the WFSA should be at the discretion of the secretary/treasurer, until funds are available this should be his house; (3) the work of the Executive Committee should be conducted generally by mail as there was no money to pay for the travelling expenses of its members; (4) it would be necessary to have a meeting in 1959, in the city in which the 1960 congress was to be held; (5) a register of the names and addresses of the officers and members of all national societies should be established; (6) an attempt should be made to keep a list of all anaesthesia journals, abstracts and digests; (7) information about anaesthesia conventions and lines of research should be collected; (8) as soon as funds are available the secretary/treasurer should visit as many countries as possible to study local conditions and to make personal contacts with the member societies.

In conclusion, the members of the Dutch organisation committee of the congress, all of them practising anaesthetists, greatly underestimated the efforts necessary to accomplish the post-congress activities, in particular the publishing of the proceedings.

Gratefully they accepted the proposal of the Anaesthesia Research Society to publish "as a contribution to world anaesthesia" the proceedings of the congress (Fig. 16) [37]. Griffith writes: "Dr. T.H. Seldon of Rochester, Minnesota, shouldered the prodigious editorial responsibility for this 320-page volume, which appeared in 1956. In so far as necessary the papers delivered at the congress were translated into English and the volume was sent without charge to those who had registered at the congress and to all members of the IARS. This represented an investment of over $ U.S. 10,000, and has been much appreciated" [26].

Indeed, for the organisers of the congress this substantial benefaction was the greatest relief possible.

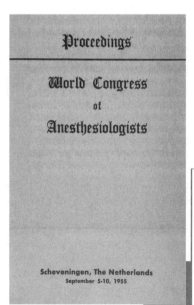

Proceedings

World Congress

of

Anesthesiologists

Scheveningen, The Netherlands
September 5-10, 1955

Fig. 16.
*The cover
of the
Proceedings
of the World
Congress 1955*

References

1. Carr EH (1985) What is history? Penguin, Harmondsworth, Middlesex, England, pp 35-36

2. Mauve M (1992) Episodes from the history of the establishment of the World Federation of Societies of Anaesthesiologists. Ned Tijdschr Anesth 5 [Suppl 1]

3. Elder RO (1952) Modern anesthesia in Argentine. Curr Res Anesth Analg 31:416-418

4. Paez VN (1991) General Secretary CLASA. Personal correspondence CLASA 074-91, 2 May

5. Poulsen H (1975) The Scandinavian Society of Anaesthesiologists 1950-1975. Acta Anaesth Scand 19:253-257

6. Ibsen B (1975) From anaesthesia to anaesthesiology. Acta Anaesth Scand [Suppl 61]:18-20

7. International Anesthesia Research Society (1925) Editorial. Curr Res Anesth Analg 4:66

8. Boureau J (1990) Personal communication. Paris

9. Monod R (1938) Rapport du Comité de Direction. Anesth Analg 4:503-505

10. Congrès International d'Anesthésiologie (1950) Presse Med 58:1300

11. Monod R (1935) Bulletin de la Société d'Etudes sur l'Anesthésie et l'Analgésie. Anesth Analg 1:61-64

12. Liste des Membres par Section (1951) Anesth Analg 8:409-411

13. Organe's archives, London. At present WFSA-Archives, G. Organe's documentation. Wood Library, Park Ridge, Illinois, USA

14. Paris Congress of Anaesthesiology. Untitled report from the meeting 2 March, 1951. Both Organe's archives, see [13]

15. Report issued by the Société Française d'Anesthésie. Draft Constitution for an International Society of Anaesthesiology. Both Organe's archives, see [13]

16. Organe's archives, London, see [13]

17. Organe's archives, London, see [13]

18. Special Meeting of Council of the Association of Anaesthetists of Great Britain and Ireland, 7 September 1951, see [13]. At this meeting J. Gillies gave a report of the informal meeting held on the previous evening, 6 September. Organe's archives, London.

19. Organe's archives, London, see [13]

20. Thalheimer M (1951) Rapport sur la création d'un mouvement international d'études sur l'anesthésie et la constitution d'une société internationale d'anesthésiologie. Anesth Analg 8:379-384

21. Archives of the Netherlands' Society of Anesthesiology. Domus Medica, Utrecht, The Netherlands

22. Monod R (1951) Translated from the French text. Anesth Analg 8:557-566

23. Personal letter from T. Gordh, 21 August 1991

24. Idem, 17 June 1990

25. Ritsema van Eck CR (1966) The World Federation of Societies of Anaesthesiologists, Founded 9 September 1955 at Scheveningen, The Netherlands. WFSA Newsletter 2:12-24

26. Griffith HR (1963) History of the World Federation of Anesthesiologists. Anesth Analg Curr Res 42:389-397

27. Organe's archives, see [13]

28. Organe's archives, see [13]

29. Goldblat A, Organe GWS, annual report WFSA 1955-1956. Organe's archives, see [13]

30. Organe's archives, London.

31. General State Archives, dossier VER 35634. The Hague, The Netherlands

32. List of Participants at the Congress. Archives Netherlands Society Anesthesiology Domus Medica, Utrecht, The Netherlands

33. Recording of Congress WFSA Scheveningen. Organe's archives, see [13]

34. Preliminary Meeting Delegates and Observers on Tuesday 6 September 1955. Archives Netherlands Society Anesthesiology, Domus Medica, Utrecht, The Netherlands

35. Report of the Committee on Nominations, Organe's archives, see [13]

36. Goldblat A. Recording of Congress of WFSA at Scheveningen. Organe's archives, see [13]

37. Proceedings on the Congress of Anesthesiologists, Scheveningen, The Netherlands, 5-10 September 1955. Edited and published by the International Anesthesia Research Society, Cleveland, Ohio

38. Goldblat A, Organe GWS, Annual Report WFSA 1955-1956. Organe's archives, see [13]

3 WITH GREAT RELUCTANCE: THE AMERICAN PERSPECTIVE ON THE WFSA

E.M. Papper†, D.R. Bacon

*E*xplaining the American perspective on the World Federation of Societies of Anaesthesiologists (WFSA) is a daunting but welcome challenge. There is something unique, and perhaps incomprehensible to those who live outside the United States, about the attitude of Americans to international organizations. Often Americans are perceived as isolationist, xenophobic, and loath to make international commitments. Yet, the truth is that Americans are not so easily categorized, having strong segments of the population that are simultaneously internationally minded and isolationists. The American contributions to the WFSA clearly demonstrate this dichotomy, with strong groups arguing for and against joining the organization.

Why did this occur? At any point in its history, the United States has been a vortex of ideas and thoughts. Every year has brought immigrants to the country, seeking one or another of the opportunities that America has in abundance. In some ways, this constant influx of people has given an international flavor to the country. On the other hand, there is equally a deep-seated desire to be rid of the ways of the "old world" and continue the American spirit of self-sufficiency. Nowhere do these values clash as elegantly as in the American decision concerning joining the WFSA.

However, before embarking on this summary of American views of worldwide events, it is necessary to enter a disclaimer. The story, as it is presented, is obviously sketchy and necessarily incomplete. There are serious oversimplifications that are necessary in a brief summary of important sociological forces. Finally, it is the height of presumption to suggest that it is possible to identify a single American way that is uniform and consistent with respect to international societies. Therefore, these suggestions of how events occurred in international anesthesiology from an American standpoint, are, at best, reasonable opinions about which other Americans may properly differ.

Roots

It may be useful to have some understanding of the background that led to the evolution of the various and complex attitudes of Americans towards international affairs. Some explanation of the origins and subsequent development of the United States as a country may be helpful to understand current American behavior. Such a presentation will be short and in broad outline to indicate some of the origins of beliefs and views that followed later. The United States, at its inception, was an extension of Western Europe. Obviously such a statement ignores the importance of Native Americans and African-American slavery. The former were characterized mistakenly by the earliest "discoverers" of this continent as Indians and were often mistreated by the various immigrants. The latter were cruelly enslaved and had neither power nor influence until well into the latter half of the twentieth century.

The Western Europeans originated from two importantly different streams of people. There were those whose purpose and mission was to seek a fortune in the New World and return home with the gold and other wealth that might be found in what became the Americas. They had little or no intention of settling nor understanding the people whom they found except to exploit them. The well-known story of the Spanish Conquistadors took place chiefly in what subsequently became South and Central America. However, their cultural influences extended to other areas of the Americas, including the southern and western parts of the future United States. These people were largely of Iberian origin, and they established an important presence of the Spanish and Portuguese monarchies in the New World. Although the earliest adventurers rarely remained in the Americas, they had an enormous impact on the establishment in the western world of the Spanish and Portuguese languages and culture. They brought with them a sense of bold adventure and displayed a marked manifestation of the entrepreneurial spirit coupled with missionary zeal to spread Christianity. They possessed an indescribable but important sense of integrated power, which overcame major obstacles to their work. Clearly some of these characteristics found their place permanently in the cultures of the New World. They were to become part of the larger American scene, including the United States.

It is generally accepted, however, that the major influence in the earliest development of this country came largely from Great Britain, Ireland, and other parts of Western Europe. Many of the colonists that settled in North America were English, Scots, Welch, Irish, Dutch, and French. Unlike the Spanish and Portuguese, they came to stay. They had no intention to "go home". These people, who were early settlers in the seventeenth century were neither aristocratic nor wealthy. Many of the immigrants were religious dissidents in Britain and Ireland who wanted to establish and enjoy freedom of worship and religion, which was crucial to them. These early settlers were most courageous to travel for long periods of time to a new world that had climates that were not salubrious, where they had to carve their homes and livelihoods in a wilderness and where they met an indigenous population that was often hostile. Some of the natives were friendly and cooperative with the new immigrants, but many were not. These religious dissidents objected to joining the established churches in Britain and France; the former Protestant and the latter Catholic. They had, in an authoritarian age, in which religion was an important part of life, suffered many disadvantages, which were sociological and economic, as well as religious. They could neither own property nor enjoy the already established rights of Anglican Christians in Britain as subjects of the monarchy. They viewed the established churches as antagonistic to their way of life and therefore sought the freedom of worship that was possible in the New World. Those who traveled to what became New England were largely Congregationalists, while others, who were Methodists or Baptists, tended to travel to other parts of the colonies, including the South. French Huguenots settled in all of the British and French colonies in North America.

There were religious dissidents other than the Protestants who came to the New World. These were Roman Catholics and Jews for the most part. The Catholics and Jews were disenfranchised and could not own property in Britain until the nineteenth century. The Catholic immigrants who arrived among the early settlers came to escape the repression they experienced and to worship in the Catholic Church. Much later, Catholic immigrants from Ireland sought refuge in America to escape the grinding poverty at home. For example, there was a large Irish Catholic immigration to escape the devastating potato famine in Ireland in the mid nineteenth century. However, not all of the Catholics were Irish nor were all of them members of the lower classes. In fact an important Catholic immigration occurred early in the colonial period of America led by the noble aristocrat, Lord Baltimore. Baltimore and the Roman Catholics sought a new life of freedom of Catholic worship. They settled in what became Maryland, in an area named for Queen Mary. The Catholic character of Maryland still exists to this day.

There was also a modest number of Jewish immigrants who came to the New World following periods of experiencing increasing hostility in Europe, culminating in their expulsion from Spain and Portugal by the Inquisition. The expulsion of the Jews in 1492 - the coincidence of the date being the same as the "discovery" of America has rarely been explored thoroughly - sent the Jews to Eastern Europe, the Netherlands, and to other parts of Western Europe, and also to the Middle East, Asia, and Africa. The Jews who went to Eastern Europe were not to become immigrants to the United States of America until their descendants sought refuge here at the end of the nineteenth and the early twentieth century. However, some of the Jews who sought religious toleration for their faith in the Netherlands went first to Britain and then went on further to escape religious persecution to the New World. There were Dutch settlements containing some Jews in New Amsterdam, later to become New York. There was also Jewish immigration to South America and subsequently from South America to North America, after they were expelled from Span-

ish territories by the Inquisition. These Jewish settlements remained permanent and evolved into an integral part of British Colonial America. They lived
without religious friction and minimal social and economic disadvantages in
the 13 British colonies.

Center stage: The American Revolution and the Fledgling United States

*"It is our true policy to steer clear of permanent alliances with any portion
of the foreign world".*

George Washington's farewell address to the people of the United States,
17 September 1796. These various peoples in the 13 colonies in America
wanted to have the normal rights and privileges of the English people of the
sixteenth and seventeenth century. The American Revolution was less of a vio-
lent upheaval than the French Revolution, and more of a change in the form
of government and social ideals. To understand American perspectives about
subsequent social attitudes, it is necessary to understand something of the
American Revolution and the character of the republic that arose from it.

The religious dissidents of New England, largely Protestant, became small
property owners. They viewed themselves as Britons overseas and expected
the same rights possessed by the people in the home country. When these
rights were not granted by the crown, they rebelled. Actually what they wanted was modest. They demanded some self-government and representation in
political affairs. These were not radicals who wished to destroy society. They
wanted to be part of that society. The writings of Thomas Paine are often
cited in this regard to support the claim of radical influence. However, there
is very much persuasive evidence to indicate that the American Revolution had
a much more British flavor than a French flavor to it. The American colonist
wished to be British. He wanted to be governed by a responsive legislature,
not one controlled by an absent ruling authority.

The decision to become a republic rather than continue as a monarchy after
the success of the revolution was a surprise to many. It was settled when
George Washington declined a proffered crown. When the loose American
Confederation, which existed after the establishment of the Republic, was
found to be ineffective, a new form of federation among the states had to be
created. The United States of America, as a nation state, depended upon the
acceptance of the newly proposed Constitution. This important document is
still effective today. It describes the rights, privileges, and attitudes that are
still currently important in understanding American behaviors in many domestic as well as international affairs. The Constitution is the bulwark that pro-
claims and assures the duties, responsibilities, and rights of the individual. It
is marked by emphasis on the protection of the action of individuals. It is the
individual who is important and not the state.

The Constitution also contains a marked emphasis on the rights and needs of the minority. It protects the individual and the minority against a "tyranni-cal majority". These emphases are descended from the essays in the Federal-ist Papers and in the prolonged and difficult debates that finally produced the Constitution. The continued emphasis upon the rights of the individual and the freedoms of the individual must be understood to grasp the nature of Amer-ican thought and behavior. The important subtleties and nuances produced by these cultural characteristics are, unfortunately, the source of puzzlement and misunderstanding of American actions and concepts in international matters.

After the successful revolution and the establishment of the United States, there was a definite wave of isolation. These early Americans did not wish "for-eign entanglement". The American hero, George Washington, as first Presi-dent, urged the new country to avoid the turmoil of foreign affairs beyond the usual diplomatic functions. He further urged that comfortable and friendly relations be established with foreign powers, largely European of course. These aspects of his advice were taken seriously and the new country attempt-ed to become as self-contained as possible. Despite these desires to be self-sufficient, there was a great need for the unstable new country to have the pro-tection, even though indirect, of the rapidly developing powerful British Navy. The unsettled conditions in continental Europe and Britain, and the long wars that began with the French Revolution and continued in the Napoleonic era, contributed strongly to the need in the young United States to develop its businesses and agriculture without involvement in European affairs. It could not afford the draining weakness of constant warfare in Europe. However, a powerful British fleet was necessary to realize this dream, despite the transient support by the French of the Americans during the revolution. Of course, these events were a tiny and unimportant American part of the Anglo-French conflicts until the end of the Napoleonic Wars. In this welter of complex forces, American isolationism was a practical and useful way of staying out of the many bloody, continuous, and enduring conflicts in Europe.

The nineteenth century

As the youthful country developed, there were several important events that help us to understand the evolution of American attitudes towards internation-al affairs, which would influence those attitudes of the twentieth century. Dur-ing the nineteenth century, the United States expanded. In 1803, Thomas Jef-ferson's administrations bought Louisiana from Napoleon, doubling the size of the country overnight. In 1846, war with Mexico resulted in additional territory. It included the Spanish-speaking settlements of California, Arizona, and New Mexico. Texas, after secession from Mexico, became a "Lone Star State" and then joined the United States shortly thereafter, as a result of the powerful presence of immigrants from the American southern states. The Northwest Territory was similarly acquired relatively inexpensively, largely by the conquest and removal of the indigenous population of Native Americans to segregated reservations.

The blood-bath of the American Civil War was a major upheaval that became the prelude to a reinforcement of the power of the Federal Government in foreign affairs of the United States. Sovereign power of foreign relations of the individual states no longer existed. There appeared to be more willingness of the United States to expand its relationship with the rest of the world at the end of the Civil War, while prohibiting foreign interference in the Americas in the proclamation of the Monroe Doctrine. Another event influencing the entry of the United States into world affairs occurred with the war against Spain in 1898. Many observers view this quarrel as a determined effort to remove important European influence from the New World. Puerto Rico became an American dependency. The United States continued its expansionist and international influence further by annexing the Philippines from Spain.

The early twentieth century

The young United States was ready to become a world power and it did so shortly after this conflict during the presidency of Theodore Roosevelt. The same American characteristics of individuality, private enterprise, and voluntary associations were the hallmarks of the coming of age of the United States as a power with which to be reckoned. They strengthened the no longer inexperienced republic as an important factor in world affairs. Entry into World War I in 1917 completed this activity of abandoning self-sufficient isolation, at least for a time. There were still surprises to come about American ambivalence toward "foreign entanglements".

At the conclusion of World War I, the American President, Woodrow Wilson, attempted to make "the world safe for democracy". The result was a sharp negative reaction in the United States that was compounded by the decision of the allied victors to punish the defeated central powers, by requiring the payment of large reparations that resulted in severe economic misfortune in Europe. The defeat of the ideals of the American President by the Senate, which has the power to accept or reject treaties, was inevitable. The associated refusal in the United States to enter the League of Nations was supported by the American people. Thus the United States then embarked on a period of political isolation in which many things foreign were viewed with suspicion. There was very little willingness to be a part of the family of nations in any significant and important way.

American medical politics between the World Wars

From the standpoint of the medical aspects of American attitudes, and particularly those of anesthesiology, there was a much more-receptive attitude toward participation in international events. There was not as much hostility to foreign relationships in medical and anesthetic circles as in other parts of American society. Despite the strong isolationism of the general public after the war, there was cooperation during the war in the intellectual as well as the practical sides of societal behavior. Anesthesia collaboration during the war were most cordial with allied opposite numbers in the armed forces. For instance, the signs of the depth of ether anesthesia developed by Arthur Guedel were described during the conflict, were made available to anesthetists in the United Kingdom and in Continental Europe, and published shortly after the war [1]. This was a major step forward in the development of the young specialty of anesthesiology and it also was a modest move in the direction of collaborative international behavior on the part of Americans. Guedel's contributions to the idea that knowledge in anesthesia was good for all people everywhere were understood at that period of the early twentieth century.

However, the interwar period clearly reflected the dichotomy of thought between the isolationists, represented by the New York Society of Anesthetists, and the internationalists, represented by the International Anesthesia Research Society. In the 1920s until the mid 1930s, the internationalists dominated the American scene in the guise of Francis Hoeffer McMechan (Fig. 1) [2]. McMechan organized the first national anesthesia organization in the United States, the Associated Anesthetists of America. By 1926, the organization had changed its name to the Associated Anesthetists of the United States and Canada [3].

Seven years before, McMechan organized the National Anesthesia Research Society (NARS). Membership was open to anyone interested in the problems associated with the specialty. Thus, dentists and basic scientists held membership on an equal footing with physicians. Beginning in 1922, the NARS published the first journal devoted to anesthesiology in the world, *Current Researches in Anesthesia and Analgesia*, with McMechan as editor-in-chief. For the first time, one place was available for the publication of articles on anesthesia. In addition, meeting announcements and matters of political interest to the physician anesthetists of the day were available. By 1925, the organization had members from across the world and changed its name to the International Anesthesia Research Society (IARS) [4].

In 1926, the IARS jointly sponsored their annual Congress of Anesthetists with the British Medical Association's Section on Anaesthetics in London. Termed the first All World Congress of Anesthetists [5], it marked the first cooperation between the British and Americans in peace time. Later that

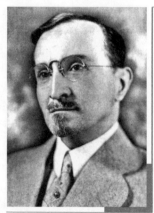

Fig. 1. *Francis Hoeffer McMechan (photograph courtesy of the Wood Library/Museum of Anesthesiology, Park Ridge, Illinois, USA)*

year, Ralph Waters (Fig. 2) of Madison, Wisconsin, who developed one of the first academic departments in the world, wrote to McMechan requesting his help in arranging the American itinerary of Dr. Helmut Schmidt of Hamburg, Germany. Waters especially wanted Schmidt to attend the 1927 Congress of Anesthetists. McMechan willingly agreed, and feted his guest during the meeting [6].

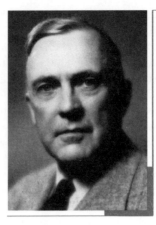

Fig. 2. *Ralph Waters (photograph courtesy of the Wood Library/Museum of Anesthesiology, Park Ridge, Illinois, USA)*

Schmidt invited McMechan to Germany and to tour Europe the following year. McMechan's French wife, Laurette, accompanied him on this trip; their stops included Hamburg, Munich, Prague, Glasgow, and Edinburgh. In 1929, McMechan would venture to Australia, where he attended the Australian Medical Congress of the British Medical Association. The meeting marked the formation of the Section on Anesthetics. In his opening remarks, Gilbert Brown, President of the section said, "Dr. Frank McMechan has done more than any other man to organize the anesthetists of the world. In fact, this section owes its existence largely to his tireless energy in persuading others to ask, and keep on asking, for a Section on Anesthetics. At this meeting he has formed the last link in his chain of groups of organized anesthetists throughout the English-speaking world." [7].

Nothing captures the flavor of McMechan the internationalist as the issue of certification does. McMechan wanted all anesthetists across the world to be certified by one organization, the International College of Anesthetists. McMechan felt that many countries did not have sufficient numbers of physicians to organize their own certifying body. Thus, for the first time, an anesthetist had credentials as a specialist in anesthesiology that were consistent from the United States to Europe to Australia [8]. It was McMechan's crowning glory.

America for Americans?

In the United States in the late 1930s nothing split American anesthetists further from McMechan than the International College. Quite simply, it had no standing and was not recognized by American medicine. Clinical criteria for the college did not conform with the criteria set forth by the American Medical Association (AMA). Additionally, McMechan had set forth as one criterion, that anesthesiologists who worked with nurse anesthetists could not be certified by the college [9]. Paul Wood (Fig. 3), John Lundy (Fig. 4), and Ralph

Waters knew that for the specialty to be recognized in
America, the AMA would have
to approve of the any efforts
at certification [10]. Working
together, Lundy, Waters and
Wood set out to create a certification scheme acceptable to
the AMA.

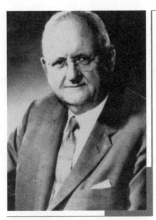

Fig. 3. *Paul Wood
(photograph courtesy
of the Wood
Library/Museum of
Anesthesiology, Park
Ridge, Illinois, USA)*

They began by using the
New York Society of Anes-
thetists, the larger of two
organizations outside Mc
Mechan's control. A new clas-
sification of membership was
created, called "fellows" that
conformed to AMA guidelines
on certification. Whereas the
International College only
required report of ten cases
anesthetized and lessons
learned from these clinical
excursions, fellows were
required to demonstrate 2,500
anesthetics given, or 3 years
post graduate training in anesthesiology and 500 anesthetics given [11].

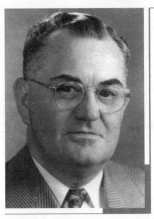

Fig. 4. *John Lundy
(photograph courtesy
of the Wood
Library/Museum of
Anesthesiology, Park
Ridge, Illinois, USA)*

Fellowship was widely popular, and soon the New York Society had
members from across the United States. For those outside of the New York
City metropolitan area, the minutes of meeting were mimeographed and
sent to them. In 1936, the New York Society changed its name to the American Society of Anesthetists (ASA) to partly reflect its national character, and
partly to conform with AMA guidelines concerning a national sponsor for a
specialty board [12]. A month later Erwin Schmidt, Chairman of Surgery at
the University of Wisconsin and nominally Ralph Waters' boss, attended a
meeting of the ASA and proposed that the American Board of Surgery (ABS)
would be willing to sponsor the American Board of Anesthesiology (ABA)
as a sub-board [13]. On 10 January 1937, Paul Wood and Ralph Waters were
invited to the Palmer House in Chicago to discuss their proposal. Given
20 minutes to speak, they discussed their plan for over 2 hours. Within a year,
the ABA had been incorporated. By 1940, for many reasons, the ABA gained
independence [14].

The offshoot of the certification process was an upheaval and a change
in the leadership of American anesthesiology. No longer was McMechan's

organization in charge, yet the ASA was wholly unprepared for this new leadership role. It would not be until well after the World War II that the ASA became comfortable as the political voice of American anesthesiology [15]. Given the antagonistic relationship that developed between the ASA and McMechan over certification, a more parochial view was in vogue.

World War II - a milestone for Americans?

The next evidence of strong international interest on the part of America was in the joining with the allies in World War II to overcome the major threat to the democratic way of life by the Nazi government of Germany. The entry of the United States into World War II was neither comfortable nor easy for this nation. There was much of the isolationist feeling at the time. There was reluctance on the part of many to enter a war in which they felt we had no important interest at stake. They felt immune to attack behind the Atlantic and Pacific Oceans. President Franklin D. Roosevelt's view was very different from that of the isolationists. He was deeply concerned after the fall of France to the Germans. His fear was that the survival of a lonely Britain against the German military might was doubtful. The Soviet Union entered the war relatively late compared with Britain and France, after Hitler unilaterally renounced the non-aggression pact and launched a massive invasion in the East after he felt sure of victory in the West.

Isolationist views in the United States dissolved automatically after the Japanese attack and the destruction of Pearl Harbor in Hawaii on 7 December 1941. American entry into the war against Japan was immediate, as was the entry into the European conflict on the side of the Western Allies. American mobilization for war was large and important to the allied cause. At its peak 22 million men and women were in the armed forces. The economy was entirely dedicated to the war effort and to the defeat of the Axis Powers. It was also the first time that a serious physical attack upon American territory had occurred. It was followed by the fear of an imminent assault upon the West Coast of the United States by Japan. The previous territorial immunity to assault unlike other nations from the continental European is crucial to the understanding of the ambivalence of American to "foreign entanglement".

The large participation of Americans in this conflict brought a good many physicians and surgeons into contact with their opposite numbers, especially in the United Kingdom and to a lesser extent with other allies. However, the attitude of Americans changed. They learned in combat in both the European and Asiatic wars how important it was to be sure that the American dream and the American way of life should be preserved by victory in the conflict. The nation closed ranks and many Americans got their first taste on a large scale of international relations.

The post-war experience

In the case of anesthesiology, a large-scale dissemination of the knowledge and methods of the newly evolving specialty from its civilian antecedents at Wisconsin, New York University, The Mayo Clinic, and The Massachusetts General Hospital, among others, took place. A new attitude became evident among young Americans, both during the conflict and immediately after its cessation with allied victory. Anesthesiologists and surgeons insisted that the lessons learned in the care of military casualties both in surgery and anesthesia must be carried into civilian life. Many young surgeons requested as well as demanded the availability of the kind of anesthesia that they saw to be so important for the care of severely injured and wounded soldiers and the many civilian casualties they encountered. Anesthesiology also engaged the interest of a good many young physicians who sought education and residency training upon their release from military service. The approximately 50 or so physicians who had meaningful anesthesia education prior to their assuming military responsibilities did a superb job, as did the civilian anesthesiologists back in the United States in providing the education that was required for young physicians who had their first major clinical experiences during the war. Many who were to become leaders in American anesthesiology had their first contact with anesthesia as very junior medical officers by being assigned to a military anesthesia service or voluntarily taking it up and continuing it upon their re-entry into civilian life.

When the war was over, many young physicians and veterans sought to complete their graduate education in their chosen fields. Anesthesiology was attractive to many because of their first-hand military experience. Associated with this increased interest in the clinical aspects of the specialty was a great desire to participate in the continued and rapid development of scientific knowledge via research. Many of the war veterans who saw an unexpected opportunity in anesthesiology also found the research opportunities very attractive. These veteran physicians were dedicated and hard working. They produced a major impetus to the enhancement of the relatively young specialty. The medical veterans engaged in a most-spectacular display of dedication, energy, and unfailing devotion to the opportunities presented by the educational experience of residency training.

As a result of the personal contacts during the war in the various armed services of the United States, as well as in the support system of civilian life, there was a strong conviction that a spirit of vengeance against the vanquished Axis Powers would be self-defeating. In a healthy and peaceful world, much more could be accomplished if the devastated and overwhelmed countries were helped back to political and economic health in the community of nations. Democracy became an achievable goal as the result of this aid. The Marshall Plan to reconstruct Europe was the result of this new American perspective.

It marked a major participation in world affairs for the United States.

A remaining problem from the American perspective was how to deal with the now unfriendly Soviet Union whose opposition to the purposes of the democratic West was very clear. This was the beginning of the Cold War, which never, despite many periods of angst, became hot, because of the awesome threat of nuclear war by either of the two remaining superpowers. All these events had major influence on Americans, including anesthesiologists, in international relations. On the positive side was the increased experience of Americans of people from other countries, much of it favorable. On the negative was the perceived constant threat of a nuclear holocaust.

This experience lead to a scenario that was very different from that after World War I. Many of the distinguished leaders in anesthesiology, e.g.. E.A. Rovenstine, Stuart Cullen, Robert Dripps, and others, who had not seen military service were very anxious to use the developments in anesthesiology in the United States to aid in the medical reconstruction of the defeated Axis nations. Rovenstine went with an American Friends group to Czechoslovakia; Cullen worked in Austria and Denmark; Dripps in Britain and many others, including Beecher, Papper, and especially Jack Moyers (Fig. 5) of Iowa, participated as instructors and visiting professors in the newly created anaesthesiology educational center in Copenhagen. All of the Americans, both World War II veterans and those who remained in civilian life, contributed selflessly and significantly to the center in Denmark, the other Scandinavian countries, and other nations in Europe. Their voluntary assignments were usually between 2 and 4 months in duration. However, Moyers repeatedly spent longer periods, (one visit lasted a year) in providing American aid to this important center. There was no longer any question about the interest of Americans in all aspects of international affairs, i.e., political, economic, medical, and of course anesthesiological.

The activities of the Copenhagen center were under the direction of Denmark's distinguished surgeon Professor Erik Husfeldt. Husfeldt directed the center and was also the university's professor of surgery. The actual anesthesia education was conducted at the various teaching hospitals in Copenhagen, each headed by its own professor and chief. The University Hospital's chief was Professor Ole Secher who has described the center and its fruitful experience elsewhere in great detail. The education, training and experience of anesthesiologists at this magnificent center was a major factor in the development of anesthesia in Europe and else-

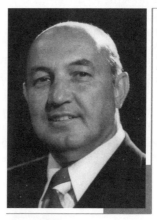

Fig. 5. *Jack Moyers (photograph courtesy of the Wood Library/Museum of Anesthesiology, Park Ridge, Illinois)*

where. Coupled with this marked interest on the part of American anesthesiologists in international activities, an informal, but very effective program developed in several American institutions. Young anesthesiologists came to the United States in large numbers after World War II to advance their experience in the clinical and scientific aspects of anesthesiology. Others came for their basic clinical training as residents. In the early post-war years, many Europeans came to Beecher's department at the Massachusetts General Hospital for either clinical or research education, or both. These visits to other departments in the United States by anesthesiologists from abroad wishing to improve their skills continued in substantial numbers immediately after the end of the war, and in some instances even before we entered the conflict. The visits to work in American institutions increased quickly and widely, especially among Europeans, but also anesthesiologists from Japan and other countries in the Far East, as well a small number from the Middle East and Africa. Some anesthesiologists from abroad made tours of several institutions on their own. Others were attracted to certain departments for the expertise they wished to acquire, and still others were advised to attend various American departments by their professors for at least a year (and often longer).

The Massachusetts General Hospital program headed by Beecher, the University of Pennsylvania department chaired by Dripps, the Columbia Presbyterian Medical Center chaired by Papper, The Mayo Clinic led by Lundy, and the more-established departments at Wisconsin and New York University, the former headed by the doyen of American anesthesia, Ralph M. Waters, and the latter headed by the distinguished E.A. Rovenstine, received large numbers of these foreign visitors. Other anesthesiologists found themselves in departments that were being formed and in sense grew up with them. During the 1950s, so common had this experience become that some of our British colleagues and friends characterized it as an earned degree-BTA-Been To America!

This process of American participation in the education and intellectual growth of our friends from abroad was significantly and favorably influenced by the extraordinary competence and skills that were acquired by American anesthesiologists in scientific research. There was a marked increase in research and clinical excellence in the United States from the end of the war through the 1960s, when important funding for research was provided for anesthesiology by the National Institutes of Health in America. Many individual anesthesiologists from abroad profited from this opportunity to learn about research and took the fruits of their knowledge back to their own countries. Many of the young people who came to study in America assumed positions of leadership in anesthesiology in their own countries, especially in Europe, in Latin America, and in Asia. The network of relationships that developed from these experiences was strong and many of the friendships became permanent. The international flavor of the fraternity of anesthesiologists is impossible to overstate. It was a very important part of the American perspective and it took advantage of the basic American instinct for voluntary assistance and association. While funded generously by the government, the international collaboration was the actions of individuals and groups. They were characterized by the American feeling of generosity toward friends, old and new, whose activities in anesthesiology would become a major force in providing good care to peoples in the entire world. The educational activities followed and overlapped important, yet different types of experiences provided by the Copenhagen center.

While all of these international collaborations were taking place, two important events in the larger American social fabric occurred that had an inevitably negative impact upon the international bent of the new American attitude. One was the intensification and continuation of the Cold War with the Soviet Union. Unfortunately, one of the unintended consequences of this problem was a marked concern in some American circles of the "infiltration" of communist influence at high levels of American government as well as other American institutions. The provocative force leading the new hysteria was Senator Joseph McCarthy, of Wisconsin, who saw a communist danger almost everywhere. In the American Congress, the leader of the anti-communists was the future President Richard Nixon. It is difficult to make clear to non-Americans how pervasive this concern and fear was. McCarthyism, as it was called, had such a major effect on American society that an entire generation of artists, writers, and performers in Hollywood's movie industry were blacklisted for alleged or real communist activities. The stain of this irrational hostility was a black mark against the previous American view of international cooperation.

American concerns about the WFSA

Americans, of otherwise good sense, reacted severely to some of the concerns of communist penetration of the American government. It was one of the reasons why there was some doubt and some antipathy toward American collaboration and participation in international organizations that freely admitted to membership the various communist countries. Among the organizations viewed with suspicion by some conservative anesthesiologists was the WFSA. There was real opposition to American participation in WFSA by the ASA by some of its leaders who felt that any society that admitted communist groups was inappropriate for American participation. It was once again "foreign entanglements" with a threat to the American ideal of freedom and the rights of individuals. *Irrational as it sounds, this was a factor in the concerns of some, perhaps many Americans, about participation with "the enemy" i.e., members of Communist countries in any organizations.*

However, the American reluctance to join the WFSA is not as simple as an anti-communist reaction. The anesthesiologists of the United States were important to the WFSA as they represented approximately 4,000 of the 6,000 English-speaking anesthesiologists in the world [18]. The soil upon which the seed of the WFSA was planted was McMechan's old organizations. In 1951, the International Anesthesia Research Society and the International College of Anesthetists, both founded by McMechan, held a joint meeting with the Associated of Anaesthetists of Great Britain and Ireland, and the Section of Anaesthetics of the Royal Society of Medicine; 422 anesthesiologists from 27 countries were present [19].

From the London meeting, a delegation went to Paris, where further discussion were held concerning the formation of the WFSA. Negotiating in earnest, a sponsor was found to help put together the organization. Jean Dalafresnaye, secretary of the Council for International Organization of Medical Societies of the United Nations Educational, Scientific and Cultural Organization was brought in to solicit support for an Organizing Committee [20]. A year later the Organizing Committee met, and Harold Griffith of Montreal was chosen as chairman. The United States was represented by members of the IARS: Drs. Friend, Sheldon, and Whitacre [21] Throughout all further Organizing Committee meetings and the first World Congress of Anesthesiologists, any official representation came from the IARS.

Back in the United States, a debate was raging in earnest. As early as 1955, editorials were written expressing opposition to the WFSA. The invitation to immediately join the organization, issued by Harold Griffith and Clarence Durshordwe (a Buffalo, New York anesthesiologist and close friend of McMechan and several of the WFSA organizers [22]) was turned down because it was felt that without a vote of the ASA's House of Delegates, the officers could not commit to the WFSA [23]. The New York State Society (NYSSA), one of the largest and oldest components of the ASA, sent a memorandum to Robert L. Patterson, who was chairman of the Investigating Committee of the WFSA outlining the NYSSA's objections. There were five points to the memorandum, and item number three is most interesting. The NYSSA was being asked for U.S. $ 450 as its dues to the WFSA. The objection was twofold, first, how was the figure arrived at, and secondly, it was thought to be "unfair and undemocratic to have a sliding scale for the determination of the number of delegates" [24].

Dueling letters to the editor continued in The *Bulletin of the New York State Society of Anesthesiologists* over the next several years. The next heated exchange occurred in 1958, when NYSSA President Vincent J. Collins wrote an open letter to the publication. Commenting upon Harold Griffith editorial in *Anesthesiology* [25] Collins argued that working through the World Medical Association (WMA), and a proposed section of anesthesia, would be better. Financial support of the WMA was purely voluntary, in contradistinction to the WFSA [26]. Collins feelings were countered by two letters published in the next edition of *The Bulletin* by E.M. Papper and M.J. Frumin, both of Presbyterian Hospital in New York City. Papper and Frumin countered the argument about representation, pointing out that the composition of the General Assembly of the WFSA was made up in the same manner as the House of Delegates of the ASA. Thus, they argued neither the New York Society in the ASA or the Americans in the WFSA could be "pushed around". Secondly, financially, both Frumin and Papper pointed out that there was a cap on the obligation and that the final assessment was well within the financial abilities of the society [27].

In the following issue Collins responded. He reiterated his stance that he was not against international cooperation in anesthesiology, but rather the forum under which it took place. Collins pointed out that there was no "fear of foreign domination", but he continued to severely criticize the "socialist structure" under which the WFSA was organized. Collins was concerned that the individual physician had no say in whether or not he joined the organization, for the physician was a member through the WFSA membership of his national society. Finally, Collins objected to the WFSA's attachment to the United Nations. He was concerned about the implications of membership in which the majority of members were socialists. Collins warned that "...medicine need not and should not have attachments with any controversial government political flavor" [28].

Within the same issue of *The Bulletin*, Collins arguments were refuted by two other anesthesiologists. B. Raymond Fink wrote supporting the position of Griffith in the *Anesthesiology* editorial of earlier that year. Fink believed that an open and honest dialog between physicians of different countries could only benefit both. Raphael Robertazzi tried to be the voice of reason in the debate. He called for reconsideration of the New York State and by implication the ASA's position concerning the WFSA. Robertazzi saw first hand at the first World Congress how hurt the world anesthesiology community was at the lack of American participation. He felt that even if a dues increase was necessary, it was well worth the increased cost [29].

In 1959, when the ASA had declined membership of the WFSA, it was divided in its decisions. Professor (later Sir Geoffrey) Geoffrey Organe (Fig. 6) who was secretary at the time of the WFSA planned to entertain a group of foreign visitors, of whom there were several American anesthesiologists. E.M. Papper was one of this group at the suggestion of the President of the ASA. Other Americans included some of the leaders of the opposition to American membership of the WFSA, as well as supporters of our proposed membership.

Professor Organe was advised to have a dinner meeting to encourage free discussion about the newly established WFSA. That dinner took place in the spring of 1959 prior to the annual meeting of the ASA. The venue was The Royal College of Surgeons in London. The British hosts put on a very warm and friendly social occasion that provided a perfect setting for the answering of questions and the

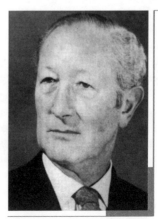

Fig. 6. *Sir Geoffrey Organe (photograph courtesy of the Wood Library/Museum of Anesthesiology, Park Ridge, Illinois, USA)*

resolution of the possible problems to facilitate the entrance of the American Society into the World Federation. Many questions were asked and satisfactorily answered by our British hosts. In fact so cordial and informative was the social and intellectual intercourse that the Americans who were opposed to American entrance into the WFSA were convinced that the previous American reasons for objecting to join the WFSA were no longer pertinent and the time of joining was clearly at hand. Such is the magic of open friendly communication!

At the annual meeting of the ASA, appropriate resolutions were introduced to join the World Federation in 1960 and were carried with almost no opposition. It was now time for Americans to participate in international affairs again. To many Americans, it was a happy relief from isolationism.

Objections resolved

Although the history of the formation of the WFSA appears, at first glance, unrelated to the American bent for isolation and its passion for anti-communism, they were, none the less, real factors in the decision of the ASA not to join an organization that appeared to some Americans to be sympathetic to communism. Many Americans were also worried that the rest of the Western world was not joining the United States in curbing the communist threat to freedom and to the democratic way of life. Unbelievable as some of these ideas now seem, they influenced the return to the earliest phases of American behavior, i.e., to cease "foreign entanglements". The reluctance of ASA to join the WFSA at that time was part of the transient isolation of Americans from international affairs. When the McCarthy era ended, Americans were more receptive to participation in world-wide matters once again.

Perhaps one of the greatest factors in the American reluctance to join the WFSA was the changing of the guard in American anesthesiology just before World War II. The ascendancy of the ASA, ostensibly around the issue of certification of specialists and in opposition to Francis Hoeffer McMechan, and his death on 29 June 1939, left American anesthesiology unprepared for international collaboration. As McMechan's close friend and anesthesiologist, Charles Wells wrote that "...Dr. McMechan ... was a born internationalist, and would not deviate from his set purpose. ...Perhaps the early competition of the national and international idealism was a prominent factor in bringing about..." [30] the tremendous growth of anesthesiology in post war America. However, in rejecting McMechan's international ideas concerning certification [10] the "new" leaders of anesthesiology were not ready for international liaisons after the war. Men like Papper, Fink, and Robertazzi were exposed to international contacts through their post-graduate programs and their careers. For Papper especially, at Bellevue with Emery Rovenstine, the world came to be trained and Papper knew the importance of international cooperation.

Leaders like Vincent Collins had yet to be exposed to the needs of the international community. However, to their credit, after years of open, and at times heated debate, they changed their minds and supported the WFSA. Learning to cooperate in international anesthesia politics as they had in the national scene so effectively, the American contribution to the WFSA has been great and equally important to the WFSA as it has been to the American anesthesiologists.

Epilog

Among the cultural exchanges that occurred were some of mutual interest to clinical medicine and the biomedical sciences. The President appointed distinguished groups of Americans in the arts, the sciences, and in other walks of life to visit China. Anesthesiology was proud to be included in this first mission. Dr. John Bonica was our representative on this American cultural mission to China. In anesthesiology, there was another mission sponsored by the National Academy of Sciences of the United States, which was sent to the Peoples Republic of China to study acupuncture for surgical anesthesia. Members of the delegation included a Chinese scholar, a physiologist, a neurologist, neurosurgeons, anesthesiologists, and a psychiatrist. In short it was a committee with an excellent background in the neurosciences. Dr. Papper had the privilege of chairing that delegation.

The experiences in China were extremely useful in changing the attitudes of Americans towards international affairs in a very significant way. The American conclusion was that whatever acupuncture did it was not reliable for surgical anesthesia. The reason had little to do with whether it provided anesthetic comfort for some patients, which it appeared to. It failed in that it did not meet the requirement of 100% success as a criterion for useful surgical anesthesia. One could understand that there might be failures in any anesthetic system, but they had to be unusual, very infrequent, and not related to the method of clinical application. The members of the United States delegation formed good and lasting friendships with our colleagues in China. We experienced many discomforts, but these were associated with the different social customs in the two countries, and the enterprise promised a collaboration that was peaceful and fruitful for the future.

As all these forces came together, it seemed that the understandable initial objection several years before the Chinese mission of some prominent American anesthesiologists to join the WFSA had been appropriately resolved in 1960. That action on the part of the ASA made it possible for Americans to work constructively on the world scene. The purpose of the World Federation, which was to bring better anesthesia to all peoples of the world, has been well accepted since 1960. Clearly an American presence was important. When the ASA joined a major force was added in providing support for the excellent missions of the World Federation.

References

1. Guedel AE (1920) Third stage ether anesthesia: a subclassification regarding the significance of position and movements of the eyeball. Q Suppl Am J Surg 34:53-57

2. Wells CJ (1948) Francis Hoeffer McMechan. Curr Res Anesth Analg [Suppl]:1-19

3. Betcher AM, Ciliberti BJ, Wood PM, Wright LH (1956) The jubilee year of organized anesthesiology. Anesthesiology 17:226-264

4. Ranney O (1939) Francis Hoeffer McMechan, AB,AM, MD, FICA, his life and work. Curr Res Anesth Analg 18:[Suppl]

5. Editorial (1926) Br J Anaesth 3:B

6. Letter from Ralph Waters to Francis Hoeffer McMechan, December 30, 1926. The Guedel Center Archives, San Francisco, California

7. Wilson G (1987) Fifty years: The Australian Society of Anaesthetists 1934-1984. Glebe, Australia. The Flannel Flower Press, p 567

8. Bacon DR (1997) The World Federation of Societies of Anesthesiologists: McMechan's final legacy? Anesth Analg 84:1130-1135

9. "Dear Frank [McMechan], I thought you told me you were sorry but you would be unable to certify me as a specialist in anesthesia. Therefore, I assume it would be kindness on our part if myself and my associates did not fill out and return the enclosed blank" Lundy's proposed response to Francis Hoeffer McMechan's request for applicants to the International College of Anesthetists. 1936. The Collected Papers of John Lundy. Mayo Clinic Archive, Rochester, Minnesota

10. Bacon DR, Lundy JS, Waters R, Wood P (1995) The founding of the American Board of Anesthesiology. Bull Anesth Hist 13:1-5

11. Application for Fellowship in the American Society of Anesthetists, The Collected Papers of the Long Island, New York and American Society of Anesthetists, Wood Library/Museum of Anesthesiologists, Park Ridge, Illinois

12. Minutes of Meeting February 13, 1936. The Collected Papers of the Long Island, New York and American Societies of Anesthetists. Wood Library/Museum Collection. Park Ridge, Illinois

13. Minutes of Meeting of the American Society of Anesthetists March 9, 1936. The Collected Papers of the Long Island, New York and American Societies of Anesthetists. The Wood Library/Museum of Anesthesiology Collection. Park Ridge, Illinois

14. Bacon DR, Lema MJ (1992) To define a specialty: A brief history of the American Board of Anesthesiology's first written examination. J Clin Anesth 4:489-497

15. Bacon DR (1994) The promise of one great anesthesia society: The 1939-1940 proposed merger of the American Society of Anesthetists and the International Anesthesia Research Society. Anesthesiology 80:929-935

16. Letter from Paul Wood to Francis Hoeffer McMechan, April 15, 1936. The Collected Papers of Paul Wood, M.D. The Wood Library/Museum Collection, Park Ridge, Illinois

17. Secher O (1978) The department of anaesthesia, Rigshospital. Personal views from 1953-78. Acta Anaesthesiol Scand [Suppl] 67:10-22

18. Griffith HR (1953) Plans for a World Federation of Anaesthesiologists. 32:S10-S17

19. Griffith HR (1951) Report on the 1951 London Congress of Anesthetists. Curr Res Anesth Analg 30:129-133

20. Griffith HR (1963) History of the World Federation of Anesthesiologists. Anesth Analg 42:389-397

21. Minutes of Meeting of the Organizing Committee of the World Federation of Societies of Anesthesiologists, 18-20 June, 1953. Wood Library/Museum Collection, Park Ridge, Illinois

22. Batt R, Bacon DR (2001) Clarence J. Durshordwe, the IARS, and the WFSA: the last true disciple of Francis Hoeffer McMechan. Anesth Analg 92:1349-1354

23. Editorial (1955) Bull N Y Soc Anesthesiol 7:1

24. Memorandum from The New York Sate Society of Anesthesiologists to Robert L. Patterson, MD, March 25, 1955. The Collected papers of Paul Wood, M.D. Wood Library/Museum Collection, Park Ridge, Illinois

25. Griffith HR (1958) On friendship. Anesthesiology 19:88-89

26. Collins VJ (1958) Comments on world friendship. Bull N Y Soc Anesthesiol 10:7

27. Papper EM, Frumin MJ (1958) Open letters to the editor. Bull N Y Soc Anesthesiol 10:2-4

28. Collins VJ (1958) Letters to the editor. Bull N Y Soc Anesthesiol 10:2-4

29. Fink BR, Robertazzi RW (1958) Letter to the editor. Bull N Y Soc Anesthesiol 10:4

30. Letter from Charles J. Wells to Sidney Cushing Wiggin, August 18, 1949. The Charles J Wells Collection. Wood Library/Museum of Anesthesiology Archive. Park Ridge, Illinois

4 WFSA - Development Between 1955 and 1972

O. Mayrhofer

Introduction

In the 1990s the Executive Committee of the Federation decided to document the first 50 years since the foundation of the World Federation of Societies of Anaesthesiologists (WFSA). Among a few others, I was approached by past President John Zorab to contribute a chapter on the early history, including regionalisation.

When Zorab retired from his function as co-ordinator, Dr. Joseph Rupreht of Rotterdam, the honorary archivist of the WFSA, took over. In a letter dated 22 February 2000, he explained to me that the editorial burden of the Jubilee Book was now on him and asked me to contribute a personal account covering the period from 1955 to 1972. I agreed but waited until the 12th World Congress of Anaethesiologists (WCA) in Montreal when I met Gullo and Rupreht personally. They reassured me that the Executive Committee had given the green light for the publication of the documentation to be presented at the 13th World Congress in Paris 2004 and he urged me to start writing my chapter.

My motivation is the fact that I was actively involved in the foundation of the WFSA and its development over the first 25 years of its existence. As the official delegate of the Austrian Society of Anaesthesiologists at the founding congress in Scheveningen 1955 and member of the first Executive Committee, my signature is on the founding charter of the Federation.

I had kept notes of most of the meetings I attended in my various capacities, but almost all of the material, including correspondence and minutes, were handed over to Professor John Bonica in 1972 when he followed me as secretary of the WFSA. I do hope that all these papers and his correspondence and meeting minutes during his term were eventually given to the Wood Library Museum after his death and are now in the WFSA archives.

Thus my story is based mainly on my reminiscences and on the ten personal issues of the WFSA Newsletter, which I edited between 1965 and 1974.

I want to point out, however, that the part of the history concerning the Latin American Regional Section is entirely based on the documentation of Dr. Ricardo Samayoa de Leon of Guatemala City, which he very kindly put at my disposal and for which he deserves full credit.

1955-1964: initial growth, the period of "childhood"

In the wake of the 1955 World Congress at Scheveningen, general disappointment was voiced that some societies had only sent observers and hesitated to join. The membership fee of U.S. $ 1 per individual member made it obviously difficult for some societies from Asia, Africa, and Eastern Europe to join. Most of all, the fact that the American Society of Anesthesiologists (ASA), with about 8,000 members, did not join, raised problems for the newly founded Federation and certainly hampered its initial activities through lack of funds.

However, the secretary/treasurer was able to find industrial sponsors and also established official links with the World Health Organisation (WHO). In addition, he tried to attend as many national and regional meetings as possible, in an attempt to popularise the idea of strength by unification. The first 5 years were certainly the most difficult and crucial in the life of the young Federation. However, the sparkling idea of the founder fathers to "provide the best possible anaesthesia to all peoples of the world" had caught on. Between the 1st and 2nd World Congress, eight additional societies expressed their wish to join the Federation, namely the National Societies of Greece (1956), Hong Kong (1956), Egypt (1957), Czechoslovakia (1958), Japan (1958), Korea (1958), South Africa (1958), and New Zealand (1959). Finally, the ASA announced that they were ready to join the WFSA at the 2nd World Congress in Toronto in 1960.

The 2nd WCA, excellently organised by a committee of the Canadian Society chaired by Professor Roderick ("Rod") A. Gordon, took place in Toronto in the 2nd week of September in 1960. It was an important milestone in the history of the young Federation. Since the ASA decided to join the WFSA during that meeting, the total attendance well surpassed 1,000, and the majority of speakers came from the two North American countries.

When, at the close of the 2nd World Congress Professor H.R.Griffith, our founding President, handed over the office to the newly elected President Professor C.R. ("Kees") Ritsema van Eck of The Netherlands, he could proudly state that the "Child-WFSA" was well on its way to adolescence. Before and during the Toronto Congress the World Federation had grown to 36 member societies, with a total individual membership of more than 12,000 in all parts of the world. This was also reflected by the composition of the board and the various committees. The four new vice-presidents came from Germany - Dr. Jochen Bark of Freiburg, the founding President of the German Society of Anaesthesiologists, from the United States-Dr. F.F. Foldes of Pittsburgh, who had been fighting enthusiastically in the ASA to join the WFSA, from the United Kingdom - Dr. John Gillies of Edinburgh, founder father of the Federation and member of its first Executive Committee, and from Brazil-Dr. Zairo Vieira of Rio de Janeiro, founding delegate and member of the first Executive Committee.

Dr. Geoffrey Organe was re-elected secretary/treasurer and - by secret ballot - half of the original members of the committee remained, whereas six were replaced by election. Thus, the members of the new Executive Committee were: Dr. Ralph S. Sappenfield, Miami, Florida,USA, chairman, Professor O.V.S. Kok, Pretoria, Republic of South Africa, vice-chairmen, Professor John J. Bonica, Tacoma, Washington, USA, Dr. Jacques Boureau, Sèvre, France, Dr. Luis Cabrera Guarderas, Santiago, Chile, Professor Enrico Ciocatto, Turin, Italy, Professor Quintin J. Gomez, Manila, The Philippines, Professor Torsten Gordh, Stockholm, Sweden, Professor Roderick A. Gordon, Toronto, Canada, Professor Otto Mayrhofer, Vienna, Austria, Dr. R. Patrick W. Shackleton, Hursley, Hampshire, UK, and Dr. Zairo E.G. Vieira, Rio de Janeiro, Brasil.

Under the influence of the ASA, the management of the WFSA became a lot more professional than it had been during the first 5 years. Following a proposal by the American delegation, the installation of four standing committees was agreed by the General Assembly. The committees on membership and on finance should primarily assist the secretary/treasurer in recruiting new member societies and in raising funds for the activities of the Federation. The Committee on Bylaws should bring the WFSA bylaws up to date and the committee on regionalisation should encourage and coordinate regional activities. It was quite evident that the organisation of World Congresses once in 4 years could not be enough to achieve the aims and goals of the Federation. Therefore, although the decision was taken to hold the next World Congress in Brazil in September 1964, it was also agreed that the WFSA should encourage and assist the organisation of regional meetings.

National and smaller regional meetings had, of course, been held before the foundation of the WFSA. The larger societies like the Association of Anaesthetists of Great Britain and Ireland (founded 1932), the ASA (1940), and the Societé Francaise d'Anesthésie (1946), to name just a few examples, organised national and regional meetings. The Asociación Argentina de Anestesiologia (founded 1943) invited in 1949 their colleagues from other Latin-American countries for the first Congreso Latino-Americano in Buenos Aires, the Swedish Society of Anaesthesia (founded 1946) held Scandinavian congesses from 1950, which lead to the foundation of the Scandinavian Society of Anaesthesiologists. The Austrian Society of Anaesthesiology (founded 1951) began in Salzburg in 1952 the organisation of so-called Central European Meetings of Anaesthetists in biannual rotation with the German and Swiss societies.

Professor T. Cecil Gray of Liverpool, attending the Central European meeting in Duesseldorf in 1959, suggested organising the First European Congress and proposed Vienna as the ideal site and 1962 as the best time, exactly between two World Congresses. When he was elected chairman of the Regionalisation Committee in Toronto this idea was officially adopted and

Vienna 1962 became the first link in the chain of - to date - 11 European Congresses. In South America the second regional meeting took place in Sao Paulo in 1954, followed by Bogota 1956, Vina del Mar, Chile 1958, Mexico City 1960, and Lima 1962. At this meeting the Confederación Latino-Americana de Anestesiologia (CLASA) was founded, which later became the Latin-American Regional Section of the WFSA.

The 3ʳᵈ WCA was held in early September 1964 in Sao Paulo, Brazil, under the presidency of Dr. Luiz Rodriguez Alves, with Dr. Carlos Parsloe acting as chairman of the Organising Committee. Although the new congress hall had not been fully completed, the meeting was a great success. About 1,300 anaesthetists, with a total of 1,800 participants from more than 50 countries, had assembled to watch, to listen, and to learn.

The national anaesthesia societies of Sri Lanka (Ceylon), the Republic of China (Taiwan), and of Yugoslavia had been provisionally admitted to the Federation in 1961 and 1962. During the Congress they became full members, together with eight new applicants, namely the anaesthesia societies of Bolivia, Bulgaria, Ecuador, Lebanon, Paraguay, Perù, El Salvador, and Turkey. This raised the count to 47 member societies, with a total membership of about 16,000.

Important decisions were taken at the two meetings of the General Assembly during this Congress. Some changes of the bylaws had to be made to keep pace with the growth of the Federation. The office of secretary/treasurer was split and the Executive Committee was enlarged to 16 members. The President of the Federation (without voting power), the secretary, and the treasurer became members ex officio, and of the 13 other members at least 1 should come from the following regions: Europe, North America, Latin America, Asia, Africa, and Australia and the Pacific Islands. Their term of office should last 8 years.

In order to increase the number of well-trained specialists in some of the developing areas, it was decided to work towards establishing regional training centres in co-operation with the WHO, national societies, and universities. The first two of these training centres should be in Latin America and in the Pacific area. Member societies and individual members should be encouraged to provide teachers, teaching material, and anaesthetic equipment for these training centres.

Finally, the organisation of regional congresses was expressly welcomed by the General Assembly as a means to bridge the gap between World Congresses. The Executive Committee would thus also be given the opportunity to hold interim working meetings between the World Congresses.

Before the close of the 3ʳᵈ World Congress in Sao Paulo, the following persons were elected to their respective offices: WFSA President 1964-1968 Dr. Geoffrey Organe, United Kingdom; vice-presidents (1964-1968) Dr. Luis Agosti, Spain, Dr. Roger Bennett, Australia, Dr. Jacques Boureau, France, Professor Enrico Ciocatto, Italy, Dr. Joseph Failing, United States, Dr. Carlos Rivas, Venezuela; secretary (1964-1968) Professor Otto Mayrhofer, Austria; treasurer (1964-1968) Dr. Henning Poulsen, Denmark; Executive Committee chairman (until 1968) Dr. Ralph Sappenfield, United States, vice-chairmen (until 1968) Professor Quintin Gomez, Philippines, members Dr. John Beard, United Kingdom (until 1972), Professor John Bonica, United States (1968), Dr. Luis Cabrera, Chile (1968), Professor Rudolf Frey, Germany (1972), Professor O.V.S. Kok, South Africa (1968), Dr. Louis Larang, France (1972), Dr. Leon Longtin, Canada (1972), Professor C.R. Ritsema van Eck, The Netherlands (1968), Dr. Luiz Rodriguez Alves, Brazil (1972), Dr. Eusebio Lopez Soares, Portugal (1972), and Professor Hideo Yamamura, Japan (1972).

At its first meeting the new Executive Committee decided to have an annual newsletter published for the information of the WFSA membership, possibly in the four main languages English, French, German, and Spanish. It was hoped that, with the help of sponsors and advertisers, the financial burden of the Federation could be kept at a tolerable level. The new secretary Otto Mayrhofer and his German colleague Rudolf Frey should act as editors.

Regionalisation of WFSA

Fore-runners in the field of regionalisation were the Latin Americans. Anaesthesiologists on the subcontinent not only had the same problems but also the same or a similar language. This probably made it easier for them to link up sooner than in other regions. The Argentinians took the lead, as they were also the first to publish a journal, *"Revista Argentina de Anestesiologia"* (1939), and to found a society, "Asociación Argentina de Anestesiologia" (1943 or 1944).

It was the Argentinian anaesthesia pioneer Dr. José César Delorme who invited his colleagues from other Latin-American countries to gather in Buenos Aires in October 1949 for the first "Congreso Latino-Americano de Anestesiologia". Although he had already spread the idea of founding a Latin-American association, this appeared to be premature at that time.

However, 5 years later when Dr. Zairo E.C. Vieira of Brazil called his colleagues to Sao Paulo in 1954 for the 2nd "CLAA", the decision was taken to hold Latin-American Congresses biannually in alphabetical order of the countries of the region. Thus the 3rd CLAA took place in Bogota, Colombia in 1956, the 4th in Vina del Mar, Chile in 1958, the 5th in Mexico City in 1960, and the 6th in Lima, Perù in 1962. This meeting marked the official foundation of "CLASA"-the "Confederación Latino-Americana de Anestesiologia". The founding members of CLASA were the national societies of Argentina, Bolivia, Brazil, Chile, Colombia, Ecuador, México, Per-Ci, Uruguay, and Venezuela. Over the years this number eventually increased to 20 member societies.

Throughout the years very good connections and relations had been maintained with the WFSA. The 7th CLAA was held in Montevideo in 1964 immediately following the 3rd World Congress of Sao Paulo, which in itself was actually dominated by a large attendance from Latin-American countries. At least in the early years CLASA had neither a President nor a board. The biannual congresses were organised by the respective host societies and the official link between the member societies was the Secretary General. At the 8th CLAA in Caracas in 1966 it was decided to shift the biannual meetings to the odd years in order not to interfere with world and major regional congresses.

Finally, in October 1987, again in Caracas, the decision was taken that CLASA should become the Regional Section of WFSA. The preliminary negotiations for this move had been held between the President Dr. Carlos Parsloe and the Executive Committee chairman Dr. Say Wan 'Lim for WFSA and Dr. Ricardo Samayoa de Leon of Guatemala City for CLASA, then its Secretary General.

Regional activities in Europe

The idea to hold European Congresses at 4-year intervals in between the World Congresses came from the British anaesthetist Professor T. Cecil Gray of Liverpool and dated back to 1959. At the time of the 2nd World Congress in Toronto in 1960, the Executive Committee agreed to this and upon Professor Gray's suggestion commissioned the Austrian Society of Anaesthesiologists to organise the 1st European Congress in Vienna in the autumn of 1962.

The Austrian Society, which at that time had only about 100 members, gladly accepted the challenge and started straight after the 2nd WCA to prepare for the 1st European Congress. Professor Otto Mayrhofer was elected chairman of the Organising Committee and President of the congress, which was to be held in the former Imperial Palace in the centre of Vienna from 3 to 9 September 1962. As this congress had the official backing of WFSA, Professor C.R. Ritsema van Eck, WFSA President, Professor G. Organe, WFSA secretary/treasurer, and Professor T.C. Gray, chairman of the committee on regionalisation, were guests of honour.

The meeting was officially opened by Dr. Adolf Scharf, President of the Federal Republic of Austria. A reception for all congress participants was given by the Mayor of Vienna, Franz Jonas, in the City Hall. There were, of course, a number of other social activities, such as a gala performance of the Lipizzan "White Horse Ballet", a special performance at the Vienna State Opera, and a ball in the Imperial Palace as the final climax of the congress.

The three main topics of the 1st European Congress of Anaesthesiology (ECA) were: recovery and special care units, anaesthesia for the aged, and problems of anaesthesia in emergency surgery. In addition, 20 symposia were held on various special topics. Well over 1,500 delegates from 48 countries of all continents participated in the congress. The WFSA Executive Committee and the committee on regionalisation held meetings during the congress. Among other matters it was decided to hold the 2nd European Congress in 1966 in Denmark.

The Danish Society of Anaesthesiologists, also one of the smaller members of WFSA, took up the task of organising the 2nd ECA. However, they summoned the assistance of their sister societies of Sweden, Norway, and Finland. The congress President was Professor Ole Secher of Copenhagen and secretary of the Organising Committee Dr. Henning Poulsen of Aarhus. The congress took place in the Congress Centre of Copenhagen from 8 to 13 August 1966 and was officially opened by His Majesty King Frederik the IX.

There were 17 symposia and 17 group discussions, about 70 free papers were presented and 16 films shown. Practically all aspects of clinical anaesthesia, intensive care, and emergency medicine were covered, research results presented, and special problems discussed, e.g., anaesthesia under primitive conditions or anaesthetic vaporising appliances. Of the 1,550 registered participants, almost 1,000 were active members. Both the scientific and the social gatherings made the 2nd European Congress of Copenhagen a most-memorable meeting.

Following intensive consultations in the years before, a General Assembly of delegates from the European member societies of the WFSA was called during the 2nd ECA., which decided to officially form a European Regional Section of the WFSA and accepted the rules and regulations of the section, which had been worked out by a preparatory committee. The most-important rules and regulations were the following:

1. The European section will consist of the European member societies of WFSA with the addition of Israel.
2. Its activities will be consistent with the aims and objects of the World Federation.
3. A regional assembly will usually be held in connexion with each ECA.
4. Each member society shall be represented by the same number of delegates as in the General Assembly of the WFSA.
5. The board of the European section shall be composed of: the chairman, two vice-chairmen, the secretary, and the treasurer. Representatives of Europe within the Executive Committee of the WFSA are ex-officio members without vote.

For the first period of office from 1966 to 1970 the following persons were elected: chairman Dr. Steven Couremenos, Athens, Greece; vice-chairman Dr. Louis Lareng, Toulouse, France; vice-chairman Dr. Borivoj Dvoracek, Prague, CSSR; secretary Professor Otto Mayrhofer, Vienna, Austria; treasurer Dr. Henning Poulsen, Aarhus, Denmark. The last two persons were elected for practical and economical reasons as they would have been members of the European board anyway as European members of the WFSA Executive Committee.

Regional meetings in Eastern Europe

The anaesthesia societies in the so-called socialist countries of Eastern Europe, which were having problems with scientific and personal exchange with their colleagues in the Western World, had started to organise regional meetings under the heading Symposia in Anaesthesiology. The first of these symposia was organised by Professors. Lothar Barth and Manfred Mayer in East Berlin in September 1959. After a lapse of 4 years, the next Eastern European meeting was held in Budapest from 25 to 28 September 1963, organised by the Hungarian Society under the presidency of Dr. Istvan Harkànyi, this time called 1st International Symposium of Anaesthesiology.

About 150 participants and speakers came from all European "socialist" countries, including the Soviet Union. In addition, there were about five guest speakers from England, Sweden, and Austria. Various topics of practical value were discussed such as anaesthesia for emergency surgery as well as for thoracic and cardiac surgery. Problems of recruiting and training anaesthetists were also on the agenda. There was general agreement among the participants that the development of the specialty throughout the whole region would gain further momentum by the continued cooperation of the anaesthesia societies. At the end of the symposium it was decided therefore to organise further meetings of the same type every other year in rotation among the anaesthesia societies of the socialist countries.

Accordingly, the 2nd International Symposium of Anaesthesiology was held in Prague from 17 to 20 August 1965 under the presidency of Dr. Josef Hoder with Dr. Pavel Schek serving as Secretary General. Apart from the various usual anaesthesia topics, I remember that problems of intensive care were on the programme for the first time.

The 3rd International Symposium took place from 21 to 26 August 1967 in Poznàn, Poland, and was organised by Professor Witold Jurcik. This one was most memorable as it had among its participants and speakers such renowned anaesthesia pioneers as Professor Robert R. Macintosh of Oxford, Professor Henry K. Beecher of Boston, Professor Torsten Gordh of Stockholm, and Professor Rudolf Frey of Mainz, Germany. In my capacity as secretary of the WFSA, I urged our East European colleagues to maintain or obtain membership of the Federation and offered special conditions for them to participate in the 4th World Congress, which was to be held in London in September 1968.

Asian-Australasian regional activities

Regional activities started in Asia and Australasia in the early 1960. It was Professor Quintin Gomez of Manila, The Philippines, who invited his colleagues from the region to his home city in 1962 to participate in the 1st Asian-Australasian Congress of Anaesthesiology. They came from Australia, New Zealand, Japan, Hong Kong, India, Malaysia, and Singapore. A number of invited speakers also came from the North American continent.

For Quintin Gomez himself, this meeting opened the door to positions within the World Federation: vice-chairman of the Executive Committee (1964-1968), treasurer (1968-1976), President (1976-1980), and director of the WFSA regional training center in Manila from 1970.

1964-1972: Consolidation, the period of "adolescence"

WFSA Newsletters

In June 1965 the first issue of the WFSA Newsletter, published by Springer in Heidelberg, Germany, was distributed to the member societies. It was printed in four languages. The English version was revised by the WFSA President Geoffrey Organe, the German by the WFSA secretary Otto Mayrhofer, the French by the WFSA vice-President Jacques Boureau, and the Spanish by the WFSA vice-president Luis Agosti. Professor Rudolf Frey of Mainz, Germany, acted as co-editor.

The contents of this first Newsletter were an introductory address by President Geoffrey Organe, in which he gave credit to the founder fathers of WFSA, the officers of the first 9-year period, and the organisers of the 3rd WCA in Sao Paulo. Organe also stressed the urgent need for supporting the development of anaesthesia in the Third World. WFSA secretary Otto Mayrhofer gave a report on the actual global situation. Dr. Robert A. Hingson of Cleveland, Ohio, chairman of the WFSA Committee on Education and Relief, described, in an article full of enthusiasm and optimism, his plans and vision for the foundation of international regional anaesthesia training centres. The aim was to improve the quantity and quality of professional anaesthesia in all developing countries. Teachers, equipment, and money would be necessary to establish well-functioning training centres. Hingson mentioned that local assistance had already been offered from places in Venezuela, The Philippines, Israel, Ethiopia, and Puerto Rico.

A congress calendar for 1965 and 1966 completed the contents of the first issue of the WFSA Newsletter. It included among others the following: 16-18 September 1965 8th Central European Meeting in Zurich, Switzerland, 1-3 October 1965 Spanish/Portuguese Meeting in Barcelona, 8-13 August 1966 2nd European Congress of Anaesthesiology in Copenhagen, 1-5 September 1966 2nd Asian-Australasian Congress of Anaesthesiology in Tokyo, and 10-15 October 1966 8th Latin-American Congress of Anaesthesiology and 3rd CLASA Meeting in Caracas, Venezuela. All these forthcoming meetings clearly demonstrated that the momentum of activities as well as exchange of information had drastically improved since the 3rd WCA in Sao Paulo.

In the second WFSA Newsletter, issued in March 1966, an account of the foundation of the World Federation was given in an article written by past-President C.R. Ritsema van Eck. The WFSA secretary Otto Mayrhofer stated in his annual report: The childhood years were now over and the Federation is progressing into its adolescence. A short passage within the annual report is also worth quoting: "The Committee for the Anaesthesia and Relief Foundation under the Chairmanship of Dr. Robert Hingson has made good headway during the past year and the first Regional Training Center, sponsored by the WFSA, is to go into operation in Caracas in October 1966. The Training

Center for the Pacific Area, which is to be established in Manila, will - it is hoped - also function very soon". The secretary, reporting on a discussion held at WHO headquarters in Geneva, with WFSA President Geoffrey Organe and the assistant director of the WHO Dr. L. Bernard, also stated, that official WHO recognition would soon be given to the Caracas training centre.

The Latin-American Anaesthesia Training Center was officially inaugurated at the University of Caracas on 12 October 1966 during the 3rd CLASA and the 8th Latin-American Congress. At the inauguration ceremony the World Federation was represented by its President, Professor Geoffrey Organe, its secretary, Professor Otto Mayrhofer, as well as by the chairman of the Executive Committee, Dr. Ralph Sappenfield, and members of the WFSA Education and Relief Committee Drs. Robert Hingson, John J. Bonica, Francis F. Foldes, E.M. Papper of the United States, and Dr. Luis Cabrera of Chile. All WFSA representatives received Honorary Diplomas of Appreciation by the University of Venezuela for their roles in the establishment of this first regional anaesthesia training centre.

In addition to 14 Venezuelan residents, three WFSA fellows from the region started their 1st year of training. For 1967-1968 five more fellowships sponsored by Pan-American Health Organisation (PAHO)/WHO were awarded to Latin-American trainees. The local faculty chaired by Professor Carlos Rivas-Larrazabal was initially assisted by two guest professors whose travel expenses were covered by WFSA and board and lodging by the University of Caracas. They were Dr. Luis Cabrera-Guarderas from Chile and Dr. Luis Orkin from New York. They were followed by several teachers from America or from Europe in the following years.

The 2nd ECA, held in Copenhagen in August 1966, during which the European Regional Section of the World Federation was officially established, has already been mentioned. Immediately thereafter, between 1 and 4 September 1966, the 2nd Asian-Australasian Congress of Anaesthesiology took place in Tokyo, organised by the Japanese Society of Anaesthesiologists. Professor Hideo Yamamura of Tokyo was congress President and Dr. Michinosuke Amano served as Secretary General. The meeting was held at the Tokyo Prince Hotel, where all foreign participants could easily be accommodated.

The total attendance was approximately 300, 150 from Japan, the other half from the Asian-Australian region, as well as from America and Europe. The WFSA was officially represented by its President Professor Geoffrey Organe, its regional vice-President Dr. Roger Bennett of Brisbane, Australia, and its secretary Professor Otto Mayrhofer. There were 48 scientific papers and two half-day panels were held at this congress. One of the panels was devoted to the present status of anaesthesiology in Asian and Australasian countries. The standard of anaesthesia in countries, like Australia, Japan, India, Hong Kong, and Taiwan, was considered very good. However, in some other countries, e.g., Indonesia, modern anaesthesia was practically non-existent, mainly because of lack of qualified physicians.

With the view to setting up a regional anaesthesia training center for Asia, a committee was elected to study the needs in the various countries and to make inquiries as to how to improve the teaching and training in the region. Members of this committee were Drs. Quintin Gomez (The Philippines), Hideo Yamamura (Japan), Roger Bennett (Australia), and Peter K. Lee (Taiwan). The formation of a Regional Section of the WFSA was postponed to the next AACA, which was to be organised by the Australian Society in September 1970.

During 1967 only a small number of medium-sized meetings could be registered. The 3rd International Symposium of the Eastern European Anaesthesia Societies held in Poznàn, Poland, from 21 to 26 August 1967 and organised by Professor Witold Jurczik, has already briefly been mentioned. From 10 to 14 June 1967 the 3rd Spanish/Portuguese Congress took place in the old pilgrim town of Santiago de Compostela in Galicia, Spain, with between 300 and 400 participants.

The 10th Meeting of the German, Swiss, and Austrian Societies in Salzburg, which had already been the site of the first German-speaking meeting in 1952, was convened and chaired by Professor Volkmar Feurstein between 21 and 23 September 1967. There were about 1,500 participants from Europe and abroad. The main topics were anaesthesia and carbohydrate metabolism, anaesthesia and renal function,and disturbances of acid-base balance.

Nothing special was reported from the 14th Brazilian Congress held in Porto Alegre from 12 to 18 November 1967, but the 9th Latin-American Congress, at the same time as the 11th Argentine Congress of Anaesthesiology, which took place immediately thereafter from 21 to 25 November in Buenos. Aires was a really big meeting, attended by more than 400 Latin-American anaesthesiologists as well as by a good number of guests from overseas.

Regional Arab Congress, 1966

Belatedly reported in the fourth WFSA Newsletter, issued in June 1968, was the fact that the 1st Arab Congress of Anaesthesiology had been held in Alexandria, Egypt, from 19 to 22 October 1966. It was held in the Chatby Maternity University Hospital under the High Patronage of President Gamal Abdel Nasser. About 200 participants attended the meeting, the majority from the host country, with the rest from Syria, Lebanon, Iraq, Jordan, Kuwait, and Sudan. Professor Sir Robert Macintosh had officially been sent by the WHO and other guests had come from Belgium, Great Britain, Germany, Holland, and Sweden.

Grouped into six sessions over 3 days, 34 scientific papers were read. The seventh session was on the status of anaesthesia in Arab countries. Following individual reports and a very lively discussion, the following recommendations were adopted.
1. Anaesthesia should be given by doctors only.
2. Training centres in anaesthesiology within the region should be encouraged.

3. Expressions used in anaesthesia should be translated into Arabic and standardised for the Arab countries.
4. An exchange of visiting anaesthetists should be started.
5. Local and regional meetings should be encouraged.
6. Anaesthetists in the region should be helped to gain higher qualifications and degrees.
7. Intensive care units, or at least recovery rooms, should be an essential part of all major hospitals in the region.

At the end of the congress the following decisions were taken.
1. The 2nd Arab Congress of Anaesthesiology was to be held in Damascus, Syria in 1968.
2. The Society of Arab Anaesthetists (SAA) was officially founded and invitations to join were directed to colleagues in countries that were not represented at the Alexandria congress.
3. A board of SAA was elected to serve for the first 2 years. It was chaired by the President of the Egyptian Society of Anaesthesiologists and the Secretary General was Professor Hashem Nassar of Alexandria. Two members each were elected to the board from the other five countries represented at the Arab Congress.

List of member societies

A list of addresses and officers compiled by the WFSA secretary was also published in the fourth Newsletter of 1968. Just prior to the 4th WCA the Federation was composed of 56 member societies with a total individual membership of approximately 18,000 anaesthesiologists in all continents. However, the societies of Egypt, Singapore, Syria, and West Africa had only provisional admission, pending approval by the General Assembly to be held in London in September 1968.

West African Society of Anaesthetists

The West African Society (WASA) is a regional body composed of members from several West African countries such as Nigeria, Ghana, Togo, Sierra Leone, and Liberia. When founded in Accra, Ghana in January 1965 there were only 15 members, but in 1968, when the application for membership of WFSA was made, the membership of WASA had grown to 35. The society held annual meetings in rotation between the above-mentioned countries. These included meetings in January 1966 in Ibadan, Nigeria - with the WFSA secretary Professor Otto Mayrhofer as guest speaker - and in January 1967 in Freetown, Sierra Leone.

Much credit for the development of physician anaesthesia in that region must be given to Dr. Shirley A. Fleming, who had originally been on the staff of the University of Toronto, Department of Anaesthesia, with Professor Roderick Gordon. Under the sponsorship of her home university she worked and taught in Nigeria between 1961 and 1967, predominantly at Lagos University Medical School, where she was appointed chair-woman of the department and first Professor of Anaesthesia. She was also essentially involved in the foundation of the WASA and became its first President. Professor Rod Gordon, Shirley Fleming's teacher, and Professor Otto Mayrhofer were elected honorary members of the young society.

The 4ᵗʰ World Congress in London, 1968

The main event of the year 1968 was, of course, the 4ᵗʰ WCA in London from 9 to 13 September. The site of the meeting was the Royal Festival Hall near the River Thames. There were 2,800 anaesthesiologists participating, with a total attendance of more than 3,700.

The congress was organised by the Association of Anaesthetists of Great Britain and Ireland. The President of the congress and of the Organising Committee was Dr. Patrick Shackleton. Dr. Douglas D.C. Howat served as Secretary General. The British mastered the task excellently and their efforts were additionally rewarded by pleasantly warm autumn weather.

The Royal Festival Hall turned out to be extremely well suited for a congress of this size. English, French, German, and Spanish were the official languages. Four major lecture halls could be used simultaneously for the sessions and in a fifth room scientific films were presented round the clock. Abstracts of practically all papers in the original language and in English translation were available at the time of registration. A complete account of the scientific papers is outside the scope of this chapter. However, all aspects of anaesthesia, intensive care, pain relief, and emergency medicine were covered, and there was much opportunity for the individual participant to listen to a lecture of his choice and for discussion. Both the scientific and the social side of the 4ᵗʰ World Congress can rightly be considered a complete success.

Administrative meetings were held by the Executive Committee and by the three standing committees on membership, on finance, and on statutes and bylaws. The General Assembly convened twice. New member societies were admitted, reports were received, and elections were held.

Professor Carlos Rivas, the director of the Ibero-American Anaesthesia Training Center in Caracas, reported on its first 2 years of operation. Five visiting professors had been teaching for periods of 2-3 months each. They had come from Chile, Brazil, Canada, and the United States. The foreign students who had been trained together with the Venezuelan residents, for minimum periods of 12 months, were from Chile (4) and Nicaragua (2) . The respective fellowships had been awarded on a 50:50 basis by the WFSA and the PAHO.

Dr. Henning Poulsen, chairman of the committee on cardio-pulmonary resuscitation, reviewing the work of his committee during the past 4 years, reported that thanks to generous anonymous donations a manual on cardio-pulmonary resuscitation, written by Professor Peter Safar of Pittsburgh, could be produced on behalf of the Federation; 50,000 copies were to be distributed in English, French, German, Spanish, and Russian to anaesthesiologists, cardi-ologists, surgeons, and other physicians all over the world. Copies of the Eng-lish version were handed out to the delegates of the WFSA General Assembly.

Finally, new officers and committee members were elected: President (1968-1972) Professor Francis F. Foldes (USA), vice-presidents Dr. Luis Cabr-era (Chile), Professor Torsten Gordh (Sweden), Professor Roderick Gordon (Canada), Professor O.V.S. Kok (South Africa), Professor Stan Pokrzywnic-ki (Poland), Dr. Ralph Sappenfield (USA), and Professor Guy Vourc'h (France); secretary (re-elected) Professor Otto Mayrhofer (Austria); treasurer (to follow H. Poulsen) Professor Quintin Gomez (The Philippines). The partly new Executive Committee was elected as follows: chairman Dr. Henning Poulsen, Denmark; vice-chairman Dr. John Beard, United Kingdom (until 1972); mem-bers Professor Rudolf Frey, Germany (1972), Dr. Josef Hoder, Czechoslova-kia (1976), Professor Douglas Joseph, Australia (1976), Dr. Louis Larang, France (1972), Dr. Leon Longtin, Canada (1972), Dr. Eusebio Lopes Soares, Portugal (1972), Professor Emanuel M. Papper, United States (1976), Pro-fessor Carlos Rivas Larrazabal, Venezuela (1976), Dr. Luiz Rodriguez Alves, Brazil (1972), Dr. Joseph Sodipo, Nigeria (1976), and Professor Hideo Yama-mura, Japan (1972).

Following a proposal by a Special Committee headed by past-President Pro-fessor C.R. Ritsema van Eck, the General Assembly voted to entrust the Japan-ese Society to organise and hold the 5th WCA in the autumn of 1972, leaving the decision of the site and the exact date to the host society.

In his closing address the outgoing President Professor Sir Geoffrey Organe paid a special tribute to his predecessor in office, Professor C.R. Ritsema van Eck, who had been active for the aims of the Federation since the very begin-ning and was now retiring from all offices and duties. He also thanked, on behalf of WFSA, the members of the Organising Committee of the 4th WCA, which had up to then been the best ever. Finally, he introduced the new Pres-ident Professor F.F. Foldes and handed over to him the new flag of the Fed-eration, which had been donated to the WFSA at the Opening Ceremony of the congress by the Association of Anaesthetists of Great Britain and Ireland. Professor Foldes thanked the General Assembly for their vote of confidence, promised to follow duely in the footsteps of his predecessors and to do every-thing in his power to advance the aims and purposes of the Federation.

Reviewing the congress calender for 1968 and 1969 it should briefly be mentioned that the Portuguese Society organised just prior to the 4th World Con-gress the 2nd Luso-Brazilian Congress of Anaesthesiology from 1 to 4 Sep-tember 1968 in Estoril, a sea resort on the Atlantic coast. The site and time were well chosen, and the meeting was very well attended. The main topics were anaesthesia for different operative specialties, humidification in anaesthesia and in prolonged artificial ventilation, tetanus, and new aspects of regional anaesthesia.

By the end of 1968 the WFSA had grown to 59 member societies, with a total individual membership of well over 20,000. This included the national societies of Ceylon, Cuba, and Korea, whose membership had been suspended by the General Assembly in 1964 because of arrears in dues, but which had meanwhile paid their membership fees to full satisfaction.

The fact that the WFSA secretariate, established in Vienna in 1964, served as a sort of clearing house for the planning of national and regional meetings, the dates of which were continuously reported in the Newsletter, proved to be particularly useful for the "in-between"-years like 1969. A good number of national and minor regional meetings were held that year, but - on the whole - overlapping could grossly be avoided.

The first of these "minor" regional meetings was the 9th Scandinavian Congress of Anaesthesiology, which took place in Bergen, Norway, from 23 to 27 June 1969. The 11th Central European Meeting of the German-speaking Societies was held in Saarbruecken, Germany, from 4 to 6 September 1969, followed by the 4th International Anaesthesia Symposium in Varna, Bulgaria, from 15 to 21 September 1969 and the 10th Latin-American Congress in La Paz, Bolivia, from 9 to 13 October 1969. To finish the list, the annual meeting of the American Society took place in San Francisco from 25 to 29 October 1969.

At all of these meetings the WFSA was officially represented by either the President, the secretary, or one of the vice-Presidents, whoever was closest to the congress site, so as to not overstrain the budget of the Federation and yet still document the interest of the "Mother-Federation" in the activities of the individual member societies.

For 1970 the largest meetings like the European and the Asian-Australasian Congress were, of course, planned well ahead so as to not clash with each other and with the annual meeting of the ASA. Welcome addresses by Dr. Josef Hoder of Prague and by Professor Douglas of Sydney, presidents of the 3rd European and of the 3rd Asian-Australasian Congress, respectively, which appeared in WFSA Newsletter 6, issued in July 1970, reminded the members of the Federation of these major forthcoming events.

The 3rd European Congress in Prague, 1970

The Czechoslovakia Society of Anaesthesiology and Resuscitation, in cooperation with the General Medical Society Purkyne, excellently organised the 3rd ECA in Prague from 30 August to 4 September 1970. The congress President was Dr. Josef Hoder, General Secretary Dr. Rudolf Jedlicka, and scientific secretary Professor Jiri Pokorny. Ten main topics were covered within a total of 72 sessions. A good number of free papers and scientific films were also presented. Some of the important topics included: neuroleptanalgesia and other new methods of anaesthesia, hyperbaroxia, muscle relaxants and their antidotes, toxicity of inhalation agents, ketamine, propanidid and other new i.v. agents, regional anaesthesia, monitoring, metabolic disorders during resuscitation, and others. The total attendance in Prague was close to 1,600, with almost 1,200 active members from 50 countries of all continents.

During the 3rd ECA, two meetings of the WFSA Executive Committee were held. Probably the most-important decision made was the transformation of the former "Anaesthesia Educational and Relief Foundation" to an "Anaesthesia Educational Foundation"(AEF) and the establishment of a WFSA Committee on Education in Anaesthesiology. The purpose of this change was the concentration of worldwide WFSA activities on educational projects in developing areas. Funds raised by the AEF from donations, WFSA member societies, individuals, companies, or philanthropic institutions were kept by the WFSA treasurer and spent only upon the order of the Executive Committee, in accordance with the recommendations of the Committee on Education. The chairman of both the Committee on Education in anaesthesiology and the WFSA AEF was Dr. Albert Betcher of New York, with trustees in all regions.

Dr. Robert Hingson, who had for many years been the chairman of the WFSA educational and relief foundation and the energy behind all fund-raising campaigns, was duely commended for his outstanding and successful efforts since the World Congress of Sao Paulo. He accepted the Executive Committee's request to serve on the EAF board of trustees and assist the new chairman with his great experience.

To maintain the operation of the WFSA training centre in Caracas - primarily for scholarships to be granted to post-graduate students from Latin America, except the host country Venezuela - an annual educational budget of about U.S. $ 20,000 was needed. Any additional money raised was to be used for the further development of the Western Pacific Training Center in Manila, to open in December 1970 under the directorship of Professor Quintin Gomez, with generous assistance from the regional WHO office.

The annual report of the WFSA secretary for 1970 stated that "The American Society of Anesthesiologists, our largest Member Society, has taken the lead in supporting the educational activities of the Federation. A voluntary donation of U.S. $ 5,000 was transfered to the AEF in 1970 and will be made again in 1971 and the following years, if satisfactory reports on appropriate spending are submitted by the WFSA treasurer. However, it should be mentioned at this point, that other WFSA member societies have also made substantial contributions to the Educational Foundation, e.g., the Anaesthesia Societies of Australia, Austria, Canada, France, New Zealand, South Africa, Kuwait, Scandinavia, and the Philippines".

As the Anaesthesia Society of the Soviet Union had meanwhile been admitted to the WFSA, the total number of member societies was now 60, with a membership of nearly 27,000 anaesthetists.

The European regional assembly also met during the ECA in Prague. A new regional board was elected for the next 4 years with the following composition:

chairman Dr. Douglas D.C. Howat, United Kingdom, first vice-chairman Dr. Emil Stojanov, Bulgaria, second vice-chairman Dr. Alfredo Arias, Spain, secretary Professor Otto Mayrhofer, Austria, treasurer Dr. August Colding, Denmark.

Finally, the Spanish Society of Anaesthesiology and Resuscitation was entrusted to organise the 4th ECA in Madrid in September 1974.

The 3rd Asian-Australasian Congress in Canberra, 1970

The 3rd Asian-Australasian Congress of Anaesthesiology, organised by a committee of our Australian member society, chaired by Professor Douglas Joseph with Dr. Judith Nicholas as its most-active and efficient secretary, was also a very successful meeting. It took place in Canberra from 19 to 23 September 1970. The total attendance of the congress was 564, of which 371 were active members, 275 from Australia and 95 from 31 other countries. The World Federation was officially represented by its President, Professor Francis F. Foldes, the chairman of the Executive Committee, Dr. Henning Poulsen, the secretary, Professor Otto Mayrhofer, and the treasurer, Professor Quintin Gomez.

In his opening address the congress President Professor Douglas Joseph pointed out that the Australian Anaesthesia Society was founded in 1934 and that Australian anaesthesia has since evolved from an empiric to a scientific discipline with a wide spectrum of activities and responsibilities.

The scientific programme of more than 110 contributions occupied 3 full days in two lecture halls. In addition, films were projected in a third room. The programme was subdivided into symposia, the subjects of which were anaesthesia and resuscitation in multiple trauma, the endocrine system and anaesthesia, pharmacological complications of anaesthesia, design and safety in anaesthesia apparatus, anaesthesia in the Asian-Australasian region, and anaesthesia and analgesia in obstetric practice.

Apart from its great scientific and social value, one of the most-important features of the 3rd AACA was the official establishment of a new Regional Section of the WFSA. Founding members of this Regional Section were the anaesthesia societies of Australia, Ceylon, Republic of China (Taiwan), Hong Kong, India, Indonesia, Japan, Korea, Malaysia, New Zealand, the Philippines, and Singapore. The rules and regulations were very similar to those of the European Regional Section and in full accordance with the bylaws of the World Federation.

The following regional board for 1970-1974 was elected: chairman Professor Douglas Joseph, Australia; vice-chairmen Professor Kenichi Iwatsuki, Japan, Professor George Tay, Singapore; secretary Professor Pritam Singh, India; treasurer Professor Quintin Gomez, Philippines; regional WFSA Executive Committee representative Professor Hideo Yamamura, Japan.

It was also decided that the next Asian-Australasian Congress of Anaesthesiology should take place in Singapore in August 1974 and that the office of the new Regional Section should be based at the home of the regional secretary Professor Pritam Singh in Amritsar, Kashmere, India.

WFSA Newsletters in difficulties

From 1970 on it became increasingly more difficult to obtain sponsors and advertisers for the WFSA Newsletter, the annual publication of the Federation. With the increase in the amount of information, the volume of the issues had been growing from year to year. Newsletter 1, which appeared in June 1965, had only 39 pages, Newsletter 6 in July 1970 already had 81 pages.

Although the advertisements had increased in number and the translations were still provided free of charge by the editors and their colleagues, the accumulated deficit could no longer be bourne by the publishing company Springer of Heidelberg, Germany. Upon recommendation of the WFSA Executive Committee, Newsletter 7, which was published in July 1971, was reduced in size to 42 pages, containing only the annual report of the secretary, the reports on the activities of the member societies, and the actual congress calender from 1971 to 1973. Newsletter , issued in April 1972, again contained more information, but by publishing it in English only its size could be reduced to 30 pages.

Other events in 1971 and 1972

For this contribution to the Jubilee Book of the World Federation the WFSA Newsletters, the publication of which continued until 1974, have remained the most-valuable sources of information. Thus it can be reported that 1971 was a rather quiet year for the Federation. The only major regional meeting was the 11th Latin-American Congress, which was organised by the Brasilian Society under the chairmanship of Professor Renato Ribeiro in Rio de Janeiro between 3 and 8 October. The General Assembly of CLASA elected Dr. Carlos C. Castanos of La Paz, Bolivia, to serve as Secretary General until 1973, and as members of the executive board for the same period Dr. Bento Goncalves, Brazil Jaime Herrera, Colombia, and Luis Cabrera, Chile.

Apart from this, only a few smaller joint meetings were organised in 1971. The 4th Spanish/Purtuguese meeting took place In Oporto, Portugal, from 9 to 12 June under the chairmanship of Dr. Pedro Ruella Torres, the 10th Scandinavian Congress was held in Lund, Sweden, from 20 to 25 June under the presidency of Professor Eric Nilsson, and, finally, the Austrian, German, and Swiss societies had their 12th biannual meeting in Berne from 1 to 4 September, organised and chaired by Professor Bruno Tschirren.

The most-significant achievement on behalf of the WFSA for 1971 was the successful initiation of the Western Pacific Anaesthesia Training Center in Manila under the direction of Professor Quintin Gomez, the WFSA treasurer. The official inauguration was in December 1970 and the first class totalled 21 doctors, 3 of whom came from outside the Philippines, namely from Korea, Japan, and Taiwan. Due to the most-active cooperation of Dr. Francisco Dy, the regional director of the WHO, four WHO fellowships could be awarded for this first course.

For the second course, starting in January 1972, two additional fellow-ships could be given by the World Federation thanks to generous financial assistance mainly provided by the member societies in Scandinavia and Australia. For this second course the recipients of these six fellowships were from Western Samoa, Tonga, the Solomon Islands, Saipan, Taiwan, and Indonesia. The stipends were designed to cover the costs of board and lodging, as well as incidental expenses. In addition, international travel tickets were provided and tuition fees paid. These courses continued into the 1980ies and gave tremendous impetus to the development of medical anaesthesiology in the Western Pacific region.

A compromise decision in Africa

With two regional training centres functioning, the question of establishing a third in Africa unfortunately remained unsolved. In 1970 Dr. Joseph Sodipo, member of the Department of Anaesthesia at the College of Medicine, University of Lagos, Nigeria, and since 1968 the representative for Africa on the WFSA Executive Committee, reported his negotiations with Dr. Adrian, the WHO regional director for West Africa. The WHO had been aiming at a physician-population ratio of 1:3,000 but in none of the West African states had this been achieved. Because of this general shortage of doctors in the region, it appeared to be unrealistic - at least for the time being - to push for training of medical anaesthesiologists. If the manpower for anaesthesia services was to be reasonably adequate within a short period, it was necessary, according to Dr. Adrian, to recruit non-doctor trainees, i.e., paramedics.

Both Dr. Adrian and Dr. Sodipo felt strongly that the candidates to be recruited from paramedical personnel to provide anaesthesia services should have medical and hospital backgrounds. The best places for the training of such paramedics would therefore be major local hospitals with existing medical anaesthesia services. WHO would fully support such paramedical anaesthesia training centres in West Africa. Dr. Sodipo promised to design a training programme for male and female nurses, but it would of course be for the WFSA Executive Committee to decide in which form the Federation could provide active support to this project. Following full information to all members of the Executive Committee, action on this matter was to be taken during the 5ᵗʰ World Congress in Kyoto in September 1972.

In his annual report for 1971 published in Newsletter 8, issued in April 1972, the WFSA secretary stated that the Federation "at the moment has 60 member societies with a total membership of close to 28,000, the regional distribution of which is the following: North America 2 societies, approximately 11,000 members, Latin America 14 societies, approximately 3,500 members, Europe 25 societies, approximately 11,000 members, Africa and the Middle East 7 societies, approximately 400 members, Asia and Australasia 12 societies, approximately 2,000 members".

The same Newsletter also contained a pre-announcement of three pages on the forthcoming 5th World Congress to be held from 19 to 23 September 1972 in the brand-new International Congress Hall just outside the City of Kyoto. A short outline of the scientific and the social programme was given, as well as information about the exhibition, travel, and accomodation.

Professor Douglas Joseph, chairman of the Asian-Australasian Regional Section of WFSA, reported in the same Newsletter on the functioning of the Regional Anaesthesia Training Center in Manila, which he had visited in the second half of the 1st teaching year. His summary read as follows: "The organization and the efforts and good will of those concerned - teachers, WHO officers, and hospital administrators - would seem to be very good. One basic difficulty is to attract sufficient overseas candidates from the region, who would benefit most from the type of training offered in this 1-year course. There are a number of factors contributing to this difficulty, amongst which is the lack of promulgamation of what is offered. If the Philippines General Hospital is to play its proper role in the training scheme there must be an increase in the standard of the facilities, and this will require contributions of essential equipment. The inclusion of basic scientists and keen clinical teachers has been achieved, but provisions must be made for a more-basic course should there be applicants from the less-developed countries. There is a serious lack of library facilities, particularly as regards the number of books and journals. It would appear that, at least for the first 3 years, finances for the reimbursement of full-time and part-time teachers is adequate, and the budgeting for this would appear to be extremely satisfactory. The organisers of the course are fully aware that teachers from within the region are necessary, and with WHO help promised for 1972 and 1973, this should be possible."

In summing up, Professor Josephs recommendations were as follows:
1. To encourage interest in the centre from amongst countries in the region.
2. To promote interest among teachers to visit the centre, in addition to encouraging other persons of high standing to pay a visit and assess the positions for themselves.
3. As it would appear that no further finances for teachers are required, support in the form of equipment, books, and journals is urgently needed. This is more important to the centre than a grant of money.

1972: WFSA fully-fledged; the step into "adulthood"

It will be remembered that, beginning with the 2nd World Congress of Toronto 1960, World Congresses on behalf of the WFSA were held at 4-year intervals, by coincidence in the Olympic years. It was also agreed from the very beginnig that European and Asian-Australasian Congresses should take place in the even years between the World Congresses. In order not to interfere with these major events, the organisers of smaller regional meetings had since the late 1950s and early 1960s been concentrating on the odd years. This had been true for the Latin-American CLASA congresses, the biannual Scandinavian meetings, and the so-called Central European congresses of the Anaesthesia Societies of Austria, Germany, and Switzerland. It did not, of course, affect the annual meetings of the major national anaesthesia societies, such as the American, Argentinian, Australian, British, Canadian, French, Italian, Brasilian, and Japanese.

The 5ᵗʰ World Congress in Kyoto, 1972

1972 was the year of the 5ᵗʰ World Congress. It was also the year of the 5ᵗʰ International Anaesthesia Symposium of the Societies in the Eastern European (socialist countries), which was held in Dresden, German Democratic Republic from 4 to 8 June 1972. The organisers of this meeting had explained to the WFSA secretary that, since only a very small number of anaesthesiologists from their respective countries would be able to travel to Japan, they had decided to stick to the date that had been agreed on by their individual societies well in advance. To demonstrate the full agreement between the Federation and this group of member societies, the WFSA secretary Professor Mayrhofer attended the symposium and addressed the audience at the Opening Ceremony. There were about 300 anaesthesiologists from the region attending the symposium.

As already briefly mentioned, the 5ᵗʰ WCA was held from 18 to 23 September 1972 in the Kyoto International Conference Hall, which was brand new and excellently suited for a meeting of that size. The main organisers were Professor Hideo Yamamura, President of the congress, Professor Akira Inamoto, chairman, Organising Committee, Professor Masao Miyazaki, Secretary General, Professor Michinosuke Amano, treasurer, and Professor Kenichi Iwatsuki, chairman, Scientific Committee.

The participants of the World Congress came from 61 countries and all continents. There were 2,087 full members and 775 associate members, giving a total of 2,862. The patron of the congress, His Imperial Highness Crown Prince Akihito - later Emperor of Japan - and the Crown Princess honoured the audience by their presence at the Opening Ceremony, during which the Crown Prince gave a short address of welcome (Fig. 1). Both Imperial Highnesses had-before the official opening of the congress - privately received and greeted the officers of the World Federation and of the Japanese Organising Committee (Fig. 2).

The scientific programme included presentations within all fields of general and regional anaesthesia, intensive and emergency care medicine, pain therapy, and problems of anaesthesia in the Third World. Besides 233 presented papers, 10 symposia and two informal round-table discussions were held; 22 scientific films were presented.

Highlights of the social programme were a concert given by the Kyoto

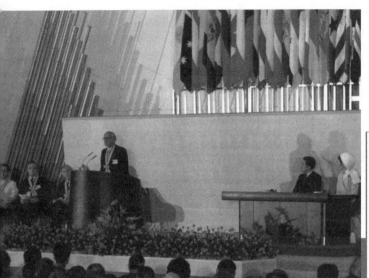

Fig. 1. *WFSA President Francis F. Foldes at the opening of the 5th WCA in Kyoto on 18 September 1972 with his Imperial Highness Crown Prince Akihito and the Crown Princess*

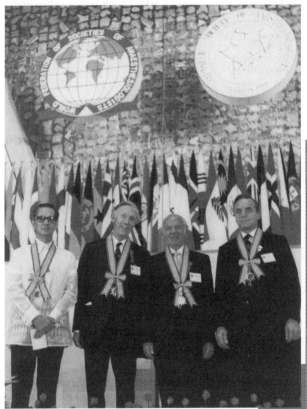

Fig. 2. *WFSA officers in front of the congress centre after the Opening Ceremony, wearing honorary badges given to them by the Japanese organisers. From left: Quintin Gomez, the Philippines, WFSA treasurer, Henning Poulsen, Denmark, chairman Executive Committee, Francis Foldes, USA, WFSA President (1968-1972), Otto Mayrhofer, Austria, WFSA secretary*

Municipal Symphony Orchestra, a reception after the official congress opening with a welcome address of the mayor of Kyoto, and the congress banquet held simultanuously in two of the major hotels, attended by more than 1,000 people, featuring folklore and geisha dancing. The closing ceremony on 23 September was followed by a most-splendid open-air farewell party, at which typical Japanese food and sake were served. The evening ended with a magnificent firework display that lit up the night of the closing day.

During the World Congress in Kyoto two sessions of the WFSA General Assembly were held, attended by more than 90 voting delegates. Some of the most-important items included admission of new member societies, namely the Icelandic Society of Anaesthetists (10 individual members), the Vietnamese Society of Anaesthetists (8), the Society of Anaesthetists of Zambia (19), the Society of Anaesthetists of East Africa (Kenya, Tanzania, and Uganda, 24 members), the Thai Society of Anaesthetists (42), and the Iranian Society of Anaesthetists (37). This brought the number of member societies to 65, with a total of well above 28,000 individual members.

Unfortunately, 5 of the member societies that had been in arrear of dues for more than 2 years had not been able to settle their accounts with the treasurer and had therefore to be temporarily suspended from membership. The Society of Anaesthetists of Paraguay, which was admitted during the 3rd World Congress in Sao Paulo in 1964, had since never responded to any letters of either the secretary or the treasurer, and had also never sent a delegate to regional or World Congresses. It was therefore assumed that this society no longer existed or at least not at that time. Of the other 4 societies, namely the Argentinian, the Egyptian, and the societies of El Salvador and Uruguay, there seemed to be hope that their financial problems would be solved soon so that they could have their full rights re-instated in due course.

In view of inflation and the increasing activities of the WFSA, the annual membership subscriptions to become effective in January 1974 were changed as follows: societies up to 100 members U.S. $ 1.50 per member, societies with between 101 and 200 members U.S. $ 1.00 per member, and societies of 201 members and more U.S. $ 0.75 per member.

The General Assembly elected at its second session the following officers and members of standing committees for 1972-1976: President Professor Otto Mayrhofer, Austria; vice-presidents Dr. John Beard, United Kingdom, Professor Louis Lareng, France, Dr. Leon Longtin, Canada, Dr. Eusebio Lopes Soares, Portugal, Professor Ferdinand Poppelbaum, GDR, Dr. Luiz Rodriguez Alves, Brazil, Professor Akira Inamoto, Japan; secretary Professor John J. Bonica, United States; treasurer Professor Quintin Gomez, Philippines; Executive Committee Dr. Henning Poulsen, Denmark, chairman (-1976), Dr. Douglas Howat, United Kingdom, vice-chairman (-1980), Dr. Steven Couremenos, Greece (-1980), Professor Marcel Gemperle, Switzerland (-1980), Dr. Josef Hoder, CSSR (-1976), Professor Douglas Joseph, Australia (-1976), Professor Jean Lassner, France (-1980), Professor Emanuel M. Papper, United States (-1976), Dr. Carlos Parsloe, Brazil (-1980), Professor Carlos Rivas, Venezuela (-1976), Professor Pritam Singh, India (-1980), Dr. Joseph Sodipo, Nigeria (-1976), Professor George Wyant, Canada (-1980); Committee on Finance Dr. Albert Betcher, United States (chairman), Professor J.J. Bonica (WFSA secretary), Professor Quintin Gomez (WFSA treasurer), Dr. H. Poulsen, Denmark, Professor C. Rivas, Venezuela; membership committee Professor H. Yamamura, Japan (chairman), Professor J.J. Bonica, United States, Dr. Alfredo Arias, Spain, Dr. J.-P. Déchène, Canada, Professor Martin Holmdahl, Sweden, Professor S.A. Oduntan, Nigeria, Professor Emil Stojanov, Bulgaria, Dr. Luis Perez-Tamayo, Mexico, Dr. George Tay, Singapore; Committee on Statutes and Bylaws Professor Jan Crul, The Netherlands (chairman), Dr. John Beard, United Kingdom, Dr. Carlos Castanos, Bolivia, Professor Douglas Joseph, Australia, and Dr. E.S. Siker, United States.

At the closing ceremony of the Kyoto World Congress the outgoing President Prof. Francis Foldes (Figs. 3, 4) handed to Professor Mayrhofer the flag of the Federation and the new presidential badge, which he had donated, designed by Dr. Juan Marin of Colombia for CLASA, showing two torches keeping alight the flame of life in darkness. This is to symbolise the task of the anaesthetist, which is also expressed by the words "Anaesthesia Deorum Ars" written around the presidential badge.

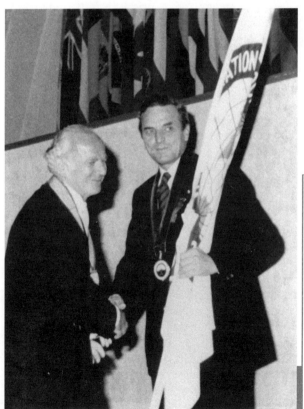

Fig. 3. *23 September 1972, closing ceremony of the 5ᵗʰ WCA in Kyoto, with outgoing President F.F. Foldes handing over the flag of the Federation to the 5ᵗʰ WFSA President Otto Mayrhofer*

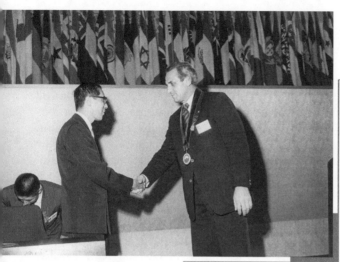

Fig. 4. *Closing ceremony of the Kyoto Congress 1972. Congress President Professor Hideo Yamamura congratulating the incoming WFSA President after his inauguration speech*

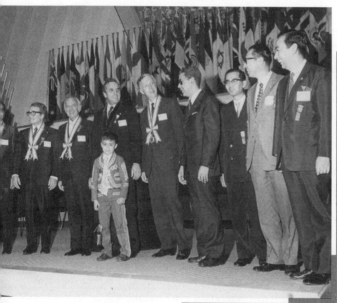

Fig. 5. *WFSA officers and congress organisers after the closing ceremony of the 5th WCA. From left: Quintin Gomez, WFSA treasurer, John Bonica, WFSA secretary, Francis Foldes immediate past President, Otto Mayrhofer, WFSA President, Henning Poulsen, chairman Executive Committee, H. Perez-Tamayo, member of the Organising Committee of the 6th WCA in Mexico City 1976, Hideo Yamamura, President, Masao Miyazaki, Secretary General, Susuma Ishii, treasurer of the 5th WCA*

The new WFSA President thanked for the vote of confidence, briefly paid tribute to his four predecessors, and promised to continue working for the Federation as he had done during the past 8 years as WFSA secretary. Finally, it was announced that the 6th World Congress will be held in Mexico City in 1976, most likely in early May (Fig. 5).

Final remarks

In his first "Letter from the President", published in WFSA Newsletter 9 in June 1973, Professor Mayrhofer listed some of his plans and intentions during his term of office, as follows: "The foremost purpose of the Federation - to make available the highest standard of anaesthesia and resuscitation to all peoples of the world and to disseminate the same amongst them (Chapter 3 of the WFSA bylaws) - should continue to be the guideline of all our actions. It is painful for me to see some societies, which had been very active in the past, temporarily excluded from the transactions of the Federation and I sincerely hope that we can soon enjoy again the full co-operation of these societies. In addition there are several areas on this globe where no anaesthesia societies exist as yet and it is one of my most pertinent aims that the Federation should give assistance in any way possible to the individual pioneers in such parts of the world".

"Having been in various parts of Africa during the past few years, I realise how much still has to be done particularily on this continent with its tremendous shortage of man power. It should be one of the foremost tasks of our Educational Foundation to give active support to existing training centres in Africa and, if possible, establish an official WFSA-sponsored training centre similar to the ones already in existence in Caracas and in Manila. Our educational and advisory committee I consider the most important of all our committees and I shall always give it my undivided attention."

"It is certainly not enough to come together every 4th year on the occasion of a World Congress. We realise how important the various regional congresses are which are being held in between. And here again, we must try to help and to sponsor regional meetings in areas where such congresses have not yet taken place. I believe that the time has come for the societies in the Middle East to start holding regional congresses and I know that our colleagues in East and West Africa are already trying to make arrangements for joint meetings."

In the course of independent professional group visits to the People's Republic of China during 1973 of the President, the secretary, and the chairman of the Asian-Australasian Regional Section Professor Douglas Joseph, contacts were established not only with some of the leading anaesthetists but also with government officials in attempts towards a future membership of the World Federation. However, this would turn out to take longer than Otto Mayrhofer's term of office, namely until 1988.

5 THE WORLD CONGRESSES OF ANAESTHESIOLOGISTS

J.S.M. Zorab

Introduction

The World Congresses of the WFSA provide significant milestones around which the organisation has evolved. The meeting in Scheveningen, in The Netherlands, in 1955, at which the WFSA was founded, is rightly regarded as the first WFSA World Congress of Anaesthesiologists, since this was the first time Societies of Anaesthesiologists from various countries sent individuals as official delegates to a world-wide meeting of anaesthesiologists. The events leading up to this historic occasion have been well documented by M. Mauve (The Netherlands) [1] (Fig. 1), a member of the original Interim Committee that created WFSA. There were 26 founding societies of WFSA and these are shown in Table 1. The United States did not feel the time was right for their society to join WFSA and the reasons behind this decision are described by Papper and Bacon (see Chapter 3). However, Dr. Oscar O.R. Schwidetsky from the United States made two generous donations because he felt that the work being done was worthy of American support [2]. The first Executive Committee decided to establish working committees and these fell into four groups as follows:

1. The Executive Committee. The statutes stipulate that the Executive Committee shall have 12 elected members. The constitution of the first Executive Committee is shown in Table 2. The WFSA officers are ex officio members of the Executive Committee. However, the bylaws state that, of the

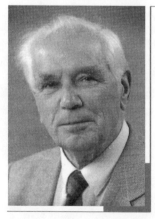

Fig. 1. *Maarten Mauve (by courtesy of Maarten Mauve)*

elected members, at least one should be from one of six defined geographical areas, i.e., (1) Africa and the Middle East, (2) Asia, (3) Australia, New Zealand, and the Pacific Islands, (4) Central and South America, Mexico, and the Caribbean Islands, (5) Europe and Israel, (6) The United States and Canada.

2. The Standing Committees. The number and nature of the Standing Committees are laid down in the bylaws. There are three Standing Committees: (1) Committee on Finance, (2) Committee on Statutes and Bylaws, (3) Committee on Education.

3. The Special Committees. The Special Committees are formed by decision of the Executive Committee for specific purposes, e.g., cardio-pulmonary resuscitation, obstetric anaesthesia, paediatric anaesthesia, etc.

4. The Ad Hoc Committees. The Ad Hoc Committees are usually formed at the time of a World Congress to assist in the conduct of WFSA business. They include the Credentials Committee, the Nominations Committee, and the Venue Committee. In recent years, an additional Standing Committee was created, the Publications Committee, and it was further agreed that the chairmen of the now, four, Standing Committees should become ex officio members of the Executive Committee.

The constitution of the WFSA was originally published in Dutch as a requirement for the organisation to be registered in The Netherlands. An English translation was prepared that became the working document for the

Table 1. *Founding Societies of WFSA*

Argentine	Denmark	Portugal
Austria	Finland	South Africa
Australia	France	Spain
Belgium	Germany (West)	Sweden
Brasil	India	Switzerland
Canada	Israel	UK
Chile	Italy	Uruguay
Colombia	Netherlands	Venezuela
Cuba	Norway	

Table 2. *WFSA First Executive Committee*

Jacques Boureau	France
Enrico Ciocatto	Italy
John Gillies	UK
Alexandre Goldblat (Ch.)	Belgium
A. Gonzales Varela	Argentina
Torsten Gordh	Sweden
Rodney A. Gordon	Canada
Harold R.Griffith	Canada
Norman J. James	Australia
Otto Mayrhofer	Austria
R. Patrick W. Shackleton	UK
Zairo E. G. Vieira	Brazil

next several years. The original constitution had a limited life and, in 1982, the Committee on Statutes and Bylaws began the task of revising the constitution. The registered address was transferred from The Netherlands to the United States of America to take advantage of benefits under United States tax law. The new constitution was approved by the General Assembly at the 9th World Congress in Washington D.C. in 1988.

1ˢᵗ World Congress in Scheveningen, 1955

The founding meeting in Scheveningen, held from 5 to 10 September 1955, was designated the first WFSA World Congress and was held under the high patronage of The Queen Juliana of The Netherlands. The Opening Ceremony was held in the Knight's Hall. Harold Griffith (Canada) (Fig. 2) was President of the congress and was elected as the first President of WFSA. Geoffrey Organe (UK) (Fig. 3) was elected secretary-treasurer and Alexandre Goldblat (Belgium) (Fig. 4) was elected chairman of the Executive Committee. An historic photograph was taken of the closing session at which WFSA was formally founded (Fig. 5). The congress provided the occasion, not only for the inauguration of the WFSA, but also for the election of its first officers. In addition, of course, as at all World Congresses, the scientific programme was the raison d'être for the congress, but the value of the opportunities provided for meetings between anaesthesiologists from all over the world should not be underrated. At the congress, a group photograph (Fig. 6) was taken of all the delegates and reproduced in the proceedings. Apart from the 5-year gap

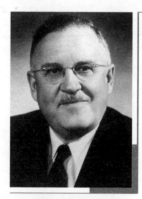

Fig. 2.
*Harold Griffith
(by courtesy
of David Bevan)*

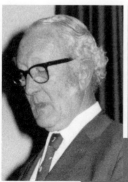

Fig. 3.
*Geoffrey Organe
(by courtesy
of John Zorab)*

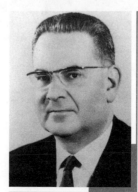

Fig. 4.
*Alexandre
Goldblat
(by courtesy of
Pierre Desbarax,
Antwerp, Belgium)*

between the first and second World Congresses, these congresses have been held at 4-year intervals ever since. Table 3 shows the venues of all the congresses, together with the leading anaesthesiologists involved in their organisation, as well as the officers elected to office within the WFSA on each occasion. In addition to the election of its officers, the World Congresses provide the occasion for a meeting of the principle committees, as well as the general assemblies at which the official delegates from member societies use their voting rights in the elections, and any other business requiring a vote. At this congress and at all succeeding congresses, the primary objective was to provide an up-to-date scientific programme to provide delegates with the news of the latest developments in the specialty. The social programme provided more opportunities for anaesthesiologists to meet one another and forge friendships, many of which subsequently became the basis of valuable exchanges both of information and personnel.

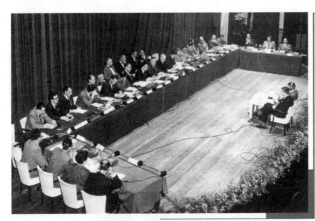

Fig. 5. *Closing session of 1ˢᵗ WCA, Scheveningen (by courtesy of Nederlandse Vereniging voor Anesthesiologie)*

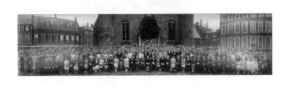

Fig. 6. *Group photograph of 1ˢᵗ WCA participants (by courtesy of International Anesthetic Research Society)*

Table 3. *WFSA World Congresses of Anaesthesiology. Congress President and/or Chairman of Org. Cttee & venues and WFSA Officers elected*

Year	Congress President and/or Chairman, Org. Cttee	Venue	WFSA President	WFSA Secretary	WFSA Treasurer	Exec Cttee Chairman
1955	CR Ritsema van Eck	Scheveningen	HR Griffith Canada	GSW Organe UK	GSW Organe UK	A Goldblat Belgium
1960	HR Griffith RA Gordon	Toronto	CR Ritsema van Eck Netherlands	GSW Organe UK	GSW Organe UK	RA Gordon Canada
1964	LR Alves	São Paulo	GSW Organe UK	O Mayrhofer Austria	H Poulsen Denmark	R Sappenfield USA
1968	RPW Shackleton DDC Howat	London	FF Foldes USA	O Mayrhofer Austria	Q Gomez Philippines	H Poulsen Denmark
1972	H Yamamura M Miyazaki	Kyoto	O Mayrhofer Austria	JJ Bonica USA	Q Gomez Philippines	H Poulsen Denmark
1976	Vasconcelos E Hulz	Mexico City	Q Gomez Philippines	JJ Bonica USA	C Rivas Venezuela	DDC Howat UK
1980	E Rügheimer WF Henschel	Hamburg	JJ Bonica USA	JSM Zorab UK	C Rivas Venezuela	ES Siker USA
1984	Q Gomez C Cruz	Manila	C Parsloe Brasil	JSM Zorab UK	R Ament USA	SW Lim Malaysia
1988	J Moyers	Washington DC	JSM Zorab UK	SW Lim Malaysia	R Ament USA	MD Vickers UK
1992	H Lip	The Hague	SW Lim Malaysia	MD Vickers UK	M Rosen UK	B Wetchler USA
1996	R Walsh	Sydney	MD Vickers UK	AA Meursing Netherlands	M Rosen UK	TK Brown Australia
2000	A Enright	Montreal	TK Brown Australia	AA Meursing Netherlands	RG Walsh Australia	D Bevan Canada
2004	P Scherpereel	Paris	?	?	RG Walsh Australia	?

2ⁿᵈ World Congress in Toronto, 1960

An informal meeting of some members of the Executive Committee had been held in London in 1956 and at that time it was decided to accept the invitation of the Canadian Anaesthetist's Society to hold the Second World Congress in Canada in 1960. Hope had been expressed that before that time the American Society of Anesthesiologists (ASA) would apply to join the Federation. This hope was realised since, in 1959, the House of Delegates of the ASA voted to apply for full membership and Ralph Sappenfield (USA) (Fig. 7) was co-opted as a member of the Executive Committee. The Canadian Anaesthetist's Society decided to hold the 1960 World Congress on 4-9 September in the Royal York Hotel, Toronto, Ontario. Roderick (Rod) Gordon (Canada) (Fig. 8) was chairman of the Organising Committee and plans got under way in 1957. A memorable congress was held with over 2,000 anaesthesiologists from 34 countries. At the general assemblies, a further 10 societies were admitted to the Federation. In addition, Griffith withdrew both as President and as a member of the Executive Committee. Meanwhile, Ritsema van Eck (The Netherlands) (Fig. 9) was elected as President, Organe was re-elected as secretary/treasurer, and Gordon as chairman of the Executive Committee. The final act of the 1960 General Assembly was to accept an invitation to hold the 3ʳᵈ World Congress in São Paulo, Brasil.

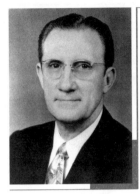

Fig. 7. *Ralph Sappenfield (by courtesy of the Wood Library Museum)*

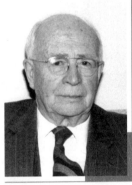

Fig. 8. *Roderick (Rod) Gordon (by courtesy of Rod Gordon)*

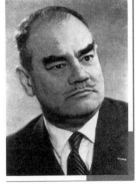

Fig. 9. *Ritsema Van Eck (by courtesy of Nederlandse Vereniging voor Anesthesiologie)*

3rd World Congress in São Paulo, 1964

The 3rd World Congress was held on 20-26 September in São Paulo. Luis Rodrigues Alves (Brasil) (Fig. 10) was President of the congress. The Opening Ceremony (Fig. 11) was held in the presence of Dr. Adhemar Pereira De Barros, Governor of the State of São Paulo. In all about 1,800 participants from more than 50 countries attended. At this congress, it was decided to change the post of secretary/treasurer, which had been held by Organe since the foundation of WFSA, into two separate posts. Both Francis Foldes (USA) (Fig. 12) and Organe were candidates for election as the next President and, after some machinations [2], Organe was elected as President, Otto (Teddy) Mayrhofer (Austria) (Fig. 13) as secretary, Henning Poulsen (Denmark) (Fig. 14) as treasurer, and Sappenfield as chair-man of the Executive Committee. The congress attracted a total registration of 1,212 active members. Eight new member societies were admitted. Included in the programme was an outstanding oration by Ralph Waters who speculated on being in that "afterplace" that most of us hope to reach and to meeting the "greats" among our anaesthetic predecessors. He closed his oration with these words: "Every gathering which brings

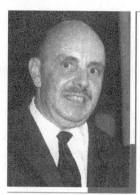

Fig. 10. *Rodrigues Alves (by courtesy of Carlos Parsloe)*

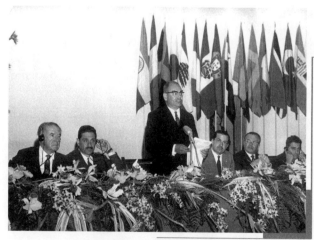

Fig. 11. *Opening Ceremony, 3rd WCA, São Paulo (by courtesy of The International Research Society)*

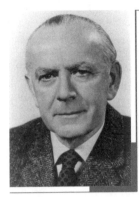

Fig. 12.
*Francis Foldes
(by courtesy
of The Wood
Library
Museum)*

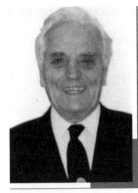

Fig. 13.
*Otto (Teddy)
Mayrhofer
(by courtesy
of John Zorab)*

together people from all parts of the earth helps a little, I believe, to hasten the day when enmity among the various nations will come to an end, and when all people can unite in a world free from animosity and misunderstanding. May this Congress continue to grow in years to come, to the benefit not only of the members who attend it, but toward the promotion of peace and co-operation throughout the world" [3].

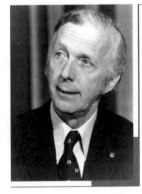

Fig. 14.
*Henning Poulsen
(by courtesy of
Henning Poulsen)*

4th World Congress in London, 1968

London had been accepted as the venue for the 4th World Congress during the São Paulo Meeting. The Association of Anaesthetists of Great Britain and Ireland (AAGBI) was the host society. Her Majesty Queen Elizabeth II honoured the occasion by agreeing to be patron.

In her message, which was included in the congress programme, Her Majesty included the following words: "I am glad that the World Federation of Societies of Anaesthesiologists decided to hold the 4th World Congress in London and it gives me great pleasure to be patron of the congress. I extend a warm welcome to all who have come to London for this occasion" [4].

An Organising Committee was appointed with George Ellis (UK)

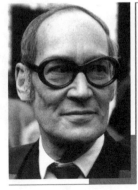

Fig. 15.
*George Ellis
(by courtesy of
St Bartholomew's
Hospital)*

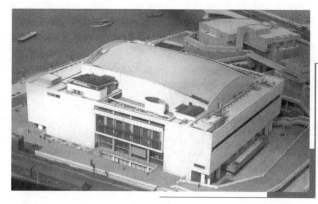

Fig. 16. *Royal Festival Hall, seat of the 4ᵗʰ WCA, London (by courtesy of Douglas Howat)*

(Fig. 15) as chairman. The congress was held in the Royal Festival Hall complex on the South Bank of the Thames (Fig. 16). Organe was President of WFSA and Patrick Shackleton (Fig. 17) was President of the congress and, in the absence of Princess Alexandra, had to make the opening speech (Fig. 18). London proved to be a popular venue and there were over 3,000 registrations - much to the relief of the Organising Committee! The full registration fee was £25 and 1-day registrations were introduced for the first time to encourage junior anaesthetists to attend. As said, the congress was due to be opened by HRH The Princess Alexandra but, sadly, she was prevented from doing so by the sudden death of her mother The Princess Marina. The General Assembly elected Foldes as the new President, re-elected Mayrhofer as secre-

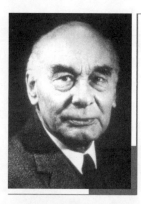

Fig. 17. *Patrick Shackleton (by courtesy of Southampton General Hospital)*

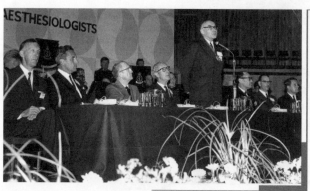

Fig. 18. *Opening Ceremony, 4ᵗʰ WCA, London (by courtesy of Douglas Howat)*

tary and elected Quintin Gomez (Philippines) (Fig. 19) as treasurer. Poulsen was elected as chairman of the Executive Committee. Nine new member societies were admitted. It was agreed that the 5th World Congress would be held in Kyoto. At the close of the congress, the outgoing WFSA President, Organe, introduced his successor, Foldes and handed over to him the new WFSA flag, which had been donated by the AAGBI.

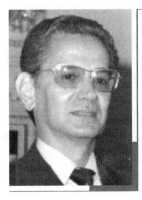

Fig. 19.
Quintin Gomez (by courtesy of John Zorab)

5th World Congress in Kyoto, 1972

The congress was held in the new, magnificent congress centre in the hills outside the city. Hideo Yamamura (Fig. 20) was President of the congress and Akira Inamoto was chairman of the Organising Committee. The congress was opened by the Crown Prince and Princess of Japan, the former giving a speech in Japanese that was simultaneously translated to the audience through headphones. It was an impressive cere-

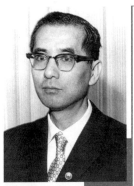

Fig. 20.
Hideo Yamaura (by courtesy of the Japan Society of Anaesthesiologists)

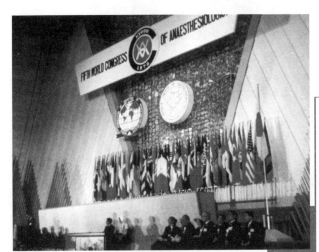

Fig. 21. *Opening Ceremony, 5th WCA, Kyoto (by courtesy of the Japan Society of Anaesthesiologists)*

mony (Fig. 21). At the end of the congress, Foldes transferred the WFSA flag
to Mayrhofer (Fig. 22) who had been elected as next President. This congress was the first time that the WFSA Presidential medallion (Fig. 23), which
had been commissioned and donated by Foldes, was used and the medallion
was also transferred to Mayrhofer. There is an interesting story behind the origin of the medallion (see Chapter 6). Other officers elected were John Bonica (USA) (Fig. 24) as secretary, Carlos Rivas (Venezuela) (Fig. 25) as treasurer, and Poulsen (Denmark) was re-elected as chairman of the Executive
Committee, the only chairman to serve two terms. The congress closed with
a magnificent party in the gardens of the conference centre, along with an outstanding firework display. A decision was taken for the next World Congress
to be held in Mexico City.

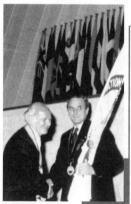

Fig. 22.
*Transfer
of WFSA flag
(by courtesy of
Otto Mayrhofer)*

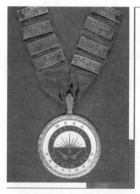

Fig. 23.
*The first WFSA
Presidential
Medallion
(by courtesy
of John Zorab)*

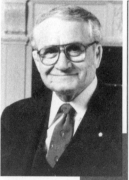

Fig. 24.
*John Bonica
(by courtesy of
the Wood Library
Museum)*

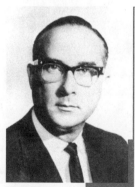

Fig. 25.
*Carlos Rivas
(by courtesy of
Señora Rivas)*

6ᵗʰ World Congress in Mexico City, 1976

The congress was held in the Mexico City Congress Centre (Fig. 26). Mayrhofer was President of WFSA, Guillermo Vasconcelos was President of the congress, and Enrique Hulsz was chairman of the Organising Committee. It had come to the attention of WFSA officials that the Mexican government had created difficulties in the issuing of visas to anaesthesiologists from South Africa. At the Opening Ceremony, which was held in the presence of the President of Mexico, Mayrhofer displayed considerable courage in voicing strong objections to these difficulties with the result that the Mexican President walked off the stage. Meanwhile, the congress proceeded and Gomez was elected as the new President. Other officers elected or re-elected were, Bonica as secretary, Rivas as treasurer, and Douglas Howat (Fig. 27) (UK) as chairman of the Executive Committee. During the congress, some discussions took place that had far-reaching effects. The so-called Medical Directives of the European Economic Community (EEC), as it was then, were about to come into force, permitting free movement of doctors throughout the member nations of the EEC. Michael Vickers (UK) and Michael Rosen (UK) (Fig. 28) had already been considering the idea of a single Pan-European anaesthetic organisation. An informal meeting was held during the congress, which included Jean Lassner (Fig. 29) (France) to discuss the creation of a European Academy of Anaesthesiology. This concept appealed to Lassner and planning continued over the next couple of years. The proposed European Academy of Anaesthesiology was duly founded at the 5ᵗʰ European Congress of Anaesthesiology in Paris in 1978. A meeting of the WFSA Executive Committee took place during this congress. The

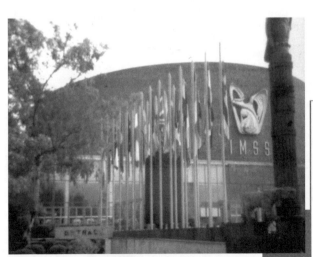

Fig. 26. Mexico City Congress Centre, seat of 6ᵗʰ WCA (by courtesy of John Zorab)

WFSA President, Gomez, expressed his concern at the founding of the European Academy, fearing that it would conflict with the WFSA. Lassner was displeased by this attitude and resigned from the WFSA Executive Committee, thereby creating a "casual vacancy". Bonica and Howat, secretary and chairman of the executive invited John Zorab (UK) to fill the "casual vacancy" which he did.

One problem that arose from the Mexican World Congress, subsequently referred to as "The Mexican Affair", concerned the disposal of the substantial surplus from the congress. Bonica played a major role in the resolution of this problem. He later wrote an editorial for the WFSA Newsletter in January 1982 saying: It is a pleasure to report on the recently achieved solution to the 'Mexican Affair' [5]. At my request, Professor Miguel Nalda Felipe participated in some meetings in October 1981 with all parties concerned. The funds derived from the 6th World Congress, which have been held in trust by the "Fundación Para la Investigatión en la Anesthesología A-C" (FUINANAC) have now been transferred to the Benjamin Bandera Foundation which has representatives from all parties and which will further the development in Anesthesiology in Mexico. Professor Nalda, supported by Drs. Castaños (Bolivia), Samayoa de Leon (Guatemala), Herrera and Sarpiento (Colombia) and Viggiano (Panama) are to be most warmly congratulated on this achievement which will benefit not only Mexican and Latin American but world anesthesiology" (see chapter 6).

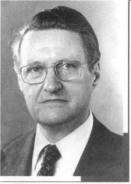

Fig. 27.
Douglas Howat (by courtesy of Douglas Howat)

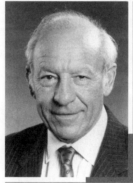

Fig. 28.
Michael Rosen (by courtesy of Michael Rosen)

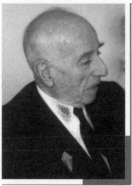

Fig. 29.
Jean Lassner (by courtesy of John Zorab)

7ᵗʰ World Congress in Hamburg, 1980

The 7ᵗʰ World Congress was held in the Congress Centre in Hamburg in what was then the Federal Republic of Germany (FRG). Gomez was President of WFSA and, during the congress, Bonica was elected as his successor. Other officers elected were Zorab as secretary, Rivas as treasurer (re-election), and Ephraim (Rick) Siker (USA) (Fig. 30) as chairman of the Executive Committee. Erich Rügheimer (Erlangen) (Fig. 31) was President of the congress and Rudolf Frey (Mainz) (Fig. 32) was appointed an honorary President. As had become the custom, there was an impressive Opening Ceremony (Fig. 33) at which there were some lengthy speeches by the Mayor of Hamburg, Rügheimer and Gomez. In his speech, Rügheimer reminded the audience that it was Henry Dunant who founded the Red Cross in 1863, thereby creating a symbol relevant to caring for human beings without regard to race, creed, colour, religion, or nationality. He explained that it was with this in mind that the Organising Committee had decided to dispense with any national symbols so that there were no national flags on display as there had been in São Paulo, Kyoto, and Mexico City. Frey, the honorary President, was a great internationalist and had friends in many parts of the world. He put together a special session that he called "Anaesthesia: Past and Future". He invited distinguished anaesthesiologists from various parts of the world to participate. Each was invited to give a five-minute talk and provide a photograph. Frey produced a booklet of this part of the session, which he called *Pioneers in Anaesthesiology*. Sadly, no copies of this seem to have survived. Amongst those that Frey invited was Shieh Yung (Fig. 34), President of the Soci-

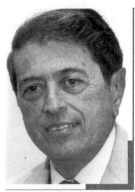

Fig. 30.
*Ephraim (Rick)
Siker (by courtesy
of Rick Siker)*

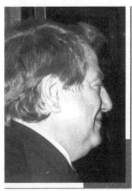

Fig. 31.
*Erich Rugheimer
(by courtesy
of John Zorab*

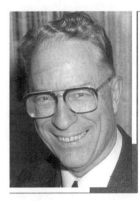

Fig. 32.
*Rudolf Frey
(by courtesy
of John Zorab)*

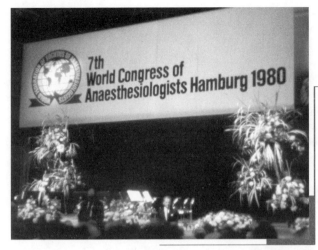

Fig. 33.
Opening Ceremony 7th WCA, Hamburg (by courtesy of John Zorab)

ety of Anaesthesiologists of the People's Republic of China (PRC). This was the first time that the PRC had been represented at a World Congress and discussions held with Shieh Yung in Hamburg ultimately led to the admission of the PRC as a member of WFSA at the World Congress in Washington in 1988. It was a very sad and huge loss to the specialty when Frey took his own life on 23 December 1981.

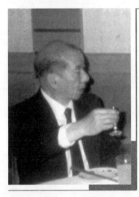

Fig. 34.
Shieh Yung (by courtesy of John Zorab)

8th World Congress in Manila, 1984

During the 6th World Congress in Mexico City in 1976, it had been agreed that the 8th World Congress would be hosted by the Australian Society of Anaesthetists. However, in the intervening years, the Australian Society had second thoughts because they thought that the facilities to host such a congress in Sydney - or anywhere else in Australia - were inadequate at that time. Therefore, at relatively short notice, The Philippine Society of Anaesthesiologists offered to host the 8th World Congress in Manila, and this offer was accepted, although not without some misgivings with regard to the ability of the Philippine Society to host a congress on this scale. Hence a preliminary visit to Manila was made by the Executive Committee in 1982, which was reassuring. In the event, all was well but not without some problems. Amongst these were the discovery of a criminal element within the Philippine postal service, which managed to intercept a number of applications for registration *and* the accompanying fees. This problem, however, was eventually overcome. The congress was held in the Manila Congress Centre. Bonica was WFSA President, Gomez was President of the congress, and Cenon Cruz (Fig. 35) was an effective Secretary General. The Opening Ceremony (Fig. 36) was attended by Imelda Marcos, since this was well before her fall from grace.

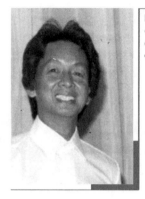

Fig. 35. *Cenon Cruz (by courtesy of John Zorab)*

One interesting episode concerned the debate by the General Assembly on the venue for the 10th World Congress scheduled for 1992. It had already been agreed that the 9th World Congress would be held in Washington D.C., in 1988. However, both Israel and South Africa had put in a bid to host the 10th World Congress. But, at that time, Israel was considered to be politically unstable and South Africa was ostracised in many parts of the world because of its apartheid policies. Thus, the General Assembly would not agree to either country hosting a World Congress. At the last minute, a bid was put from the floor by the delegates from The Netherlands. However, The Netherlands, at that time, barred entry to some individuals from selected countries, and, particularly after the problems at the Mexico Congress in 1976, the WFSA

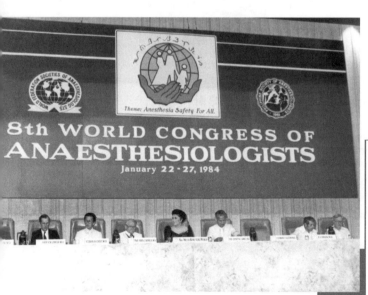

Fig. 36. *Opening Ceremony of 8th WCA, Manila (by courtesy of John Zorab)*

Executive Committee wanted reassurance that *all* anaesthesiologists from any country would be permitted to attend. This was a sensitive issue, since several South Africans, having had visa problems in being admitted to the 6th WCA in Mexico City, had again experienced similar problems in entering Manila-some had to collect their visa in Hong Kong en route. Thus telegrams were exchanged between the delegates from The Netherlands and the Dutch Foreign Office in The Hague and, with suitable reassurances being offered, the bid from The Netherlands was accepted.

Meanwhile, there was an interesting meeting of the Nominations Committee at which the next President was to be nominated. There were two "hot" candidates, Carlos Rivas (Venezuela) the current treasurer and Carlos Parsloe (Brasil) a vice-president. Opinions were sharply divided. Eventually a vote was taken and Rivas was narrowly defeated. Thus, Parsloe was duly elected President by the General Assembly. Richard Ament (USA) (Fig. 37) became treasurer and Saywan Lim (Malaysia) (Fig. 38) was elected chairman of the Executive Committee. Zorab was re-elected as secretary. Sadly, not very long after the Manila congress, Gomez became seriously ill and had major surgery. He never really recovered and, at the time of writing (18 years later), is still in hospital. Despite the anxieties of both the congress organisers and WFSA officials, it was gratifying to learn that the Manila congress eventually made a surplus of U.S. $ 230,000, of which U.S. $ 115,000 was returned to WFSA. Meanwhile, Washington D.C. had been selected as the venue for the 9th World Congress in 1988 and Jack Moyers (USA) had been appointed chairman of the Organising Committee.

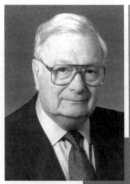

Fig. 37.
Richard Ament
(by courtesy of
Richard Ament)

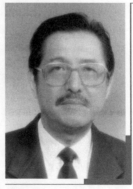

Fig. 38.
Saywan Lim
(by courtesy of
Saywan Lim)

9th World Congress in Washington D.C., 1988

The 9th World Congress was held in the relatively new congress centre in Washington D.C. Moyers had done a marvellous job as chairman of the Organising Committee. C. Everett Koop (Fig. 39), Surgeon General of the United States, gave a stirring address at the Opening Ceremony before a colourful backdrop of Washington monuments (Fig. 40, 41). There was an audience of many thousands at the Opening Ceremony and two elderly Kodak cameras had been

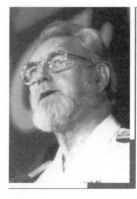

Fig. 39.
C Everett Koop (by courtesy of Chad Evans Wyatt, Photography, Washington D.C.)

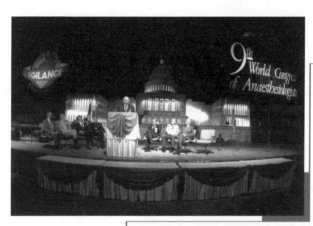

Fig. 40, 41.
Opening Ceremony, 9th WCA, Washington D.C. (by courtesy of Chad Evans Wyatt Photography, Washington D.C.)

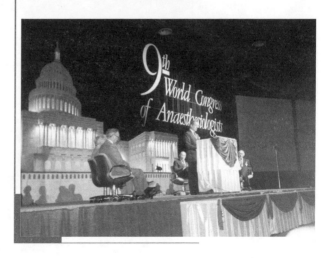

mounted on the top of ladders either side of the auditorium and, whilst the audience were requested to remain motionless, each camera swept one half of the audience each, producing a photograph of amazing clarity (Fig. 42), which makes an interesting comparison with the photograph of all the delegates taken at the 1st World Congress in Scheveningen in 1955 (Fig. 6). Parsloe was President of WFSA and, during the congress, Zorab was elected as the next President. Lim was elected secretary, Ament was re-elected treasurer, and Vickers was elected as chairman of the Executive Committee.

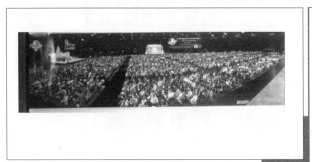

Fig. 42. *Group photograph of 9th WCA participants (by courtesy of Chad Evans Wyatt Photography, Washington D.C.)*

10ᵗʰ World Congress in The Hague, 1992

For the 10ᵗʰ World Congress, WFSA returned to the country of its birth. The congress was held in the congress centre in The Hague and Harm Lip was chairman of the Organising Committee. Zorab was President of WFSA and the congress was opened by Prince Bernhard (Fig. 43), who was representing Her Majesty, Queen Beatrix, who was unable to be present. In an entertaining Opening Ceremony, a professional magician joined with Lip (Fig. 44) in some spectacular illusions. During the congress, Lim was elect-

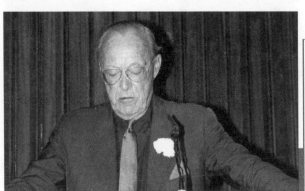

Fig. 43. *Prince Bernhard (by courtesy of Hans Koreman fotographie, Leiden)*

ed as the new President, Vickers as secretary, Rosen as treasurer, and Bernard Wetchler (USA) (Fig. 45) as chairman of the Executive Committee. A pleasant surprise awaited the participants at this congress who, on opening their congress bag, found a complimentary copy of an illuminating book describing some episodes from the early days of WFSA [1]. The author was Professor Maarten Mauve and reference to this book has been made in the opening part of this account. The fall of communism during the 1980s and 1990s had a major effect on WFSA. Until 1988, the USSR was represented by a single Anaesthetic Society, the "All-Union Society of Anaesthesiologists and Reanimatologists", which represented all the 15 republics of the USSR. Elena Damir and Armen Bunatian were the WFSA representatives. However, each of the 15 republics had its own anaesthetic society. After 1990, the 15 individual societies became independent and

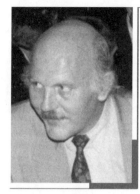

Fig. 44.
Harm Lip (by courtesy of Hans Koreman fotographie Leiden)

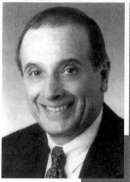

Fig. 45.
Bernard Wetchler (by courtesy of Bernard Wetchler)

some of them applied to become members of WFSA in their own right. The sequence of events was as follows. Some of the 15 societies formed a single larger society known as the Federation of Anaesthesiologists and Reanimatologists (FAR). These included the societies from Armenia, Azerbaijan, Georgia, Kyrgistan, Moldova, Russia, Tajikstan, and Ukraine. At the 1992 World Congress in The Hague, the 8 FAR societies and the other 7 applied for membership of WFSA. FAR then comprised Russia and the following 7 societies: Belarus, Estonia, Latvia, Lithuania, Kazakstan, Turkmenistan, and Ukraine. Later, almost all other societies of the former USSR became independent members of WFSA. However, since the 11th World Congress in Sydney in 1996, FAR only represents the Russian Federation and its more than 80 regional societies (there are 89 regions in Russia!).

11ᵗʰ World Congress in Sydney, 1996

The 11ᵗʰ World Congress was held in the congress centre in the spectacular setting of the redeveloped Darling Harbour in Sydney. There must have been many who were grateful to the wise decision by the Australian Society to decline to hold the congress in 1984, as originally decided, and to wait for the superb accommodation that the delegates were able to enjoy to the full and that was able to accommodate what was the biggest World Congress in the history of WFSA. Lim was WFSA President. Sir William Deane, Governor General of Australia, formally opened the Congress. His speech was followed by one from Richard Walsh, chairman of the Organising Committee. Then, all eyes looked upwards as James Morrison, a famous Australian trumpeter was slowly lowered from the roof on to the stage whilst playing his trumpet. The Opening Ceremony continued with a stage show with many colourful dancers (Fig. 46). Then, the audience was entertained to a live television transmission showing the well-known Australian anaesthetic historian, Gwen Wilson (Fig. 47) being interviewed in the Ether Dome in Boston (USA). At the end of the week, a further spectacular brought the congress to a close in which

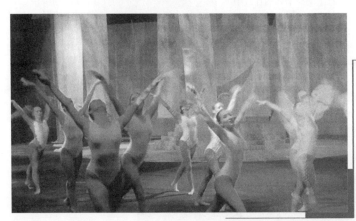

Fig. 46.
*Opening
Ceremony, 11ᵗʰ
WCA, Sydney
(by courtesy of
the Australian
Society of
Anaesthetists)*

Australian riders on horseback rode on to the stage and handed responsibility for the next World Congress in Montreal to other riders from the Canadian Mounted Police. During the congress, Vickers was elected as the new President with Anneke Meursing (The Netherlands) (Fig. 48) as secretary. Rosen was re-elected as treasurer and TC Kester Brown (Australia) (Fig. 49) was elected as the chairman of the Executive Committee.

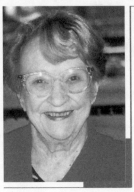

Fig. 47.
*Gwen Wilson
(by courtesy
of the Australian
Society of
Anaesthetists)*

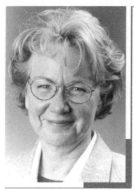

Fig. 48.
*Anneke
Meursing
(by courtesy
of Anneke
Meursing)*

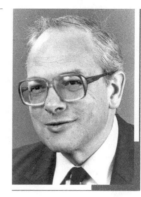

Fig. 49.
*Kester Brown
(by courtesy
of Kester Brown)*

12ᵗʰ World Congress in Montréal, 2000

The 12ᵗʰ World Congress was held in the congress centre in Montréal and excellently organised by Angela Enright (Canada) (Fig. 50). As in Sydney, there was a spectacular stage show as part of the Opening Ceremony (Fig. 51). Vickers was President of WFSA and, during the congress, Brown was elected President and Meursing was re-elected as secretary. In addition, Richard Walsh (Australia) (Fig. 52) and David Bevan (Canada)

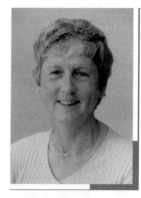

Fig. 50.
*Angela Enright
(by courtesy
of Ruth Hooper)*

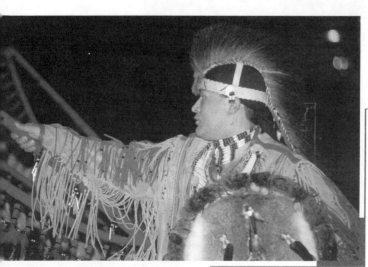

Fig. 51. *Opening
Ceremony, 12ᵗʰ WCA,
Montreal (by courtesy
of the Canadian
Anaesthesiologists Society)*

(Fig. 53) were elected as treasurer and chairman of the Executive Committee, respectively. During the congress, the decision was confirmed to hold the 13th World Congress in Paris and Philippe Scherpereel (France) was appointed as chairman of the Organising Committee.

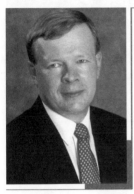

Fig. 52.
Richard Walsh (by courtesy of Richard Walsh)

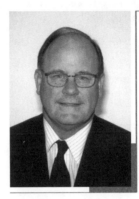

Fig. 53.
David Bevan (by courtesy of David Bevan)

Conclusion

In closing this account of 12 World Congresses, I should like to quote from the address I made at the closing ceremony at the 9th World Congress in Washington D.C. after having been elected President of WFSA. "It is my belief that WFSA stands for something which is, perhaps, of more fundamental importance than even its educational programmes. I believe that our specialty has created an international family of anaesthesiologists which is without parallel - certainly in other medical specialties and, perhaps in all other professions... And that is how it must continue. For, I believe that all of us, irrespective of colour, creed, religion, or political persuasion, share the common goal set out in the objects of the Federation - to make available the highest standards of anaesthesia and resuscitation to all peoples of the world."

References

1. Mauve M (1992) Episodes from the history of the establishment of the World Federation of Societies of Anaesthesiologists. Nederlands Tijdschrift voor Anesthesiologie 5 [Suppl 1]

2. Griffith HR (1963) History of the World Federation of Societies of Anesthesiologists. Anesth Analg 42:390

3. Waters R (1967) Editorial. Surv Anesthesiol 11:3

4. Progress in Anaesthesiology (1970) Proceedings of the Fourth World Congress of Anaesthesiology. Excerpta Medica Foundation. Amsterdam

5. Editorial (1982) WFSA Newsletter

6 WFSA Presidential Medallion

J.S.M. Zorab

The Presidential Medallion has an interesting history that is recorded in full below. I am indebted to Mayrhofer and Parsloe for the following details. The original design was made by Dr. Juan Marín Osorio from Colombia. Dr. Marín was born in 1907 in the rural community of Sonson, near Medellin, Colombia. He entered the Medical School of Bogotá in 1928, but dropped out in 1932/1933 to become a "chloroformist" in a local paediatric hospital, where he remained until 1946. In 1947, he founded a private school for non-medical anaesthetists. In 1949, he founded the Colombian Anaesthesia Society. He had, meanwhile, re-entered medical school, but did not graduate until 1956. He described the inspiration for the design of his logo in a booklet, a translation of which follows.

Dr. Marín Osorio originally designed his logo for the graduates of his own anaesthesia school in 1947 and, in 1949, used it as the logo of the Colombian Anaesthesia Society. In 1971, at a meeting in Rio de Janeiro, a committee comprised of Drs. Jose Silva Gomez (Colombia), Juan Koster (Peru), Izo Grunwald (Uruguay), and Ricardo Samayoa de Leon (Guatemala) recommended that the logo should be formally adopted as the official logo of the Confederation of Latin American Societies of Anaesthesiologists (CLASA), and this was agreed. However, later, Professor Foldes sought the permission of Dr. Marín to "convert" what was then the CLASA President's Medallion into a Presidential Medallion for WFSA (Fig. 1). However, it was not until the 5th World Congress in Kyoto in 1972 that this new WFSA Presidential Medallion was presented by Professor Foldes, outgoing President, to Professor Otto Mayrhofer, the new President.

In 1984, following his election as President of WFSA at the Manila Congress, Carlos Parsloe travelled to Africa in his presidential capacity. As he was on an official visit, he took the Presidential Medallion with him. When he came to leave Africa, to his horror he could not find the medallion and assumed it must have been stolen. This was in about 1986. On his return, he reported the loss to the WFSA secretary (Zorab). The secretary and chairman of the Executive Committee (Vickers) consulted and concluded that as no detailed photographs were known to exist, making a replica was impossible. Therefore a new Presidential Medallion was designed (Fig. 2) and made so that it would be available for the next World Congress in Washington in 1988. At the same time, the opportunity was taken to order a number of smaller versions of the medallion to be presented to past Presidents when they had completed their term of office. Thus it was at the 9th World Congress in Washington D.C. in 1988 that Carlos Parsloe became the first President to receive the new President's Medallion. After the ceremony of transferring the medallion to Zorab, as the incoming President, Parsloe received the new past Presidents' Medallion, as did other past Presidents who were present. As Geoffrey Organe was unable to be present, Zorab received a medallion on his behalf and, on his return to England, had the

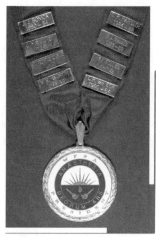

Fig. 1. *CLASA President's Medallion is converted into a Presidential Medallion for WFSA, in 1971*

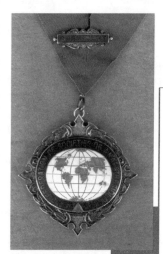

Fig. 2. *A new Presidential Medallion was designed before 1988*

pleasure of presenting it to him personally at his home. He died not long after. It was only several years later that we learnt from Professor Mayrhofer that Dr. Marín had had a replica of the original medallion made, which he had given to Mayrhofer, who has since generously lodged it in the WFSA office in London. But the story did not end there.

Parsloe later told me that the "stolen" medallion had, in fact, been found in his hotel room in South Africa. It was returned to the South African Society and in due course, much to his relief, was returned to Parsloe and thence to the WFSA office in London. Thus the WFSA now has three Presidential Medallions. The recovered original, the replica of the original, and the new, different one commissioned before the existence of the replica of the original was known.

World's emblem of anaesthesiology *(by Juan Marín Osorio, Fig. 3)*

Origin

On 5 March 1947, I delivered the inaugural lecture of the first School of Anaesthesiology in Colombia, S.A. under the auspices of Saint Joseph's Hospital Society of Surgery in Bogotá. The School's first term commenced shortly afterwards. Prior to this time, lectures on anaesthesiology had been given at the Faculty of Medicine, only for students and for their general information. However, none of these students showed any special interest or intention to specialise in the subject. During the first term, it was suggested that the school should have an appropriate emblem. This idea appealed to a fertile Latin imagination, and from a search of ancient mythology our symbol was born. From Greek mythology we have the Dream represented as an adolescent sleeping in perfect quietness. From the Romans a much more-interesting symbol was obtained, namely Dream and Death, the twin sons of Night, which are represented by two nude adolescents walking towards the sunset, with flaming torches held in their hands pointing to the floor, lightening the dark of the path. The latter is a beautiful scene but contains too many figures to be distributed in the small space of a shield without having the gift of a Cellini, whose work both in gold and silver along these lines has never been surpassed. It was therefore necessary to simplify the theme, which we did by taking only the flambeaus with their meaning.

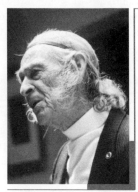

Fig. 3.
*Juan Marín
Osorio
(by courtesy of
Carlos Parsloe)*

Explanation

The upper part of the circle, in white, represents the integral life of the human organism and the sun of Consciousness, sinking or emerging from the horizon of Mystery. The lower part of the circle in blue represents the Unconsciousness, rarely seen, and the two flaming torches.

Our profession and our emblem

The anaesthetist must completely darken the sun of Consciousness and keep lit, but in careful watchfulness, the torch of Dream, so that its flame will not be extinguished, permitting his sister, Death, to grow and vivify and vanish to that unknown, fascinating, mysterious, and impenetrable land.

Anesthesia deorum ars

The original shield's legend was local and non-transcendent anaesthesia H.S.J. 1918. For 4 years I searched for a universal and eternal sentence that condensed in two or three words the essence of its meaning. In 1950, the Professor of Semantics began his lecture with this magnificent aphorism of Hippocrates "Dare dolorem opus divinum est". I had, of course, known it long since, but on that day, something similar to what must have happened to Newton, when at the sight of a falling apple, he discovered the Law of Universal Gravitation, happened to me. I also saw clearly at that instant and reasoned in the following manner: if alleviating pain is a divine task, we, the anaesthetists that not only prevent pain but also alleviate it and cure it, sometimes when our patients die, we are definitely doing divine work. Therefore anaesthesia is the art of gods. To say it in Spanish is far too long. I then looked for help in the most elegant of all dead languages, Latin, which allowed me to say Anesthesia deorum ars.

Comments

The anaesthesiological myth was born and is developing in a continent that does not tolerate anything other than what it considers the Truth, it's small truth. Hence, when lecturing before selected groups I ended my exposition with the former lemma, more than one risen eyebrow let it be known that I had offended the sentiments of some of my listeners. Sienkiewics says in his immortal novel *Quo Vadis* that in the restless world of Neron's tome and through the enchanting Libia-Vinicio romance, the Doctor of the Gentiles had the fortune of conversing with Petronius and after a long interview in Ancio the great question of a superior being or beings arose. St. Paul asked Petronius what was his conception of God and the arbiter with his exquisite elegance gave, to my understanding, the most-beautiful and least-compromising definition the human mind has ever yielded. To my understanding, the poet said, the Gods are no more than a figure of speech. This definition may possibly lack any transcendental meaning, even in the philosophical field, but the literary man has, through poetic fiction said so many and wonderful truths that God might be, as an example of universal beauty, the Summun of Literary Beauty. As the arbiter elengantiarum, I also love the Gods, in a literary way. However, should we approach the Bible, we read in Genesis chapter 11 verses 21 and 22:

> 21. *And the Lord God caused a deep sleep to fall upon Adam and he slept: and He took one of his ribs and closed up the flesh instead thereof.*

> 22. *And from the rib, which the Lord God had taken from man, he made a woman and brought her unto the man.*

Hence our Lord God, causing drowsiness in His most beloved creature, before a costotomy, accomplished the first anaesthesia in the Universe and thus my lemma, Anesthesia deorum ars, should not be considered irreverent, but the recognition of one more title of Anaesthetist Magnus, which, until now, has been lamentably ignored.

Translated from the original Spanish version by Juan Marín Osorio in about 1972. Note the English translation of Dr. Marín's description of his inspiration could be improved but this cannot be done without access to the original Spanish version.

7 WFSA REGIONAL SECTIONS

J.S.M. Zorab

WFSA Regional Sections

It was not long after the foundation of WFSA that there was a widespread feeling that 4 years was too long between major international congresses. Mayrhofer recalls that it was Cecil Gray (UK) who, whilst attending the Central European Meeting in Düsseldorf in 1959, suggested that WFSA should hold a European Congress half way between its World Congresses. This idea was readily accepted. As a result, the 1st European Congress of Anaesthesiologists was held in Vienna in 1962. At the congress, the European Regional Section (ERS) was formally established; 35 years later, this was to become the Confederation of European National Societies of Anaesthesiologists (CENSA), maintaining its connection with its "parent", WFSA. The 2nd European Congress was held in Copenhagen in 1966.

Asia was not far behind and, also in 1962, the 1st Asian-Australasian Congress was held in Manila and the Asian-Australasian Section (AARS) of WFSA was similarly established. Both Regional Sections flourished and 4-yearly congresses were held in the intervening even year between World Congresses. However, WFSA was not the first or only organisation to organise regional congresses.

Confederación Latinoamericana de Sociedades Anestesiología (CLASA)

In 1949, the Latin-American Congresses Protocol was signed by five Latin-American national societies in Buenos Aires, and six of these societies became founder members of WFSA. During the 6th Latin-American Congress in Lima in 1962, the same year as the Regional Sections of WFSA were founded, CLASA was founded. CLASA remained an independent organisation until 1988 when, at the 9th World Congress of WFSA in Washington DC, it was formally admitted as a Regional Section, similar to the ERS and AARS. The African Regional Section of WFSA was not founded until 1997.

The 3ʳᵈ European Congress in Prague, 1970

The 3ʳᵈ European Congress in Prague was, for many delegates from Western Europe, their first experience of coping with communist immigration and customs officials. It was tiresome, to say the least, but delegates eventually reached their hotel. Stephen Couremenos (Athens) was chairman of the ERS board and Jiri Pokorny was chairman of the Organising Committee. The congress was memorable, not so much for the scientific content, but for the opportunity to meet anaesthetists from different parts of Europe and, particularly, from Eastern Europe, from which, at that time, travel was difficult or impossible for anaesthetists in the Warsaw Pact countries.

One episode from that congress is particularly memorable. An English-speaking tourist group was sitting in their coach about to leave on an excursion. A young Czech lady of 18 or so was the tour guide. Just after the coach started, she asked if the tourists were all from England. She was assured that we were and she proceeded to discard her prepared "tourist commentary" and began to tell us what it was like trying to live under the communist system and how she and her compatriots hoped desperately that Dubcek would help Czechoslovakia towards democracy. It was a fascinating but very sad account of the reality of her life. After we returned, we all thanked her for trusting us and telling us so much. She then invited one or two of us to join her and her student friends at a Bierkeller that evening. It was an underground get-together in more ways than one and a hugely enjoyable evening was spent with many toasts to Dubcek, albeit in hushed tones.

4ᵗʰ European Congress in Madrid, 1974

The officers of the ERS that had presided in Prague had finished their term of office and new officers were elected. Dr. Alfredo Arias (Spain), who was President of the congress, was elected as chairman, Jean Lassner (France) was elected secretary, Augustus (Gus) Haxholdt (Denmark) was treasurer, and John Zorab was elected a vice-chairman. In those days, the ERS had an income of its own derived from a small supplement to the WFSA dues paid by the ERS member societies. The amount was not great and the 1981 annual report records the ERS dues as being U.S. $ 0.50, making the total WFSA dues U.S. $ 1.75 per active member. Nevertheless, collecting these dues was a nightmare as several societies declined to pay dues to *both* WFSA *and* the ERS. The ERS income was only used to fund the members of the board to hold an annual meeting, usually in conjunction with some other meeting. It was at a meeting of the ERS board in Salamanca in 1977 that the board faced the truth that it served no useful purpose other than organising the venue of the next European Congress. Having accepted this, it was clear that there was no justification for a separate income, and expenses for an occasional meeting of the board could be met from the surplus made from the previous European Congress. Thus, at the 6th European Congress in 1982, it was agreed to abolish the separate ERS dues.

5th European Congress in Paris, 1978

The European Academy of Anaesthesiology was inaugurated at this meeting at which the Executive Committee of WFSA was holding one of its interim meetings. At the first meeting of the ERS General Assembly, Gomez (now WFSA President) made a speech voicing his concern about the foundation of the EAA, fearing that it would weaken the influence of WFSA in Europe. Lassner, who was at that time the new President of the EAA, did not agree with these sentiments and resigned from the WFSA Executive Committee. As a result, a "casual vacancy" on the executive was created. After discussion between John Bonica (WFSA secretary) and Douglas Howat (chairman of the Executive Committee), John Zorab (UK) was invited to fill the vacancy until the next World Congress in 1980. Following this, Bonica and Howat had further discussions and Zorab was asked if he would be willing to stand for the position of WFSA secretary, the election of which would take place at the next World Congress meeting.

6th European Congress in London, 1982

At the European Congress in Paris in 1978, it had been agreed that the next one would be in London in 1982. Zorab, already secretary of WFSA, had been appointed by the AAGBI as Secretary General of the Organising Committee. The chairman was Philip Helliwell, the current President of AAGBI. Derek Wylie was appointed President of the congress, which was opened by HRH the Princess Margaret, Countess of Snowdon.

There was an interesting incident at the Opening Ceremony. Arrangements had been made for the Presidents of all the European societies of anaesthesia to be assembled at one side of the stage and, one at a time, to walk over to Her Royal Highness to receive a commemorative scroll to mark the occasion. All went according to plan but it was the time when Poland was striving to escape from the communist yoke and implement a democracy. The struggle that involved the Gdansk dock workers under the leadership of Lech Walesa was intense. Professor Marek Sych was President of the Polish Society at the time and, as he crossed the stage, the entire audience rose to their feet and applauded. Her Royal Highness mentioned later that she found it a most-moving experience.

On a lighter note, there was a minor crisis when the Czechoslovakian lady concert pianist due to play that evening, wished to rehearse on stage. Only then was it discovered that the lift which takes the Steinway Concert Grand from the basement to the stage had broken down. Steinway sent some strong men and the piano had to be carried up an emergency winding staircase to the stage. As Zorab returned to his hotel over the other side of the Thames, he thought he would buy a nice bouquet for presentation to the pianist after the concert. Just across the Thames foot-bridge, there was a typical London flower barrow. There were plenty of flowers but, asked for a presentation wrapping, the barrow boy replied that all his wrapping paper is "up the street" in his shed and he couldn't leave his barrow. A compromise was reached and, for 20 minutes, Zorab took on the role of barrow boy, and sold flowers to passers by (including some Congress participants) and the barrow boy returned, wrapped the flowers appropriately and all was well!

7ᵗʰ European Congress in Vienna, 1986

The Egyptian affair

An interesting episode in the history of WFSA about this time concerns the Egyptian Society of Anaesthesiologists. The full correspondence is lodged with the WFSA archives. Early in the 1980s there were two Egyptian societies of anaesthesiology. Both wished to become members of WFSA. However, WFSA regulations specify that only one society may become a member from any one country. It was clear that one society was completely inactive and provided no services to its members. The other was recently formed and active. The matter was left to the two relevant societies to resolve for themselves. It was at a meeting of the Executive Committee at the European Congress in Vienna in 1986 that Professor Shaker from Cairo was invited to attend the committee and he explained that the "inactive" society had now been persuaded to disband and that the new society, of which Shaker was secretary, would be the representative society within WFSA.

African Regional Section

Whilst Africa was high on the list of areas in which WFSA might have a role to play, not a great deal happened in the early years. In the 1960s and 1970s, much thought was given to establishing an African training centre on the lines of those in Caracas and Manila. Indeed, Henning Poulsen, among others, travelled to Africa for WFSA to explore the possibilities. However, the absence of any educational infrastructure meant that these ambitions went unfulfilled. Nevertheless, after many discussions, an African Regional Section of WFSA, similar to the European and Asian-Australasian Regional Sections, was eventually established in 1997 and the first African Regional Congress was held in Durban in that year. The growing pains are of some interest. The decision to establish an African Regional Section was taken by the Executive Committee at its meeting at the 11th World Congress in Sydney in 1996. Kester Brown, chairman of the Executive Committee, met with representatives of the African delegates and formed a steering committee. There were three nominations for chairman for the proposed African Regional Section. Dorothy Ffoulkes Crabbe (Nigeria) and Hannes Loots (South Africa) tied. Hannes Loots then withdrew so that Dorothy Ffoulkes Crabbe became the first chairman. It was agreed that the organisation should be for the whole of Africa, without domination by any one country. Kester Brown and Anneke Meursing assisted in the drawing up of a constitution. At the meeting for election to the board, Lawrence Marks (Zimbabwe), David Morell (South Africa), and Hannes Loots were elected. No representative from Egypt attended, but this left Dorothy Ffoulkes Crabbe isolated with no representative from Francophile West Africa. Lawrence Marks decided to withdraw in favour of Martin Chobli (Benin) to achieve a better balance. These generous acts by a South African and a Zimbabwean augured well for the future.

Publications

One of the educational initiatives of WFSA was to provide various publications. One type was low-cost clinical training manuals. Several of these were published as follows.

Manuals

Cardiopulmonary resuscitation - 1st edition 1968, Peter Safar.
Cardiopulmonary cerebral resuscitation - 2nd edition 1981, Peter Safar
Cardiopulmonary cerebral resuscitation - 3rd edition 1988, Peter Safar
Obstetric anaesthesia and analgesia - 1st edition 1972, John Bonica
Obstetric anaesthesia and analgesia - 2nd edition 1982, John Bonica
Basic techniques of nerve block, Bruce Scott
Paediatric anaesthesia, Anneke Meursing et al.
Critical care in the tropics, Iain Wilson et al.
WFSA career guide, John Zorab

WFSA Lectures in Anaesthesiology

This series comprised written "lectures" on a variety of topics by well-known experts. These were published by Blackwell. John Zorab and Jack Moyers were co-editors, Robin Weller followed Moyers later. Two issues a year were produced from 1984 to 1988 when publication ceased, as Blackwell did not find them sufficiently profitable.

WFSA Newsletters

The first WFSA Newsletter was introduced by Professor Mayrhofer and was published from 1972 to 1977. They have been described in details elsewhere and all copies are now in the WFSA archives. However, as Mayrhofer has described, this newsletter had to cease publication owing to rising costs. Following the Hamburg congress, a new simplified newsletter was introduced by the new secretary (John Zorab). This was a folded sheet of A4 paper. It had the advantage of being cheap to produce and, in fact, each issue was "sponsored" by a medical or equipment company so no costs fell on WFSA. This newsletter was translated by anaesthetists in various countries and either distributed through national societies or reproduced in a national journal. The first newsletter (January 1981) was reproduced in 12 anaesthetic journals in a total of eight languages. This newsletter continued, with two issues a year for the next 12 years. A full set is lodged with the WFSA archives.

The WFSA annual report

Prior to 1980, the WFSA annual report appeared as a number of stapled A4 sheets. Constitutionally, the secretary is required to produce an annual report, but the existing style was not conducive to easy reproduction or distribution. The new simplified newsletter paved the way for a similar booklet-style of annual report, which contained the following:
a) The report
b) The address lists of committee members
c) The WFSA directory of member societies
d) An international congress calendar.

This format was adopted in 1981 and has continued ever since. All annual reports from 1981 to 1992 are available in the archives.

Statutes and bylaws

The original constitution of WFSA was registered in The Netherlands in 1955 and had a "life" of 30 years, after which it was due to expire. Thus, in 1981, the Statutes and Bylaws Committee, under the chairmanship of Professor Vickers, embarked on re-writing the statutes and bylaws of WFSA. This was a major task and the revised constitution was eventually accepted by the General Assembly at the World Congress in Washington in 1988.

8 WFSA AND THE CHANGING WORLD: 1982-2002

M. Vickers

Introduction

To attempt to define boundaries in a continuum is to risk creating artificial entities. Organisations do not exist in a vacuum but change and evolve continuously according to the circumstances in which they find themselves. Perhaps the greatest change over the last 20 years has been the increasing financial strength of the Federation, allowing the practical development of ideas that had evolved over the previous years but could not be afforded. Even so, their implementation also depended on technological changes, notably electronic communication and the compact disc.

At the same time, one must not overlook the influence of the worldwide expansion in the number of specialist anaesthetists, associated with the great expansion of the role. This is still evolving and there is a developing recognition of the important role of anaesthetists in acute services - particularly in the prevention of unnecessary complications of accidents - a major problem in developing countries. In parallel there has been the acceptance of the concept of the anaesthesia team, and the continuing need for a non-medical element in the delivery of services.

The financial environment

In 1976, when I was elected to the Education and Scientific Affairs Committee, the income from the membership fees (about U. S. $ 40,000 per annum) was only sufficient to run the organisation. In the 21 years of its existence WFSA had accumulated reserve assets worth less than one and a half times its annual expenditure - a knife-edged existence. The Hamburg Congress in 1980, however, was considerably larger than its predecessors (5,695 registrants) and the WFSA received U. S. $ 60,000, almost equalling the existing reserves.

The Washington Congress in 1988, however, initiated a step change.

Organising the Congress on behalf of the American Society of Anesthesiologists (ASA) was a redoubtable figure, not only in the ASA but also already within the WFSA, Dr. Jack Moyers (Iowa, USA). He persuaded the ASA that as the biggest and wealthiest national society they should give a lead. They already held annual meetings that were almost as big as a World Congress, ensuring them a regular income and did not need a big "profit" from the World Congress. At his prompting they agreed in advance to donate half of any surplus to the WFSA.

What surprised us all, even him I suspect, was the fact that professional financial control created a much greater surplus than expected, the WFSA share being U. S. $ 500,000. As the treasurer (Dr. Richard Ament, Buffalo, USA) had obtained tax-exempt status in the United States in 1986 this sum, when invested, started to produce an income exceeding that from membership dues. The Federation was thus suddenly able to tackle its objectives more vigorously.

The 50% share of any surplus was written into the contract between WFSA and host societies for all subsequent World Congresses. Without exception, so far, they have all produced useful surpluses, thus steadily increasing the funds invested (almost U.S. $ 3 million by 2000) and producing a rising investment income. The prolonged stock market rise of the 1990s magnified even more the investment income now available for educational activities, funding of educational publications and, later, an office to handle the great increase in the administrative work generated.

Unfortunately, this increasing affluence also had a negative effect. The late 1980s and early 1990s was an era in which there was still significant inflation and the running costs of the WFSA were bound to increase without the added cost of the extra work. Whereas these factors would previously have meant a rise in annual dues (which had been unchanged since 1980), this politically unpopular move could be safely postponed. The burgeoning activities of the Federation meant that the WFSA was no longer covering running costs by member's subscriptions. In 1998 the treasurer invited societies to increase their payments voluntarily by a modest U. S. $ 0.25 per member (which many did) and in 2000 it was agreed that in 2004 the rise would become mandatory.

Almost simultaneously a prolonged downturn in world stock markets drastically reduced the investment income, several years before the rise in subscriptions would come into effect. This enforced a considerable "belt tightening", principally in office costs and travelling. The budget was expected to be in balance by 2003, but until then there had to be some draw down of capital to fund committed educational expenditure.

The WFSA Foundation

One of the hidden problems with expansion was the lack of transparency about what elements of the total income were being spent on which functions. It is inherently unsatisfactory to use charitable income to fund routine expenditure, as the above sequence demonstrated. A decision was therefore taken at the 2000 General Assembly to set up a legally independent Foundation to raise funds for charitable WFSA activities. In due course, investments arising from congress surpluses would be transferred to the Foundation. The long term objective must be for the expenses of running WFSA to be met by member Societies and the educational work (in its broadest sense) to be funded by the Foundation.

Education

The enhanced income from invested congress surpluses had its greatest impact on the education budget-as indeed it should have. Development affected both the management and control and the type of educational activities.

Management and control

In 1982 any educational event was administered by a cumbersome process in which the treasurer paid claims that had received the signed approval of the chairman of the Education Committee, confirming that he had authorised the event, and the counter-signature of the chairman of the Executive Committee. All three of these individuals were often living in different continents. It was a prudent system, necessary, perhaps, when funds were tight, but cumbersome when the level of activity increased. The evolution of different types of activity also demanded simpler methods.

The first essential development was the creation in 1988 of a delegated 4-year education budget when Dr. Kester Brown (Melbourne, Australia) became chairman of the committee. A parallel change was his "appointment" of a designated committee member for each region, with an identified share of that budget and autonomy over its use. This released a lot of enthusiasm and generated much activity. As chairman of the Executive Committee, I opted out of the loop believing that we had to trust the Education Committee chairman to only approve expenditure within the agreed parameters and not to exceed the budget.

Scope. For the quadrennium 1980-1984 the visiting educational team was the predominant concept but for a variety of practical reasons was replaced by visiting "professors" in 1986. This, too, failed to generate much interest and was replaced by the concept of refresher courses, approved by the Executive Committee in 1986 and which progressively became the predominant educational activity.

Refresher courses. Although the first WFSA refresher course was in 1987 (Nairobi) the level of activity accelerated due to the increased budget from 1988. These were organised by (usually) two or three visiting lecturers, sometimes working alone but progressively supported by local teachers, lasting 3-

5 days, with heavy emphasis on questions and answers and small group discussions. The feedback showed them to be well attended and tremendously appreciated, and demand rose. By appealing to some wealthy member societies [notably the Dutch, and the German societies, and the Association of Anaesthetists of Great Britain and Ireland (AAGBI)] to fund one or more of the lecturers, additional courses could run - as many as 5-6 a year in 12 English-speaking African countries. (This stratagem was even further extended by the AAGBI who persuaded local regional societies throughout the UK to take on this commitment in rotation! This was also beneficial in raising the profile of the needs and in enthusing additional volunteers outside the programme.) At the same time, financial support was given to Philippe Scherpereel (Lille, France) to support and expand similar courses in 15 French-speaking central and West African countries.

If there was a weakness in the early years it was that the WFSA refresher courses operated an "open door" policy and, in Africa, the bulk of the audience consisted of non-medical anaesthetists. These were very enthusiastic, often travelling very considerable distances to attend. This was obviously desirable, but there was inevitably a tendency to teach at an appropriate basic level, and the few local medical anaesthetists felt that they had not had the fullest possible benefit. In 1991, refresher courses (for physicians only) spread to Russia and the sending of a speaker to their annual meetings led to an onward spread to the Baltic States, the Ukraine, and even as far as Archangel and Khabarovsk (Siberia), the later being organised from Japan by Fuji Mori (Osaka). New ground was broken with a course to teach anaesthetists how to service their equipment (in Tanzania in 1998), lack of servicing being one of the major problems in some areas.

Scholarships. During this period of expansion, WFSA worked on the principle that it was more cost effective to take a few teachers to lots of learners rather than financing the long-distance travel of a few learners. A case, however, could also be made in special circumstances for individuals to be sent some distance for concentrated training, but it needed strict financial control. For instance, in 1990, the Executive Committee set aside U. S. $ 5,000 per annum to fund (at U. S. $ 1,000 a head) a few potential leaders from eastern bloc countries for short, intensive visits to Western Europe.

The Standing Committee on obstetric anaesthesia pressed for either a professorship or a training centre for obstetric anaesthesia over many years and a considerable sum was earmarked without any viable proposal being put into effect. Two possibilities gradually emerged and in 1990, Trevor Thomas (Bristol, UK) was asked to chair a working party to try and bring matters to a conclusion. In the event, they recommended an arrangement to take potential high flyers (one at a time) from developing countries in sub-Saharan Africa for 3 months residential training in obstetric anaesthesia in Durban (South Africa) under Professor Rocke. The first trainee was accepted in 1997. This was given a high priority because of the dreadful maternal mortality rate in many such countries in sub-Saharan Africa, emergency caesarean section being the commonest surgical operation. Another training centre for paediatric anaesthesia was funded in the late 1990s in Santiago, (Chile) to take an anaesthetist from a less affluent South American country.

Training centres. When there is an on-going programme to train other nationals, scholarships shade into training centres. Notable has been the Beer Sheva project, a scheme set up in 1990 by Gabriel Gurman (Tel Aviv, Israel) to accept three young trainees from East European countries for 1-2 months each. Over 90 have benefited over the first 11 years of the programme. WFSA support in 2001 was U. S. $ 16,000. The programme was originally limited to Romanian anaesthetists and it is particularly gratifying that a similar programme is now to be mounted in Cluj (Romania) for Moldavian anaesthetists. Another "spin-off" has been a training programme for Albanian anaesthetists in Milan, Italy.

In 1996 formal financial support was approved for doctors from Cambodia and Laos to train for a year in Bangkok under Thara Tritrakarn (Thailand), which later spread to take trainees also from Vietnam, Myanmar, and Siberia.

In summary, one can see that there has been a steady increase in the number, scope, and types of educational ventures undertaken by WFSA, either alone or in co-operation with others. This naturally depended on, and was reciprocally stimulated by, a steady increase in the budget, which increased from roughly U. S. $ 40,000 per annum in 1984 to over U. S. $ 150,000 per annum by 2000.

Publications

Educational publications were the second main development related to increased income, but this overview draws attention to a wider remit than purely educational. There were also internal publications that helped the organization to cohere.

Internal publications

Newsletters. Otto (Teddy) Mayrhofer (Vienna, Austria) produced a secretary's newsletter that ran for ten issues from 1964, but folded because of cost. In 1980 John Zorab (Bristol, UK) became secretary and he soon used his talent for putting pen to paper by reviving this venture in a less costly way. After the first issue he got it sponsored, and produced it in four languages, with translations by volunteers recruited by him. (The WFSA has been indebted to several commercial companies for such support that was being acknowledged as late as 1992.) Zorab's successor (Dr. Say Wan Lim, Kuala Lumpur, Malaysia) developed a quarterly report, which included information on regional events as well as Federation business.

In 1991 Dr. Patrick Foster (Toronto, Canada) proposed that the newsletter should be upgraded and become more professionally styled as a quarterly with a wider remit. He was keen to be editor and it was agreed in 1992 to give it a try. He collected, edited, and produced camera-ready pages locally under the title "*Anaesthesia Worldwide*" and sent them electronically to the secretary where a local printer produced the copies for distribution. The first issue was for the final quarter of 1993.

It has to be admitted that it was not a success. The editor was too remote from the sources of WFSA news and did not receive enough copies. Indeed, there really was not enough "news" to fill four issues a year. Dr. Foster commissioned articles, including profiles of the principal officers and editorials by them and others, but after five issues it was generally felt not to be a very effective way of proceeding. An alternative, combining it with *The World Anaesthesia Newsletter*, seemed a more-attractive option.

Annual reports. Although these were required under the constitution they had not appeared in printed form until Zorab became secretary. His format, a report of Federation activities, a directory of member societies, the composition of committees, and a congress calendar has persisted to the present day, with the addition of an address list of committee members and a personal homily from the secretary.

External publications

Handbook of obstetric anaesthesia. The Federation had published a handbook by Peter Safar on cardiopulmonary resuscitation in 1968 when the late John Bonica (Seattle, USA) was secretary. He initiated another handbook, on obstetric anaesthesia, written in collaboration with Gertie Marx. These had been economically feasible because his university had acted as publisher. These handbooks filled a great need in the developing world and were much in demand when exhibited at congresses. A second edition of 3,000 copies of the *Obstetric Anaesthesia Handbook* was prepared in 1991 (printed cheaply in Kuala Lumpur) and continued to be popular, although the transport from Malaysia to congresses and to storage for unsold copies increased the real cost.

Lectures in Anaesthesiology. Zorab also started a new twice-yearly venture under the above title in 1984, consisting of topics of particular value in underdeveloped regions, subsidised by Blackwells, and edited by himself and Moyers, the latter subsequently replaced by Dr. Robin Weller (Bristol, UK). It ran until 1988 when sponsorship dried up. Even though the contributors were unpaid and there were no "frills" such as photographs, it was not economically viable and depended on sponsorship.

Career guides. Zorab also drew on his experience as secretary of the AAGBI and prepared recruitment-orientated career guides, paid for by Ohmeda, in several languages.

Handbook of paediatric anaesthesia. The model of the two previous handbooks dominated thinking and their success was the stimulus and model for this third handbook, but its genesis was less straightforward. Indeed it would probably never have been successfully completed as envisaged as a multi-authored work written by the members of the committee on paediatric anaesthesia. Fortunately it was taken in hand as a virtual solo endeavour by Anneke Meursing (Rotterdam, the Netherlands) and published in time for the 10th World Congress in The Netherlands in 1992. The cost of printing was defrayed on this occasion by generous donations: the Asian-Australasian Regional Section donated $7,500 and two member societies (Japan and the Netherlands) also contributed. This venture fully revealed that the business of not only printing, but storing and distributing books was really beyond the capability of the WFSA, in the way that it was then being managed by individual officers.

Update in Anaesthesia. In 1991 I was approached by Dr. Iain Wilson, (Barnstable, UK) who had spent time working in Africa, with a request for WFSA help in starting a publication that, he believed, would fill a great need. *Update in Anaesthesia* would consist of two types of articles: straightforward "how to do it" articles and simple explanations of relevant basic science-physiology, pharmacology, and physics. It was conceived as a "part work": the issues would accumulate to form a textbook. In many ways it resembled Zorab's *Lecture Notes* initiative, but was not to be solely directed to a medical audience. Furthermore, he had innovative ideas on how to get it to where it was most needed.

It was clear that the readership could well be mostly non-medical anaesthetists attempting to provide basic anaesthesia services in the most-primitive circumstances and without access to any educational resources. The World Federation has always been a strictly medical organisation but the Executive Committee was persuaded that the outlay was small and the benefit potentially considerable. Accordingly we offered sufficient funds for a year's trial. This venture soon confirmed Dr. Wilson's predictions and with the help of the British Council got wide distribution. In 1992, the Executive Committee authorised a further £2,000 for 2 more years. It was soon being requested in other languages, thus demonstrating that, at least as far as anaesthesia services are concerned, a lot of the world is still under-developed. In 2002, 14,000 copies of *Update in Anaesthesia* were published twice a year in Mandarin Chinese, Russian, Spanish, French, and English, distributed in over 100 countries, and although it is now supported by others WFSA is still an important source of income.

This is where technological change made its first obvious impact on this aspect of WFSA activities. Dr. Michael Dobson (Oxford, UK) started putting accumulated copies onto floppy diskettes. The contents could be printed locally - a considerably easier and cheaper method of distribution. At the same time the contents of each issue were also made available via an early educational satellite venture from which they could be downloaded. When the World Wide Web was sufficiently developed, Dobson put the contents in

English, French, and Russian on a dedicated web-site and the material is now also available on compact disc.

World Anaesthesia. This started life as a private initiative by Dr. Roger Eltringham (Gloucester, UK) and was registered as a charity in the United Kingdom. It was funded by relatively small personal subscriptions and made available free to deserving cases. Its focus was as a communication organ rather than an educational function. It published newsletters from a variety of places in what was then called the "third world". There were some more educational articles - useful tips, simple trials of techniques or appropriate equipment designed for primitive conditions.

By 1996 it was becoming a victim of its own success - greater demand than its subscriber base could support. It was my view that there could be a saving of effort and expenditure, and gain in coverage if the Federation's newsletter (*Anaesthesia Worldwide*) combined with *World Anaesthesia* by paying for copies for member societies. This would inject WFSA resources into a going concern serving a relevant function and widen the interest in the newsletter. It continued publishing two issues a year as *World Anaesthesia Newsletter* from 1997 until the end of 2000, with continuing WFSA financial support. Unfortunately, the proportion of the contents relating to WFSA was very small in relation to the proportion of the costs that the Federation was bearing. The economic downturn in 2000 forced WFSA to re-think its priorities and it was decided to restart its own low-cost newsletter.

Too much or too little?

By 1990 the problems of what written material the WFSA should be producing really needed a fresh look and a policy. It was, for example, difficult to keep to a consistent policy on who should receive what material and at what cost. Those who really needed the books could not afford even the highly subsidised price and those who could afford them did not need or buy them. The handbooks also needed new editions, which no longer found ready volunteer writers. As this was fast becoming a major part of the Federation's activities, I recommended that there should be a Standing Committee on publications. Dr. Bernie Wetchler (Peoria, USA), as chair of the Executive Committee, set up a publications working party in 1990 under Moyers to consider the options and make recommendations. In 1992 they recommended, amongst other things, that there should be a Standing Committee on publications and in 1996 the General Assembly agreed to this with a separate budget of U.S. $ 40,000. Eltringham was appointed chairman.

Educational packages

For some time the International Anesthesia Research Society (IARS) had generously been mailing their annual revision lectures to a list of "deserving cases", which was started by Zorab and which successive WFSA secretaries had attempted to maintain. In 1996, Wetchler set up a literature distribution working party to direct educational aid, particularly to teaching "centres" in developing countries by sending them packages of books, journals, videos, refresher course lectures, etc., tailored to the individual teaching centres' requirements, costing up to U.S. $ 500 each. An initial budget of U.S. $ 10,000 was established. The Publication Committee subsumed this work after it was established. By the end of 1998, 133 packages had been sent to centres in 85 developing countries. The programme continued at roughly the same rate before being suspended as one of the economy measures of 2002-2004.

World Congresses

Seen over a 25-year span, there have been relatively few changes in the structure of these, the most-obvious development being the considerable growth in size, no doubt related to the increase in the number of practising anaesthesiologists worldwide. Following the death of Harold Griffiths, the first President, a special Griffiths Symposium has been made a feature, dedicated to his memory. Practical workshops have been added and more small group discussions. The congresses have also remained fairly expensive: as the host society is liable for any loss it naturally takes a cautious view on the numbers likely to register when setting up its budget. This has been a regular cause for dissatisfaction, particularly from those priced out of attendance. In an attempt to ameliorate this, organisers have developed aid programmes, appealing to more-affluent societies to donate basic fellowships covering registration and student-type accommodation. The WFSA has always set its face against subsidising registrants: apart from the impossibility of fairly selecting the lucky few, the effect is to reduce the congress surplus. As the Federation's share is devoted to educational activities that benefit many more people than the few free attendees, the overall effect of subsidising registrations is perverse. This stance was significantly weakened in 2000 when it was decided to contribute to a fund set up by the host (Canadian) society for this purpose.

As well as the increase in size, there has been an unwelcome evolution in the attitude of speakers. In 1980 any expert would have naturally regarded an invitation to speak at a World Congress as a great honour. In 2002 there were invited speakers who refused to speak unless free registration was offered: there were those who required accommodation, those who expected travel costs to be met, and even one who wanted first-class air travel!

Regions, Regional Sections, and regional congresses

Regions and Regional Sections are often confused. The constitution of WFSA defines six regions solely for the purpose of ensuring an equitable representation of all parts of the world on key committees. The list perpetuates some historic anomalies: Israel is listed as part of "Europe", while Lebanon and Jordan are in "Africa and the Middle East", which also includes South Africa.

The first Regional Section (European) was set up in 1962 by a local initiative to provide a major congress 4-yearly, interspersed between the World Congresses and followed WFSA geographical grouping. However, the next, the Asian-Australasian Regional Section (AARS), also set up by local initiative in 1962 for the same purpose, combined the countries of two WFSA regions. The third, the African Regional Section (ARS), did the reverse, being based on only part of the Africa and Middle East region. It is these Regional Sections that organise the regional congresses and are therefore not constitutionally actually anything to do with WFSA, except for the fact that they "trade" on the logo. They also get some support from the practice of the Executive Committee holding its mid-term meeting at one of the regional congresses, providing quite a few potentially low-cost, high-value speakers. The Confederation of Latin American Societies of Anaesthesiology (CLASA), another pre-existing independent grouping, and the AARS have continued to hold their congresses throughout the review period. The European Regional Section became embroiled in the competition between the European Society of Anaesthesiologists (ESA) and the European Academy of Anaesthesiology (EAA) and derogated from being a WFSA Regional Section to a become a fully independent Confederation of European National Societies of Anaesthesia (CENSA) and a partner in the new European Federation of Anaesthesiologists. The Regional Section for Africa (ARS) was formed (in 1997) and has since held its first post-formation congress.

The WFSA has always encouraged the Regional Sections, and three have modelled their constitutions on it. The AARS donated U.S. $ 7,500 towards the cost of the *Paediatric Handbook* from its surplus from their meeting in 1988, partly in response to the decision by the host society (Hong Kong) to devote most of the surplus to founding a College of Anaesthetists of Hong Kong. This produced a general feeling that WFSA educational funds should gain some benefit from regional surpluses, once the legitimate needs of the host society and the Regional Section had been met. It is a matter of regret that a formal agreement on surplus sharing has not been achieved, despite lengthy negotiations.

World Health Organisation

WFSA has long been a body officially recognised as a non-governmental organisation (NGO) "in relation" to the World Health Organisation (WHO). However, the relationship was in desuetude until resuscitated by Zorab in 1984. A series of meetings led to a request for WFSA to provide expert input on anaesthetic agents and adjuvants for a WHO list of "essential drugs" and a decision to prepare a basic manual on anaesthesia. Dobson was asked to be author of the resulting book - *Anaesthesia at the District Hospital* - which was published by WHO in 1988. It was subsequently translated into French, Spanish, Portuguese, Russian, Arabic, and Indonesian.

An obvious topic for further joint efforts related to the problem of oxygen supplies in rural Africa and other developing countries. Oxygen concentrators were an obvious potential solution. However, most concentrators then available had been developed for domestic use in western countries, and no information was available about whether they would be suitable for use in anaesthesia in the tropics. WHO was responsive to the idea of jointly developing a performance standard and delegated the task to WFSA. A 2-day workshop was organised in London in 1989 and a performance standard was produced. Based on this, WHO subsequently produced a specification of the characteristics required for an oxygen concentrator for use in developing countries. Despite initial problems, a number of very effective and successful machines were subsequently developed. Dobson was involved in the field testing of 30 machines.

The officers wisely saw that Dobson's effectiveness within WHO might be enhanced by granting him some official title, and the Executive Committee agreed in 1991 to his being described as the Special WFSA Liaison Officer with WHO, a title he still retains. This bore fruit in several ways. The "umbrella" of WFSA was used to advise WHO on the production of "*The Clinical Use of Blood*," a handbook for clinicians aiming to improve the availability and safety of blood supplies in developing countries. WHO published a second edition of "*Anaesthesia at the District Hospital*" in 1998 and discussion arising from this led to the amalgamation of the two handbooks under the title "*Surgical Care at the District Hospital*", which will be published shortly. This also incorporates the primary trauma care (PTC) manual, thus effectively adopting PTC as the WHO recommended method for the care of severely injured patients.

This liaison has proved very helpful in negotiations with the United Kingdom Department for International Development who have funded two projects. One was the cost of making distance learning materials and testing them in Zimbabwe, mostly from *Update in Anaesthesia* (again led by Dobson), whilst also making a contribution to its publication, translation, and distribution costs. The second was the purchase and field trial in Mozambique of 30 "Glostavents", designed by the late Roger Manley with the needs of the developing world in mind. Our standing as a partner of WHO with a proven track record should provide more opportunities to work for the good of anaesthesia services in developing countries. (Dr. Dobson's chapter covers the relationship with WHO in more detail).

Facilitation

WFSA officers need to be adept at spotting good ideas originating outside the organisation where the Federation can materially assist. Examples have already been touched on: the initial support for *Update in Anaesthesia*, supporting Scherpereel with cash to extend teaching in French-speaking Africa, and supporting the New Zealand and Australian societies in their work in the Pacific Islands. Some others come to mind over this period.

Task force on safety

This was an independent group of experts from many countries, brought together by Communicore and funded by industry. They made contact when their work was nearly completed, wanting some authoritative endorsement for their recommendations and wide publicity. They had completed a task that WFSA could (perhaps should) have undertaken and their recommendations were quite consonant with the Federation's stance. Accordingly, it was possible to arrange for them to have a special symposium at the 10th World Congress, endorse their recommendations, and arrange for their publication in *The European Journal of Anaesthesiology*.

Primary trauma care

Trauma is not only a major cause of disability in the developing world, it has devastating economic consequences for those affected and their extended families. Basing their ideas on the widely accepted model of cardiopulmonary resuscitation training, Haydn Perndt (then chairman of the Education Committee) and Dobson encouraged Dr. Douglas Wilkinson (Oxford, UK) and Marcus Skinner (Australia) to develop a PTC course specifically tailored for use in developing countries. The WFSA Education Committee funded the first courses, which started in Fiji in 1997, followed by Uganda, Nigeria, Nepal, and India. The Australian government added its support for work in the Pacific and Michael Rosen (Cardiff, UK) obtained funds from British Petroleum to mount the course in Vietnam. It has developed in 17 countries in four continents and has been incorporated into the forthcoming WHO handbook *"Surgical Care at the District Hospital"*.

Translation copyright purchases

When Eastern Europe was opened up, there was a great need for modern textbooks in Russian, but local publishers could neither afford the cost of translation nor the copyright to publish such translations. Officers or committee members have been able to find volunteer translators and WFSA has negotiated to buy the rights to two major British textbooks and donated them to a Russian publisher.

Joint training fellowships in pain

Rosen used the leverage of the treasurership to extend the idea behind the Eastern European fellowships to persuade the (UK) Pain Society and the German Society of Anaesthesiology and Intensive Care to contribute to a fund obtained by him from the Soros Foundation to bring Eastern European anaesthesiologists to Germany or the United Kingdom for training in pain management.

Office administration

John Bonica (secretary 1972-1980) carried out the secretarial work within his university department. Zorab had no department and it was agreed that the WFSA should employ his wife part-time. Subsequent honorary secretaries (and treasurers) all employed part-time secretarial help.

The need to develop a permanent office increasingly became a matter for discussion. There were contrasting views on this. Unless the secretary and the treasurer were both located fairly close to the office-and this was not the sort of coincidence that had ever occurred - the other would still need secretarial support. Whose need was greatest? Also, there seemed to be no basis for deciding the best place to locate the office and wherever it was, it would eventually be inevitable that there would be no officer living close to it. On the other hand, the electronic revolution was under way and the "paperless" office was being predicted. It seemed likely that before long it would be immaterial as to where such an office was physically located: it could be a cyber-office, accessible to all. If that proved to be true, then it really became a question of where was most likely to be most convenient. It really came down to a choice between New York, where the New York Society of Anesthesiologists offered to find space in their premises, and London, where unofficial "feelers" suggested that the newly formed Royal College of Anaesthetists (RCOA) might be willing to provide space.

In 1992 the General Assembly gave the officers authority to set up a permanent office. Contrary to all previous experience, both the secretary and the treasurer were actually working, not only in the same country, but in the same university department. Under Ament the Federation had American-based auditors and financial advisers and because of the tax-free status in the United States, and the fact that the dues were calculated and paid in dollars, Rosen the new treasurer decided to keep these. However, for many practical reasons, a sterling account was needed and so both dollar and sterling accounts in the United Kingdom, as well as the dollar investment account in the United States, were in use. This alone expanded the bookkeeping role, but the expansion of the whole field of publications and the increase in activity of the Education Committee progressively expanded the secretarial work as well.

The current treasurer and secretary (Rosen and Vickers) were the obvious officers to decide on the needs for space, staff, and overall budget. Furthermore, if it were to be set up within the next 6-8 years, they were very well placed to get it up and running if it were in the United Kingdom. There were two deciding factors: the first was that Zorab, now in charge of the running the European Diploma in Anaesthesiology (EDA), was also needing to find premises and staff. Not only might it be possible to share space, but John West, his intended part-time administrator, could also work part-time for the WFSA. Secondly, we estimated that WFSA's share of the expenses would be the same or less than we were already spending. Everyone, it seemed, would be a winner.

Thus it came about that in 1995 the WFSA and the EDA jointly rented space in the RCOA. To counter some of the initial misgivings we attempted to manage our affairs through the London office without necessarily visiting it. If that could be achieved then subsequent officers would be able to do so too. Accordingly all WFSA files and some past officers' papers were transferred to the new office. It was intended that Mr. West could attend to all WFSA business part-time, 2-3 days per week. However, he soon pressed for some part-time secretarial help.

In 1996, in Sydney, the incoming secretary, Meursing, discovered that the administrative secretary of the Australian Society of Anaesthetists, Ms. Karen McMurchy, was intending to work in London for 2-3 years and she decided to employ her full time as part of the office staff. Despite this unplanned expansion, in the 1st full year of the office (1996) the expenses only rose slightly (about 7%). However, things soon started to go wrong. For a variety of reasons that are not relevant, it became apparent that the joint arrangements were not working well and seemed unlikely to improve. In 1997 it was concluded that WFSA would have to have a separate office with dedicated staff, and the office moved to Imperial House under the administrative direction of Ms. McMurchy.

Because of the need to satisfy the United States tax authorities, the American auditors required accounts for which a part-time bookkeeper was necessary. Because the Honorary Secretary was now much more remote in Malawi, a very comprehensive system of recording all inward and outward correspondence, fax, e-mails, and telephone calls was set up, which generated a lot of secretarial work, initially coped with by extra temporary staff. As the Montreal Congress approached, the "temporary" secretarial help came to be almost full time. Most unfortunately this second secretary resigned at this point. Ms. McMurchy fell ill on return from the Congress and was advised to change to a less-stressful job. Suddenly, there was only a part-time bookkeeper in the office. A very expensive time ensued trying to induct locums and then a new administrator who turned out to be quite unsuitable and had to be dismissed after only 4 months. Her replacement, Mrs. Ruth Hooper, however, was a trained bookkeeper. Drawing on the experience of previous officers, she and the secretary were able to streamline the work so that she could manage the office single-handedly.

This experience showed that it is possible to do much of the work electronically. The financial control and management generates the bulk of the routine work, but the preparation of the annual report and meeting papers (particularly preceding and following the World Congress) necessitates extra secretarial help at times of peak activity.

Constitution

The original constitution of the WFSA was time limited and legally needed to be replaced after 30 years. On the advice of Dr. Rick Siker (Pittsburg, USA) chairman of the Executive Committee, the Statutes and Bylaws Committee worked on the basis that the constitution was working satisfactorily and that minimal changes should be made, merely correcting a few problems that were already apparent. There were two such matters. Rules of procedure for the General Assembly were brought in, which could be adopted or amended at the start of the first meeting. These made provision for any contentious or unprepared matter to be referred to an ad hoc Reference Committee. This has certainly ensured that these potentially difficult meetings could be handled more smoothly.

The second major change has, I believe, been unhelpful. There was a feeling that there was a "democratic deficit" in that the Executive Committee was solely responsible for nominating the members of the ad hoc Nominations Committee at the World Congress which, in turn, nominated members for the vacant places on the Executive Committee. This was felt to be altogether too cosy. To break this cycle a postal ballot was introduced for membership of the Nominations Committee. The Executive Committee nominates 10 (recently increased to 16) national societies from which all full member societies could ballot for 8. The members of the Nominations Committee were to be one of the delegates from each of the 8 chosen societies plus a chairman nominated by the Executive Committee. According to the bylaws, the delegate was to be selected from the society's delegates (if they were entitled to more than 1) by the Executive Committee.

Whatever the supposed ill effects of the old system, one thing it did ensure was that the Nominations Committee contained mostly delegates who were knowledgeable about Federation affairs. They also tended to have been regular attendees and thus with an international outlook. Under the new system, the Executive Committee has always accepted whoever the society nominated. This was often their current President who might only have been in post for some months and never have attended a World Congress before. The task of nominating half the Executive Committee and the next President of the WFSA has thus been entrusted to a group with a sometimes hazy appreciation of what they were trying to achieve, putting great influence in the hands of its (Executive Committee) appointed chairman.

With this change another attempt to improve the nomination process has come in. It was always open to societies to nominate for membership of the Executive Committee, but nominations were very rarely made. The old Nominations Committee never lacked for ideas, but with a less-expert group it was felt that they needed more information and so nominations have been actively canvassed by the secretary. This has involved societies in submitting full curricula vitae plus photographs plus covering citation and statement of willingness to serve, on behalf of numbers of delegates who might have no realistic chance of being selected. Copies have to be made for all members of the Relevant Committee. It has become a major administrative burden.

The exercise has perhaps been of more value when it comes to the newly elected Executive Committee's task of filling vacancies on the various other committees, but it has also had an ossifying effect. The constitution distinguishes between Standing Committees, whose functions are always going to be needed, and Special Committees that are intended for transient functions and purposes. Despite strenuous efforts by successive chairmen of the Executive Committee, some Special Committees have never proved their value. Asking for nominations to a potentially Defunct Committee merely serves to perpetuate it. In the whole period covered by this review, although a few committees changed their function, no Special Committee was ever wound up, even if it had achieved nothing in the preceding 4 years and the outgoing chairman advised winding it up.

Electronic communication

This rapidly changing field has had a considerable impact on WFSA, in the attitude to meetings, committee communications, and office practices.

Meetings
In 1990, the officers started to utilise the opportunity presented when at least two of them were going to be independently funded to attend some event, to arrange a meeting of officers. These meetings developed into an annual meeting of officers from 1991 onwards. However, electronic advances have now made it quite easy to conduct telephone conferences between the officers, which enable them to reach a consensus more quickly than waiting for an annual meeting. Further technical advances look set to render this facility more useful, for example, video conferencing by mobile phone is just around the corner.

Committee communications
The Executive Committee only meets every 2 years. Siker introduced sequentially numbered "round robins" to all members, which usually enclosed a return form asking for an opinion or a decision, or both. However, the system depended on international postal services, and those in some countries are, to say the least, unreliable. Unfortunately, so were some members of the Executive Committee. The advent of e-mail has speeded up the response time, improved the response rate, and vastly reduced the cost of communicating regularly. All the officers and Major Committee chairman now conduct most of their business by e-mail, with great saving in cost and improvement in efficiency.

Communicating with societies
2002 saw the first use of e-mail as an alternative to conventional printing and posting for communication with member societies by way of the annual report of the secretary. This is in flux, as about half the societies do not have the means to accept, download, and print bulky e-mail attachments. The electronic dissemination and return of the annual survey and request for dues must surely follow.

Web site

The compilation of the annual report, never mind the cost of printing and distributing, is a major staff expense, and yet the information is never fully up-to-date, with constant changes in the composition of member societies. Paradoxically, some information only changes every 4th year. What is clearly needed and is under active development is a properly designed and maintained web site to carry, amongst other things, much of this information. Relatively little would then need to be posted annually to member societies.

Office practices

Far from reducing the use of paper, e-mail initially led to an increase, as the office felt the need to print hard copy for record purposes. Routines for sorting out what can safely be discarded are urgently needed. Whilst regular electronic back-up allows one to rely on this for archiving, the "filing" presents novel problems and encourages retention of paper copies of what is often only of transient interest.

Archives

The above leads on to consideration of archiving. Successive Presidents and other officers left their papers to their successors and by the time Zorab took office as secretary, it was obvious that this was unsatisfactory. There was often duplication of material, conflicting filing systems, and retention of a lot of correspondence with no permanent value. In 1986, Zorab reported to the Executive Committee that storage space was going to be available in the new headquarters of the AAGBI and in 1988 he appealed for relevant material. This arrangement did not materialise and in 1990 he arranged for the Wood Library Museum to become the official repository of WFSA archives for a relatively modest payment.

That, however, did not resolve the problem of what to keep in the archives. Vickers attempted to tackle this by drafting guidance to future incoming officers as to what to keep. This, however, got swallowed up in the parallel decision to appoint an honorary archivist (Joseph Rupreht, Rotterdam, The Netherlands), who also made proposals. Both were considered at the Executive Committee meeting in 1996 and, in time-honoured fashion, referred to a working party. There is no evidence that this ever did any work: no report or recommendations emerged and this omission was overlooked in subsequent meetings of the Executive Committee. One major unresolved problem was that whilst the intention was excellent, the necessary financial under-pinning was ignored. The archivist needed to visit the site of the papers before transfer, have them sent to him and have their onward transfer funded, or be funded to visit the Wood Library regularly. None of these options was delineated or officially recognised for funding. Not surprisingly, not a lot was done, despite the archivist's willingness.

Ignoring these "problems" was facilitated by the development of the office. Unlike the situation when the need for an archive site was conceived, WFSA now had a logical permanent place in which to house archive material. In consequence, a parallel archive has developed in the office - indeed has recently replaced the Wood Library for recent material. This is an important matter requiring some clear thinking to define what is appropriate for each location and what, if anything, needs to be duplicated in both.

Conclusion

The last 20 years have been an exciting time in which to have the opportunity to work for the good of the world community in anaesthesia. Rising income has allowed activities to be started or expanded by WFSA to a considerable extent. One can, at last, see some improvement as a result of the Federation's efforts, and at the same time a clearer picture of how much more needs to be done. The efforts of the developing world to catch up with the developed world's systems are frustrated by the constantly increasing sophistication that the developed world employs. The gap between the two, if anything, grows rather than shrinks.

The structure of the organisation has struggled to cope with the changes imposed by the increased and more varied activities: the need to ensure greater continuity, the separation of charity funds and business funds, more-realistic budgeting and more monitoring of expenditure between the 4-yearly general assemblies, all seem to the writer to have lagged behind the enthusiastic expansion of "front-line" activities. I have no doubt of the capacity of the current generation of officers to get a grip on these.

Reference sources

WFSA newsletters, General Assembly minutes, Executive Committee minutes, and Standing Committee files.

9 WFSA AND THE WORLD HEALTH ORGANISATION

M. Dobson

*W*FSA had for some time been collaborating with the World Health Organisation (WHO) when in 1982 a request came to John Zorab from WHO Pharmaceuticals to comment on possible inclusions of anaesthetic drugs in the WHO list of essential drugs. John realised that it would be much more helpful to give advice not only on the drugs but on the ways in which they should be used - with implications for both equipment and the training of users. It was clear from the beginning that this would be an initiative aimed towards anaesthetists in developing countries - colleagues in the west already benefit from strong professional associations with associated educational opportunities, and do not look to WHO for guidance on clinical issues. In consequence, WHO convened a meeting in 1984 to discuss anaesthesia, at which WFSA was represented by John Zorab, Patricia Coyle, Say Wan Lim, Howard Zauder, and Mike Dobson. As a result of this and similar meetings, WHO decided to prepare manuals on anaesthesia and surgery at district hospitals. Mike Dobson was asked to be author of the anaesthesia manual and prepared a draft that was approved by the same group. Publication of the book *(Anaesthesia at the District Hospital)* was financed by WHO and it appeared in 1988 in time for the World Congress in Washington; its publication was shortly followed by companion manuals, the first covering general surgery and the second obstetrics and traumatology. The anaesthesia manual proved to be popular and helpful, and was subsequently translated into French, Spanish, Portuguese, Russian, Arabic, and Indonesian. Because of our experience in working on the anaesthetic manual, WFSA was also invited to contribute to the surgical manuals.

Largely as a result of the good contacts thus developed, WHO was responsive to our suggestion in 1989 that we work on a joint performance standard for oxygen concentrators. WFSA was aware of the poor availability of medical oxygen in many district hospitals in the world, and the potential of oxygen concentrators to supply some of these hospitals in a reliable and economic way. Most concentrators then available had been developed for domestic use in western countries, and no information was available about whether they would be suitable for use in the rigorous circumstances of the tropics. A joint performance standard was therefore produced, and because this involved consultations with the manufacturers, WHO delegated the job to WFSA. A workshop took place in London in 1989, attended by anaesthetists with relevant experience, independent technical experts, and representatives from manufacturers. Within 2 days they produced a specification of the characteristics required of a concentrator for use in developing countries. These specifications were incorporated by WHO into a performance standard, with supervised testing. As a result a number of concentrators were submitted by manufacturers; all of these failed the performance tests but as a result of their failure a number were subsequently improved and modified by the manufacturers to produce what have been shown to be very effective and successful machines. In addition to the laboratory testing described, WHO also helped to organise and finance a field testing project in which 30 concentrators were installed in small hospitals in Upper Egypt, and their use and performance closely monitored. The machines selected proved to be very successful in use and the project was subsequently the subject of a publication in *The Lancet*.

WFSA has for many years been sponsoring refresher courses in developing countries, the majority of these in Africa, and it was following a refresher course in Tanzania in 1995 that Dobson and Wilkinson began to develop the concept of primary trauma care (PTC). This is a system of management of patients suffering from severe trauma of which there is an epidemic in the developing world. PTC differs from other trauma management systems in that it is simplified and capable of being adapted to local situations. A proposal was made to further develop PTC in conjunction with WHO, but no response from WHO followed and PTC was therefore developed independently in subsequent years, with considerable support from WFSA and other professional groups such as the Australian Society of Anaesthetists, the Royal College of Anaesthetists, and the Association of Anaesthetists of Great Britain and Ireland.

Also in 1995 WFSA was invited by the Assistant Director General (Dr. Antesana) to participate in a formal review of the overall programme for health technology of WHO. As a result of this review a number of changes were made in WHO structures and Dr. John Emmanuel was appointed as Head of Blood Safety and Clinical Technology. With the AIDS epidemic in full flow, the availability of safe blood became an extremely important issue in which WHO and WFSA had shared concerns, and a number of anaesthetists worked under the WFSA umbrella with WHO on the production between 1997 and 2000 of *The Clinical Use of Blood* (Richard Page, Anthony Chisakuta, Laurie Marks, Henry Bukwirwa, Mike Dobson, Dixon Tembo, Paul Fenton, and Meena Cherian). *The Clinical Use of Blood* is a detailed handbook for clinicians aimed at improving the availability and safety of blood supplies in developing countries throughout the world. It was launched in India at a joint meeting of the Indian Society of Anaesthetists and WHO early in 2001, and a further launch in Africa took place in Durban in September of the same year.

The second edition of *Anaesthesia in the District Hospital* had been published by WHO in 1998, incorporating a number of changes from the original, and this time WHO also wished to review the surgical manuals that had been produced in the past in association with it. An editorial group was therefore established containing a number of anaesthetists, including Mike Dobson, Paul Fenton, and Douglas Wilkinson, as well as representatives of surgical disciplines. A revised manual covering both anaesthesia and surgery has now been produced under the title *Surgical Care at the District Hospital* and this will be published later in 2003. During the preparation process it became clear that in order to assist in the management of trauma at district hospitals it would be appropriate to incorporate the PTC manual within this document, thus effectively adopting PTC as the WHO recommended method for the care of severely injured patients.

WHO has also given moral support to proposals WFSA has made for joint projects with other groups, most especially the United Kingdom Department for International Development (DfID) in 1997. It became clear from an informal conversation that DfID might support a WFSA project, and subsequently a joint project was developed that received moral (but not financial) support from WHO. The support of WHO was very important in persuading DfID to provide the funding needed. The projects aimed to increase the availability of safe anaesthesia in Africa; the first by creating a set of distance learning materials, developing existing educational materials derived from *Update in Anaesthesia* and making these the core of a learning system that would then be available for use in other developing countries. The Distance Learning Project has been hampered by the appalling political and economic situation in Zimbabwe that developed after the project started, but a great deal of progress has been made and a draft set of materials is now within our grasp.

The second project was set up to introduce and study the use of a lung ventilator designed specifically by the late Dr. Roger Manley to meet the needs of developing countries. Machines were supplied to a umber of countries (the largest number to Mozambique) and the effects of their introduction studied-many valuable lessons have been learned not only about the supply of technology but also about the support required to ensure the availability of spare parts and to train technical staff and clinical users in safe use of the equipment.

Most of the liaison work since 1984 has been organised through Mike Dobson, who in 1991 was granted the official title of WFSA Liaison Officer with WHO, a title I still retain. The amount of liaison activity has increased, and in 2000 at the Executive Meeting in Durban the Committee agreed to appoint Professor Mohammed Ben Ammar as Assistant Liaison Officer. Currently we have active contact with a large number of WHO departments including Blood Safety and Clinical Technology, Integrated Management of Childhood Illnesses, Reproductive Health, Injury Prevention, Pharmaceuticals, and Publications. WHO has also appointed Mike Dobson in a personal capacity to expert panels on Blood Safety, and a new expert panel on District Hospital Services.

Working with WHO can be both rewarding and frustrating. It is always necessary to bear in mind that WHO's overall view relates more to public health and community health than to acute medicine and surgery. Furthermore, WHO is limited by its United Nations' status, in that it can only work through governments and Ministries of Health. This means that we can never regard WHO as a solution to the anaesthetic needs of the world. However, it can at times be an extremely useful tool and has been of inestimable help to WFSA over the last 20 years. Relations of course do vary, and with the appointment in 2003 of a new director general and a new WHO link person for us within the organisation, we will have to wait and see how things develop. Our standing as a partner of WHO with a proven track record will certainly provide further opportunities in the future to work for the good of the specialty and it is our responsibility to help provide safe anaesthesia for all the peoples of the world.

10 HISTORY OF THE WFSA ASIAN AND AUSTRALASIAN REGIONAL SECTION

C.H. Hoskins

In the photo below (Fig. 1), the flag raising ceremony for the 1st Asian and Australasian Congress of Anaesthesiology (AACA), is pictured the New Zealand delegate, Dr. James Church of New Plymouth. It was he who had previously, first stimulated my interest in the practice of anaesthesia during my initial hospital internship. Little did I realise at that time what a profound effect that would have on my own and my family's life. Some 23 years after working with Jim Church I attended the 5th AACA in New Delhi, India as President of the New Zealand Society of Anaesthetists. This began an 18-year association with the Asian and Australasian Regional Section (AARS) and the WFSA. In that time not only was I privileged to work with highly motivated colleagues but also established life-long friendships throughout the world. As a tribute to these associations it is my pleasure to present the history of AARS of the WFSA.

In 1960, during the 2nd World Congress of Anaesthesiologists in Toronto, Canada, the Executive Committee of the WFSA agreed to promote regional

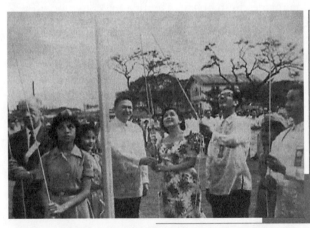

Fig. 1. *Flag raising ceremony of the 1st AACA, WHO grounds, Manila, 6 November 1962. From the left: James Church (New Zealand); two staff members; Emmanuel Pelaez, Vice-President of the Philippines; Betty Gomez (the Philippines): Quintin Gomez (the Philippines); a staff member; Cenon Cruz (the Philippines) (by courtesy of Florian Nuevo)*

congresses to be staged in between the World Congresses. This would enable those who could not attend the world meetings to discuss their mutual problems, exchange scientific information, and promote the objectives of the WFSA.

Accordingly, the 1st AACA was held in Manila, Philippines, on 6-10 November 1962 (Fig. 2). Records of this historic occasion show that nine countries of the region were represented: Australia (7 delegates), Hong Kong (2), India (1), Japan (5), Malaya (7), New Zealand (1), Philippines (144), Republic of China (2), and Thailand (2). Dr Geoffrey Organe (secretary/treasurer, WFSA) and Dr. Francis Foldes (vice-President, WFSA) were invited guests.

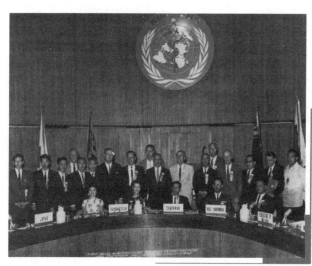

Fig. 2. *House of Delegates - the "First Regional Assembly". First AACA, Manila, 7th November 1962 (by courtesy of Quintin Gomez)*

The first business meeting of this AACA (thus the first regional assembly) was held on 7 November 1962, with Dr. Quintin Gomez (chairman of the congress Organising Committee) in the chair. The first executive board was elected, namely: Dr. Quintin J. Gomez (Philippines) President, Dr. Hideo Yamamura (Japan), Dr. J. McCulloch (Australia), and Dr. Tandan (India) vice-Presidents, and Dr. Luista de Castro (Philippines) Secretary General. Dr. Russell Cole (Australia) was appointed chairman of the membership committee and Dr. Kwong Li Yee (Republic of China) as chairman of the special projects committee. At the subsequent executive board meeting, Dr. Geoffrey Organe spoke of the possibility of an anaesthesia training centre in Asia, similar to those already established in Copenhagen and Vienna. The World Health Organisation could recruit seminar lecturers from overseas and with government aid, the training centre could undertake a broad programme of advanced studies in anaesthesia for all Asian countries. Dr. Francis Foldes concurred with this and proposed that the training centre be in Manila. The board approved this.

Panel discussions on muscle relaxants and spinal anaesthesia, as well as 22 free papers constituted a stimulating scientific programme. However, to indicate that the first AACA was not all work and no play, many social activities were liberally interspersed to enliven the congress and to formulate many ongoing friendships (Fig. 3). Although the number of participants and the number of societies represented were not large, this congress was a significant first step towards the future development of the AARS of the WFSA. The effort and enthusiasm of the Philippine Society of Anaesthesiologists who organised the congress was greatly appreciated.

The Japan Society of Anaesthesiology hosted the 2nd AACA in Tokyo, 1-5 September 1966. On this occasion more than 350 delegates from 19 countries, including the United States, Great Britain, Austria, and Brazil participated in the congress. Dr. G. Organe (President, WFSA), Dr. R. Bennett (vice-President, WFSA), and Dr. O. Mayrhofer (Secretary General, WFSA) attended as honoured guests. Interestingly the registration fees for this congress were delegates U.S. $ 10 and associates U.S. $ 5!!!

At the General Assembly (Fig. 4) the following were elected: Dr. Hideo Yamamura (Japan) President, Dr. Michinosuke Amano (Japan) secretary, and

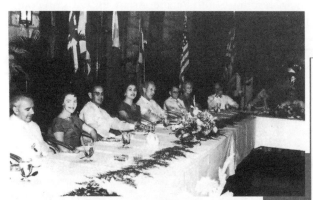

Fig. 3. *Farewell Reception, First AACA, Manila Polo Club, Manila, 10th November 1962 (by courtesy of Quintin Gomez)*

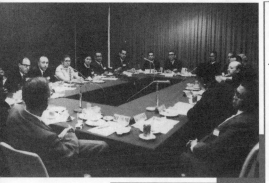

Fig. 4. *General Assembly, Second AACA, Tokyo, Japan, September 1966. From the left: Mayne Smeeton (New Zealand); Martin Isaac; Nancy Butt (Hong Kong); Douglas Joseph (Australia); Patrick Maplestone (Australia); Margaret McLelland (Australia); Luisita de Castro (the Philippines); Joseph Briz (the Philippines); Quintin Gomez (the Philippines); Hideo Yamamura (Japan); Michinosuke Amano (Japan); Akira Inamoto (Japan); Kenichi Iwatsuki (Japan); Otto Mayrhofer, WFSA Secretary; Geoffrey Organe (UK); Roger Bennett (UK); Dong Shik Rhee; Peter Lee (ROC) (by courtesy of Hideo Yamamura)*

Dr. Yukata Inada (Japan) treasurer. Dr. Gomez (previous President, Philippines), together with the delegates of the Japan Society of Anaesthesiology, proposed the establishment of an Asian and Australasian Federation of Societies of Anaesthesiologists. A committee was formed to proceed with this matter and the objective of the establishment of the Regional Section by 1970. Dr. Gomez, Dr. Bennett (vice-President of WFSA, Australia), Dr. Lee (Republic of China), and Dr. Yamamura (Japan) were elected to this committee. Also on the agenda was the idea of an anaesthesia training centre. This was unanimously supported and further implementation was left to the above committee.

The increase in the number of participants and the represented societies indicated a bright future for the Asian and Australasian region of the WFSA. In all, 48 free papers were presented during the scientific sessions as well as two panel discussions: (1) Present status of anaesthesiologists in Asian and Australasian countries and (2) Anaesthesia for poor-risk patients.

Following the congress, a post-congress meeting was held in Kyoto on 7-8 September. The majority of members participated in this event (Fig. 5).

The 3rd AACA, hosted by the Australian Society of Anaesthetists, was held in Canberra, Australia, 19-23 September 1970. On this occasion there were more than 700 participants representing 12 of the societies of the region, as well as delegates from neighbouring South Pacific, Asian, and African countries. There were 11 other countries, including Great Britain and the United States. Dr. Francis F. Foldes (President, WFSA), Dr O. Mayrhofer (Secretary General, WFSA), and Dr. H. Poulsen (chairman, Executive Committee, WFSA) were among the invited guests.

At the meeting of delegates, Dr. Douglas Joseph of Australia was elected as President of the congress. The members of the executive board were elected as follows: chairman Dr. Douglas Joseph (Australia), vice-chairmen Dr. Kenichi Iwatsuki (Japan), Dr. George Tay (Singapore), secretary Dr. Pritam Singh (India), and treasurer Dr. Quintin J. Gomez (Philippines). Representative of the WFSA Executive Committee was Dr. Hideo Yamamura.

During this congress, on 22 September 1970, the Regional Section was for-

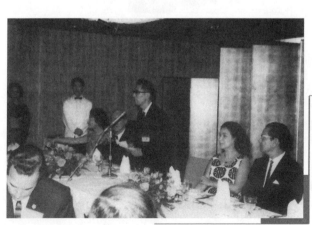

Fig. 5. *Banquet, Second AACA, Tokyo, September 1966 (by courtesy of Hideo Yamamura)*

mally adopted, together with its bylaws. The official name, "The Asian and Australasian Regional Section of the World Federation of Societies of Anaesthesiologists" and its domicile in the country of residence of the secretary were agreed to. In keeping with the World Federation's constituent five regions, the term Regional Section was considered more appropriate. The Asian and Australasian region was defined as embracing Asia, Australia, New Zealand, and the Western and Central Pacific Islands. Membership of the Regional Section was open to national societies and associate members of the WFSA within this region.

Following the report from the Ad Hoc Committee on the anaesthesia training center, it was agreed that such a center based in Manila, Philippines would be established. The scientific sessions consisted of 70 free papers, 14 film presentations, and 6 symposia on: (1) anaesthesia and resuscitation in multiple trauma, (2) endocrinology and anaesthesia, (3) pharmacological complications of anaesthesia, (4) design and safety of anaesthetic apparatus, (5) anaesthesia and analgesia in obstetrics, and (6) anaesthesia in the Asian and Australasian region.

A post-congress meeting, including a scientific session on paediatric anaesthesia and resuscitation, was held in Melbourne on 25-26 September. The Singapore Anaesthetic Society (as then named) also presented a post-congress seminar from 30 September to 2 October.

During the 4th World Congress of Anaesthesiologists in Kyoto, Japan, in 1972, the AARS held an assembly. Eleven countries attended, namely Australia, Hong Kong, India, Japan, Korea, Malaysia, New Zealand, Philippines, Republic of China, Singapore, and Thailand. At this assembly Dr. Gomez presented a report on the anaesthesiology training centre, Western Pacific, Manila. Dr. Singh proposed a sub-committee to investigate the feasibility and funding of an exchange programme for anaesthetists.

The 4th AACA was held in Singapore on 22-26 September 1974. Twenty-four countries were represented, 14 being from the Asian and Australasian region. There were about 700 participants. The WFSA President, Dr. O. Mayrhofer addressed the Opening Ceremony as an honoured guest. At the regional assembly, Dr. George Tay was unanimously elected as President of the 4th Congress. The following were elected as members of the executive board: chairman Dr. Hideo Yamamura (Japan), vice-chairmen Dr. Kenichi Iwatsuki (Japan), Dr. George Tay (Singapore), secretary Dr. Pritam Singh (India), and treasurer Dr. Thelma S. Tomelden (Philippines). Representatives of the WFSA Executive Committee included Dr. Quintin J. Gomez (Philippines) and Dr. Douglas Joseph (Australia).

The minutes of the regional assembly of the AARS held in Kyoto in1972 were adopted. Dues of members were increased from U.S. 20 cents to U.S. 25 cents. By vote, the site for the next congress was agreed to be New Delhi, India. At the scientific session 185 papers were presented together with 7 symposia on: (1) training in anaesthesia in the Asian and Australasian Region, (2) dental anaesthesia, (3) new techniques, (4) new drugs, (5) respiratory failure and its management, (6) organ transplantation, (7) acupuncture anaesthesia. Approximately 250 participants attended the post-congress meeting organised by the Malaysian Society of Anaesthesiologists in Kuala Lumpur, Malaysia on 27-29 September. This was followed by a similar meeting in Jakarta, Indonesia on 30 September to 5 October. All these meetings greatly contributed to the mutual understanding of member societies.

The 5th AACA was held in New Delhi, India on 23-27 September 1978. About 800 delegates and 400 accompanying persons attended the congress, which was inaugurated at a colourful ceremony by the President of India, His Excellency, Shri N. Sanjiva Reddy.

Delegates from 10 societies as well as Dr. Quintin J. Gomez (President, WFSA) attended the regional assembly. At the assembly Dr. Pritam Singh was unanimously elected President of the 5th Asian and Australasian regional congress. Members of the board were elected as follows: chairman Dr. Cedric Hoskins (New Zealand), vice-chairmen Dr. Cenon Cruz (Philippines) and Dr. Saywan Lim (Malaysia), secretary Dr. Venkata Rao (India), and treasurer Dr. Masao Miyazaki (Japan) (Fig. 6). Representatives of the WFSA Executive Committee included Dr. Quintin J. Gomez (Philippines) and Dr. Pritam Singh (India). Better communication between the board and member societies was strongly urged at the regional assembly and the secretary was asked to distribute widely the minutes of meetings, etc. By this better communication, it was hoped to actively interest member societies in regional activities and training. Some delegates were outspoken on financial matters and explained that their societies were withholding dues payments until better financial control was evident. It was agreed that the Regional Section should operate its own bank account and that the section would collect the subscriptions.

Dr. Quintin Gomez reported on the WFSA Western Pacific Anaesthesia Training Centre. Points of note were that the sixth annual class would graduate at the end of 1978, that so far, 184 students had graduated, of whom 47 came from countries outside the Philippines, and that faculty staff had come from 12 different countries, with Australia providing the biggest external contribution.

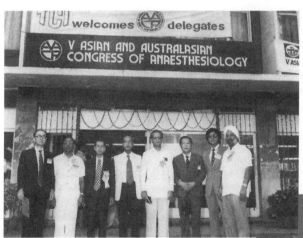

Fig. 6. *AARS Regional Board, Fifth AACA, New Delhi , 24th September 1978. From the left: Masao Miyazaki (Japan); Venkata Rao (India); Hideo Yamamura (Japan); Kenichi Iwatsuki (Japan); Quintin Gomez (the Philippines); George Tay (Singapore); Saywan Lim (Malaysia); Pritam Singh (India) (by courtesy of Cedric Hoskins)*

Scientific sessions were held at The All India Institute of Medical Sciences. Attendance at nearly every session was overwhelming, with some standing in the lecture theatre passageways. There were 250 paper presentations as well as six special lectures, an oration, and symposia on: (1) anaesthesia for developing countries, (2) anaesthesia and clinical pharmacology, (3) shock, (4) closed circuit anaesthesia, (5) anaesthesia for neurosurgery, and (6) monitoring in anaesthesia.

During the 7th World Congress held in Hamburg, West Germany, a meeting of the board of the AARS was held on 18 September 1980. Plans for the next regional congress, to be held in Auckland, were presented by Dr. Tony Newson (New Zealand) and agreed upon. To improve communication between the widely distributed societies of the region it was agreed to institute a Regional Section newsletter. The resignation of Dr. Venkata Rao (India) as secretary was noted and, as a consequence, Dr. Cedric Hoskins (chairman) took over this additional responsibility.

The first AARS newsletter was published in mid 1981. The printing and distribution to member societies was underwritten by the Malaysian Society of Anaesthesiologists. This most-welcome contribution to regional affairs continued for several years.

The 6th AACA was held in Auckland, New Zealand on 18-23 January 1982. There were 410 delegates and 180 associates. They were from 30 countries world wide, including 11 regional member societies and 2 of the South Pacific.

This congress, which was held in excellent summer weather and marked by the festive spirit that prevailed at all social functions, had several notable highlights. It was the first time that a WFSA Executive Committee meeting was held during an AACA. It was the first time an AARS chairman had relinquished his position on home ground and the four stalwarts of the WFSA and the AARS maintained their record of never missing an AACA. Dr. Nancy Butt (Hong Kong), Drs. Kenichi Iwatsuki and Hideo Yamamura (Japan), and Dr. Quintin Gomez (immediate past President, WFSA, Philippines) were all in Auckland at the congress banquet to receive their well-deserved rewards. Drs. Noel Cass and John Marum delighted everyone at the banquet with their duet "in praise of their colleagues in anaesthesia".

The congress was opened by the Queen's representative, His Excellency the Governor General, Sir David Beattie. The scientific programme that followed commenced with a plenary session entitled "Towards rest from pain" co-chaired by the WFSA President, Dr John Bonica and the President of the New Zealand Society of Anaesthetists, Dr. David Wright. There were 111 free papers, as well as symposia on: (1) obstetrical regional anaesthesia, (2) paediatric anaesthesia, (3) the heart and anaesthesia, (4) regional anaesthesia, (5) selected controversies in intensive care, (6) pain control in surgical patients, and (7) the lung and anaesthesia.

Two regional assemblies and three board meetings were held during the congress. These were enhanced by the presence of officers of the WFSA, namely the President, Dr. John Bonica, the secretary, Dr. John Zorab, the

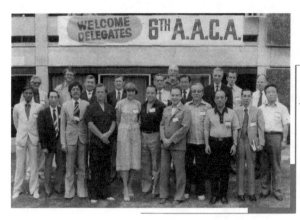

Fig. 7. *Sixth AACA, Auckland, New Zealand, January 1992; AARS Regional Assembly delegates with the WFSA Executive Committee (by courtesy of Cedric Hoskins)*

treasurer, Dr. Carlos Riva, and the chairman of the Executive Committee, Dr. Rick Siker. Dr. David Wright (New Zealand) was unanimously elected President of the 6ᵗʰ AACA. A new board of the AARS was elected with officers as: chairman Dr. Saywan Lim (Malaysia), vice-chairmen Dr. Cenon Cruz (Philippines) and Dr. Nubuo Nishimura (Japan), treasurer Dr. Masao Miyazaki (Japan), secretary Dr. Cedric Hoskins (New Zealand), and representative on the WFSA Executive Committee Dr. Ben Barry (Australia) (Figs. 7,8).

Communication, education, and finance were discussed fully at the business meetings. Under the stewardship of Dr. Miyazaki, not only were the finances in an efficient order, but a strong financial base was being secured to promote regional affairs. Agreement that a proportion of the profit from the AACAs be returned to the Regional Section to maintain this financial base was reached and the probability that future annual capitation fees could be waived was envisaged.

The anaesthetic training centre in Manila was continuing to provided a high standard of training, but it was noted to be less attractive to those from other centres because of their own local training programmes. The Australian and New Zealand Societies of Anaesthetists were promoting local training of anaethetists from the South Pacific Islands.

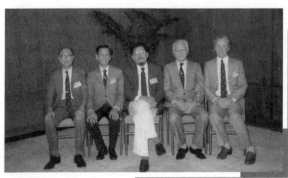

Fig. 8. *AARS Board 1982-1986. Taken in Hong Kong, 23ʳᵈ September 1986 (by courtesy of Cedric Hoskins)*

A logo for the AARS was accepted. This was in two parts, the WFSA logo and a logo to represent the Asian and Pacific Basin. The colour was blue to symbolise the oceans and sky that bound and link our vast region. A similar logo had been used at the 3rd AACA in Canberra. In addition, at that 3rd Congress, the AACA flag was first flown. This flag was designed by Mrs. Roberta Lomaz of Sydney and presented to the region by the Australian Society of Anaesthetists. It has been flown at all subsequent congresses. During the 6th AACA banquet, in keeping with tradition, the flag was handed over to the next host society, the Hong Kong Society of Anaesthetists (Fig. 9).

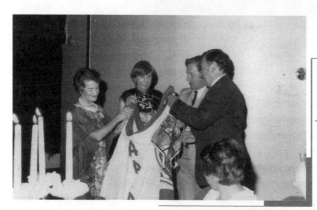

Fig. 9. *Handing over the Congress Flag at the Sixth AACA Congress Banquet, Auckland, January 1982 (by courtesy of Cedric Hoskins)*

Many of the delegates to the 6th AACA proceeded on to Christchurch to attend the General Scientific Meeting of the Faculty of Anaesthetists of the Royal Australasian College of Surgeons.

A meeting of the AARS board was held on 25 January 1984 during the 8th World Congress in Manila. One of the functions of the Regional Section, namely promoting communication, was again emphasised. Continuation of the newsletter and other avenues to encourage the development of anaesthesia and patient care with active participation by all members was confirmed. Whilst there were still some problems with collection of dues from some societies, the finances were in a sound state. Continuation of the annual capitation fee was to be reviewed during the 7th AACA in Hong Kong. Dr. Jean Allison (Hong Kong) reported on progress for this congress. The theme for the congress was to be "New directions in anaesthesia" and it would be held 1 week after the European Congress to enable delegates to attend both. Such an arrangement was to be promoted in the future.

The 7th AACA was held in Hong Kong on 20-25 September 1986. At the inaugural ceremony His Excellency The Governor, Sir Edward Yourde, in officially opening the congress carried out the traditional "eye dotting" of the Lion prior to the Lion Dance to bring good luck and success to the congress (Fig. 10).

Some 670 delegates from 35 countries attended. Of these, 14 were AARS member societies and 2 were from South Pacific Islands. A forerunner of things

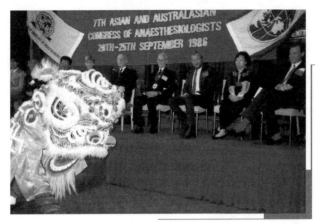

Fig. 10. *Seventh AACA, Hong Kong, 20ᵗʰ September 1986 Opening Ceremony and traditional Lion Dance (by courtesy of Cedric Hoskins)*

to come was the attendance of 19 delegates from the People's Republic of China.

The skills of delegates were revisited by the extensive scientific programme, "New directions in anaesthesia", commencing with 3 PEARLS (personally arranged learning sessions). Then followed 5 plenary sessions, 7 symposia, 4 clinical symposia, 10 computer workshops, 50 poster sessions, 6 videos, plus 3 films together with 270 free papers.

This only briefly indicates the considerable programme provided to enable practitioners to keep abreast with the latest advances in the art and science of anaesthesia and patient care. The social programme was equally extensive and exciting.

So this congress followed and added to the achievements of those previous congresses by advancing knowledge and enabling friendships to flourish by the social interaction of professional people from all over the world, irrespective of their race, creed, or political persuasion.

Two regional assemblies and three board meetings were held. Each was again honoured with the attendance of WFSA officers, Dr. Carlos Parsloe, President, Dr. John Zorab, secretary, and Dr. Richard Ament, treasurer.

Dr. Jean Allison was unanimously elected President of the 7ᵗʰ AACA. To ease matters of protocol, it was decided to change the constitution to allow the congress President to be elected well in advance of the congress.

Following a joint proposal from the Japan Society of Anaesthesiology and the Philippine Society of Anaesthesiologists with relation to the members of the board, the constitution was amended. This amendment increased the board to seven elected members and formalised a previous ad hoc arrangement by including representatives of the AARS, during their term of office on the Executive Committee of the WFSA as ex officio members, without vote. The following officers were subsequently elected: chairman Dr. Il-Yong Kwak (Korea), vice-chairman Dr. Manuel Silao (Philippines), secretary Dr. Robert Hare (Australia), treasurer Dr. Ryo Tanaka (Japan), and board members Dr. Jean Allison (Hong Kong), Dr. Chana Buakham (Thailand), and Dr. K. Vignasan (Malaysia). Representatives of the WFSA Executive Committee included Dr. Cedric Hoskins (New Zealand), Dr. Saywan Lim (Malaysia), and Dr. Nubuo Nishimura (Japan) (Fig. 11).

Minutes of business meetings record the improved state of the finances of the section. With a positive balance of U.S. $ 14,000 and the expected revenue from the 7th AACA (as agreed at the 6th AACA, U.S. $ 10 per registrant), the annual capitation fee on member societies was abolished from 1 January 1987. During discussions on aid to the South Pacific Islands, it was noted that the New Zealand Society of Anaesthetists had extended its membership as associates to anaesthetists from these islands. Therefore, the way was open for the WFSA to grant financial assistance to provide educational aid such as refresher courses and visiting educational teams to these anaesthetists. The need for a technician to be a member of the visiting team was stressed.

The Korean Society of Anaesthesiologists was elected unanimously to host the 8th AACA in 1990 (Fig. 12). To enable a society adequate time to

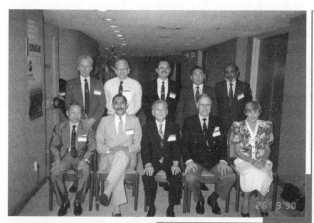

Fig. 11. *AARS board 1986-1990. Taken in Seoul, 26th September 1990. Top row, from the left: Cedric Hoskins (New Zealand); Kester Brown (Australia); Saywan Lim (Malaysia); Chana Buakham (Thailand); K. Vignasan (Malaysia). Bottom row, from the left: Mitsugu Fujimori (Japan); Manuel Silao (the Philippines); Il-Yong Kwak (Korea); Robert Hare (Australia); Jean Allison (Hong Kong) (by courtesy of Robert Hare)*

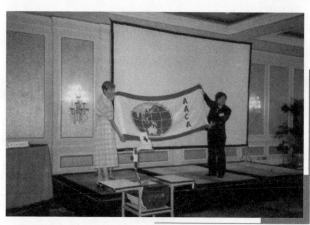

Fig. 12. *Keeping up the tradition of the handing over of the Congress Flag to the next host society, the Korean Society of Anesthesiologists; Hong Kong, 25th September 1986 (by courtesy of Cedric Hoskins)*

prepare for a successful congress it was agreed that this be done for the 9th AACA. Consequent upon this decision, the Thai Society of Anaesthesiologists was elected to host the 9th AACA in 1994. At the regional assemblies of the 6th AACA in Auckland, much discussion had taken place on "Guidelines to be implemented by the host society for an AACA". Before the meeting in Hong Kong these guidelines had been circulated. It was expected that they would greatly assist host societies to stage a congress worthy of anaesthesia in the region, as well as improve the base of funds to be available for regional educational activities, etc. At this regional assembly of the 7th AACA these "guidelines" were approved (Fig. 13).

Following the 7th AACA, a post-congress meeting was held in Beijing, People's Republic of China. This historic event, the Beijing Symposium of Anaesthesiology, 29-30 September 1986, was the first international symposium of anaesthesiology ever held in China. The Chinese Society of Anaesthesiology under the chairmanship of their President, Dr. Shieh Yung, organised the congress in association with the China Association for Science and Technology and assisted by the Hong Kong Society of Anaesthetists. Over 60 delegates and their families from all parts of the world attended, including officers of the WFSA, Dr. Carlos Parsloe, President, Dr. John Zorab, secretary, and Dr. Saywan Lim, chairman, Executive Committee. Mornings were devoted to plenary sessions. In the afternoon visits were paid to the Beijing hospitals and medical schools. This symposium paved the way for the Chinese Society of Anesthesiology to be admitted to the WFSA in 1988 (Fig. 14).

The next meeting of the regional board on 28 May 1988 was in Washington (USA) during the 9th World Congress of Anaesthesiologists. Minutes record the admission of the Chinese Society of Anesthesiologists to the WFSA and to the AARS, and the influential part played by Dr. Peter Tan of the Chinese Taipei Society of Anesthesiology (previously the Society of Anesthesiologists of the Republic of China). Presentation of the final report of the 7th

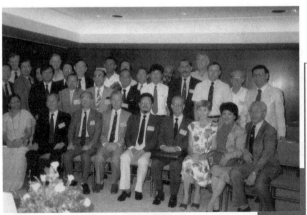

Fig. 13. *Second Regional Assembly delegates, Hong Kong, 23rd September 1986 (by courtesy of Cedric Hoskins)*

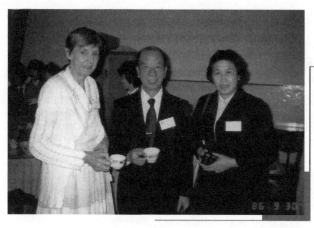

Fig. 14. *First Beijing Symposium of Anaesthesiology, Beijing, 30th September 1986 (by courtesy of Cedric Hoskins)*

AACA included notification that U.S. $ 20,000 from the profit would go to the AARS account. The report on progress for the 8th AACA in Seoul, Korea, with the main theme being "Better understandings in anaesthesia" was agreed upon. As a consequence of previous discussions in Hong Kong, it was agreed to recommend to the next regional assembly, which would be held in Seoul, that the constitution be amended to allow, on the advice of the host society, the election of the President of the next AACA before that AACA. Prospectively, Dr. Hung Kun Oh of the Korean Society of Anesthesiologists was then nominated as President of the 8th AACA. As part of the educational role of the AARS, it was agreed that the sum of U.S. $ 7,500 would be donated to the proposed publication of the WFSA *Manual for Paediatric Anaesthesia*. The Japan Society of Anesthesiology also contributed financially.

At a meeting of the board held during the 6th ASEAN Congress of Anaesthesiology in Manila on 9 November 1989, Dr. Kwang Woo Kim (Korea, chairman Organising Committee) and Dr. Robert Hare (Australia, AARS board secretary) reported on the excellent progress towards the 8th AACA. The document "Guidelines to be implemented by the host society for the AACA" was discussed, with general agreement that some of the profit be used by the AARS/WFSA for education. However, the means of implementing this was subject to much discussion. Consequently, acceptance of the document in its original form was deferred for further study. The role of the AARS in the WFSA was also broadly considered. One responsibility was the 4-yearly AACAs. However, it was recognised that a more-important and ongoing function was the dissemination of scientific information and promotion of education. Following the suggestion of Dr. Kester Brown (Australia, chairman, WFSA Committee on Education), it was agreed that WFSA Standing Committee members, resident in the AARS, should discuss with their societies ways and means to use AARS funds to the best advantage in their area. It was accepted that this ongoing challenge be again considered during the next AACA in Seoul September 1990. The Australian and New Zealand societies have continued to provide a wide range of aid to anaesthetists of the South Pacific region. Most important has been the contribution of technical help in the servicing and repair of equipment. The secretary, Dr. Robert Hare (Australia), outlined his proposed visit and teaching courses in Hanoi. As planned, this visit took place from 6 to 10 December 1989. Dr. Hare took with him an overhead projector and a photocopier that were presented to the anaesthesists at the Viet Duc Hospital by the AARS. Dr. Hare delivered several lectures and "round-table" discussions that were attended by some 50 anaesthetists and nurse anaesthetists, some of whom had travelled up to 300 km or more from their provincial hospitals. These were translated into Vietnamese by Dr. Khoa and the Director of Anaesthesia, Dr. Ton Duc Lang. Overall this initial visit was considered to be most successful and Dr. Lang requested closer association with the AARS and further aid in the form of textbooks, journals, and teaching. For Dr. Hare the most-striking impression was the very high standard of anaesthesia practised under the most-basic conditions.

The 8ᵗʰ AACA was held in Seoul, Korea on 23-28 September 1990 (Fig. 15). The election of Dr. Hung Kun Oh of the Korean Society of Anaesthesiologists as President of the congress was ratified at the first regional assembly; 1,350 delegates and accompanying persons, of whom 650 were from "off shore" attended this vibrant congress. In keeping with the founding principals of the WFSA, anaesthetists from Bangledesh, China, Nepal, Papua New Guinea, Sri Lanka, and Vietnam were invited and funded by the Organising Committee.

Three AARS board meetings were held in Seoul. In delivering the chairman's report, Dr. Il-Yong Kwak sadly noted the deaths of the treasurer of the board, Dr. Ryo Tanaka (Japan), and a former chairman, Dr. Douglas Joseph (Australia). The death of Dr. Nancy Butt (Hong Kong) was also recorded. Following discussions on the use of the considerable funds available to the AARS, it was resolved that these be apportioned over the next 2 years for books and travelling scholarships. Consequent upon the worthwhile visit of Dr. Hare to Vietnam in 1998 and a proposal by the chairman of the WFSA Education Committee, Dr. Kester Brown (Australia) it was recommended that a

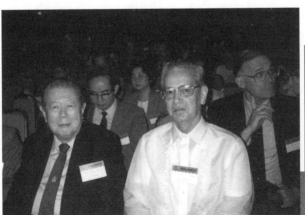

Fig. 15. *Opening Ceremony, 8ᵗʰ AACA, Seoul, September 1990 (by courtesy of Robert Hare)*

refresher course be held in Vietnam with teachers from Thailand. Dr. Chana Buakham (Thailand) welcomed his society's involvement. The suggestion that anaesthetists from surrounding countries, i.e., Laos and Cambodia, should be invited to attend was accepted. The secretary, Dr. Hare reported on his discussions with Dr. Halpern (Davis University, California) concerning the availability of a considerable quantity of textbooks. Dr. Halpern would arrange for these to be transported to a seaport, for the AARS to then distribute them to selected countries in the AARS. A report was presented concerning a planned workshop for a group of South Asian societies (Bangledesh, India, Nepal, and Pakistan) to be held in 1991. Reference was made to the publication of the 1st edition of the *"History of the AARS"*. This had been funded by the ARRS and was written by Dr. Cedric Hoskins (New Zealand). This history would be distributed to all at the congress, as well as WFSA societies, the WFSA executive, and the Wood Library/Museum of Anesthesiology in Washington.

Two regional assemblies were held in Seoul. Here agreement was reached that congress profits more than U.S. $ 20,000 be split between the WFSA and the host society. It was emphasised that this was to enable the WFSA to fulfill the aim of aiding needy societies in terms of education and training. New societies, namely the Chinese Society of Anaesthesiology, the Society of Anaesthesiologists of Nepal, and the Society of Anaesthetists of Papua New Guinea, were welcomed to the AARS. At a secret ballot, the Chinese Society of Anaesthesiologists Taipei was selected as host for the 10th AACA. New board members were elected as follows: chairman Dr. Manuel Silao (Philippines), vice-chairman Dr. J.H. Lee (Taipei), secretary Dr. Robert Hare (Australia), treasurer Dr. Ryo Ogawa (Japan), and board members Dr. Deepthi Attygalle (Sri Lanka), Dr. S.N. Samad Choudhury (Bangladesh), Dr. Kwang Woo Kim (Korea), and representatives of the WFSA Executive Committee Dr. Kester Brown (Australia), Dr. Cedric Hoskins (New Zealand), Dr. Saywan Lim (Malaysia), and Dr. Kenjiro Mori (Japan) (Fig. 16).

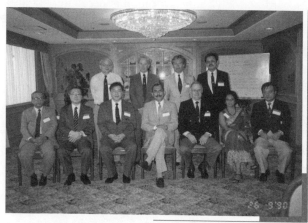

Fig. 16. *The AARS board 1990-1994, Seoul, 26 September 1990. Top row, from the left: Kester Brown (Australia); Cedric Hoskins (New Zealand); Saywan Lim (Malaysia). Bottom row, from the left: Samad Choudhury (Bangladesh); Ryo Ogawa (Japan); J.H.Lee (Taipei); Manuel Silao (the Philippines); Deepthi Attygalle (Sri Lanka); Kwang Koo Kim (Korea) (by courtesy of Robert Hare)*

The extensive, high-quality scientific programme more than adequately covered the main theme of the congress, namely, "Better understandings in Anaesthesia" with 14 pre-congress refresher seminars, 8 special lectures, 10 scientific symposia, 6 panel sessions, and 10 workshops, as well as an extensive range of free papers. To further enable delegates to renew past friendships and to make new ones there was a wide-ranging programme of social events.

The highlight was the official banquet at the Little Angels Performing Arts Center. This, together with the trip to and from the banquet for delegates in a motorcade of over 40 coaches with a full police escort to assist the ease of passage through the dense Seoul traffic, created a lasting impression.

At the 10th World Congress in The Hague, Netherlands, a regional board meeting was held on 15 June 1992. The report of the Organising Committee for the 9th AACA to be held at the Central Plaza Hotel in Bangkok was presented by Dr. S Pausawasdi, who noted excellent progress. Dr Salard Tupavong (Thailand) was elected as President for the 9th AACA. The admission of the Pacific Society of Anaesthetists into the WFSA and the AARS was recorded. The secretary, Dr. Hare, reported that nearly 5 tonnes of textbooks from the United States had been distributed by courtesy of the of ACPAD (an Australian Government Organisation) to Bangledesh, Indonesia, Papua New Guinea, and Vietnam. Books and journals had been sent to Sri Lanka at the recipients' expense. He also outlined the formation, by the societies of Bangledesh, Butan, India, Pakistan, Nepal, and Sri Lanka, of the South Asian Confederation of Anaesthetists. Dr. S Choudhury (Bangledesh) announced that the 1st SACA Congress was to be held in Bangledesh in October 1993. The board agreed that the AARS advance up to U.S. $ 5,000 to support visiting lecturers who were travelling through the region to attend and speak at the AACA.

During this period, the AARS facilitated a visit to Laos by Dr. Hadyn Perndt to make contact with the few anaesthetists in that country and to initiate aid. These developments in the AARS were highlighted by Dr. Hare in the secretary's regional newsletter, 1992. He discussed the diversity of the member societies of the AARS with regard not only to their location and culture, but also to the range from affluence to extreme poverty. The teaching and practice of anaesthesia in some countries was a monumental task by virtue of the huge population, as in the Indian subcontinent, China, Indonesia, and the Philippines, and in others such as the Pacific Islands and Papua New Guinea, because of their remoteness. He concluded that the AARS had graduated from an organisation of anaesthetic societies holding a regional congress every 4 years, to one that was busily concerned with the teaching of anaesthesia and the support and encouragement of our colleagues throughout the whole region.

The 9th AACA was held in Bangkok, Thailand on 6-11 November 1994. The congress, hosted by the Royal College of Anaesthesiologists of Thailand, was officially opened by Her Royal Highness Maha Chakri Sirindhorn. The extensive scientific programme provided many educational opportunities for the 1,350 delegates (including 20 from China) and accompanying persons who attended from some 54 countries worldwide. Delegates from the nearby developing countries of Cambodia, Laos, Myanmar, and Vietnam were invited and funded by the congress, further fulfilling the educational aim of the AARS. Leading anaesthetists from nine countries of the region took part in the congress theme symposium "Anaesthesia by the year 2000, present status and future prospects in the AARS", to outline the challenges lying ahead.

During the congress, AARS regional assemblies and board meetings were held, as well as a WFSA Executive Committee meeting. In his report, the chairman, Dr. Manuel Silao, emphasised that the first priority of the board was the continued promotion and enhancement of anaesthesia in the region. He also acknowledged the presentation of funds to the AARS from the 8th AACA held in Korea.

The AARS committee on education had been very active, i.e., Dr. Hare's visit to Vietnam, 1989, followed by refresher courses in Hanoi in October/November 1991. This 8-day course funded by the AARS was conducted by Dr. Thara Tritrakarn (Thailand), Dr. Abdul Raksamani (Thailand), and Dr. David McCuaig (Australia). Of the Vietnam refresher courses, the secretary, Dr. Hare said "one important side benefit of these courses is that avenues have now been opened up for cooperation that would end years of isolation and that this would apply to other countries." The chairman of the committee on education, Dr. Mitsugu Fijimori reported that in September 1991 Dr. Prithvi Raj (Atlanta, USA) and Dr. Tat-Leang Lee (Singapore), with AARS support, visited the Peoples Republic of China to conduct refresher courses in Beijing and Shanghai. There were educational visits to Papua New Guinea (Dr, G Gordon, Australia), as well as to other centres. In February 1993, Dr. Thara Tritrakarn and Dr. Nguyen Thu organised a refresher course in Ho-Chi-Minh City funded by the WFSA. Dr. Bernard Wetchler (chairman, Executive Committee, WFSA) reported that the WFSA was exploring proposals to establish regional centres for training throughout the world.

The regional assembly ratified changes to the regulations following a review undertaken by the chairman, Dr. Manuel Silao. The revised regulations would facilitate reporting of the region's finances to the regional assemblies.

Dr. Silao outlined a proposal for an Asian Board of Anaesthesiology, similar to the European Board, with the aim of establishing standards of training and equipment. He suggested that a committee be established to carry this further and to report to the next board meeting in Taipei. The theme for the 10th AACA to be held in Taipei, Taiwan in May 1998 was confirmed as "Safe and save".

Two societies presented bids for the 11th AACA. The Malaysian Society of Anaesthesiologists was elected to host this congress in Kuala Lumpur in 2002. The new regional board for the next 4 years was elected as: chairman Dr. J.H. Lee (Taipei), vice-chairman Dr. S.M. Samad Choudhury (Bangledesh), secretary Dr. John D. Richards (Australia), treasurer Dr. Ryo Ogawa (Japan), and board members Dr. Kwang Woo Kim (Korea), Dr. Tat-Leang Lee (Singapore), and Dr. M. Roesli Thaib (Indonesia). Representatives of the WFSA Executive Committee included Dr. Kester Brown (Australia), Dr. Mitsugu Fujimori (Japan),

Dr. Cedric Hoskins (New Zealand), Dr. Saywan Lim (Malaysia), Dr. Kenjiro Mori (Japan), and Dr. Manuel Silao (Philippines) (Fig. 17).

Again, delegates were entertained to a lavish and extensive social programme highlighting the wonderful friendliness and hospitality of the host society and the Thai people. The official reception at the Saranram Palace was hosted by the Deputy Minister of Foreign Affairs. This was the first time that any medical congress had been so recognised by the Thai Government - one up for anaesthesia. For this visit, as with others, not only were the coaches accompanied by police escorts to speed the way through the traffic, but each had as a tour guide, a Thai anaesthetist to provide a knowledgeable commentary of the history and architecture of Bangkok. The closing ceremony at the Rose Garden Country Resort was a magnificent show with a banquet dinner, for over 1,200, outdoors under the stars in the balmy evening air, a fireworks display, and then the delegates, in Thai tradition, placing opened flowers carrying glowing candles on the river to transport their dreams and best wishes.

"Mini" board meetings were held during the SASA congresses in Colombo, 1995, in Karachi, 1997, and in Madras in 1999. In keeping with the principal of initiating and establishing aid from within the region, Dr. Thara Tritrakarn (Thailand) was noted as being instrumental in coordinating teaching in the nearby countries of Indo-China.

The 10th AACA was held in Taipei, Taiwan on 10-16 May 1998. At the regional assemblies the chairman, Dr. J.H. Lee, outlined the initiatives of the Royal College of Anaesthesiologists of Thailand in establishing a training scheme for Laotian and Cambodian anaesthetists. This had been running for 2 years with good results. Draft standards for anaesthetic practice, which had previously been outlined by Dr. Manuel Silao (Philippines), were again discussed, as well as the proposed Asian Academy of Anaesthesiology. It was hoped that eventually visiting exchange examiners could be arranged. In addition, each member society could use these standards as a basis on which to develop their own principles of excellence in training and anaesthetic practice.

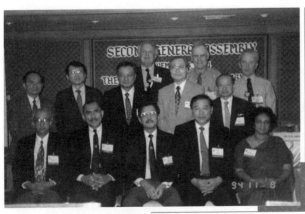

Fig. 17. *The AARS board for 1994-1998 with the previous board, Bangkok, 11 November 1994. Top row, from the left: Roesli Thaib (Indonesia); Tat-Leang Lee (Singapore);); Kwang Koo Kim (Korea); John Richards (Australia); Ryo Ogawa (Japan); Robert Hare (Australia); Mitsugu Fujimori (Japan); Cedric Hoskins (New Zealand). Bottom row, from the left: Samad Choudhury (Bangladesh); Manuel Silao (the Philippines); Saywan Lim (Malaysia); J.H.Lee (Taipei); Deepthi Attygalle (Sri Lanka) (by courtesy of Cedric Hoskins)*

On behalf of the 10th AACA Organising Committee, Dr. Peter Tan (Taipei) reported that due to the then current Asian financial situation, only 384 delegates had registered but that the support from the industry was high. Dr. Sylvian Das (Malaysia) informed the board of the satisfactory progress towards the 11th AACA to be held in Kuala Lumpur, Malaysia, in July 2002 with the theme of "Anaesthetists as the perioperative specialist".

The new regional board was elected as: chairman Dr. Tat-Leang Lee (Singapore), vice-chairman Dr. Sylvian Das (Malaysia), secretary Dr. J.D. Richards (Australia), treasurer Dr. Kazuo Hanaoka (Japan), and board members Dr. Alan Merry (New Zealand), and Dr. Florian R. Nuevo (Philippines), Dr. Roesli Thaib (Indonesia). Representative of the WFSA Executive Committee included Dr. Deepthi Attygalle (Sri Lanka), Dr. Kester Brown (Australia), Dr. Kwang Woo Kim (Korea), Dr. J.H. Lee (Taipei), and Dr. Haydn Perndt (Australia).

AARS board meetings were held in Sydney during the 11th World Congress in April 1996 and in New Delhi in November 1999 at the AOSRA meeting. An informal meeting was held in Montreal at the 12th WCA in June 2000.

The 11th AACA was held in Kuala Lumpur, Malaysia on 10-13 July 2002. This was again an opportunity for the AARS board to meet and for member societies to play a part in discussions concerning the development of safe anaesthesia and resuscitation for the people of the region. Dr. Sylvian Das, vice-chairman of the board and chairman of the congress Organising Committee, reported that despite the apprehension following the events of 11 September 2001, there were 905 registrants for the congress, of whom 350 were from 36 overseas countries. He noted that great difficulties had been experienced in contacting member societies and disseminating publicity. Dr. Kester Brown (WFSA President) pointed out that although the WFSA has a newsletter, key journals, and a website, personal communication remains one of the best methods for promotion. The presence of leading invited speakers, hands-on practical workshops, and local hospital visits are also important attractions for a successful congress.

Prior to the AARS meetings, the board had met with the WFSA executive during which the role of the AARS was discussed at length. The board agreed with the WFSA proposal to formalise recognition of the Regional Sections. The AARS board chairman, Dr. Tat-Leang Lee, drew attention to the disparity in standards throughout the region and to the proliferation of other regional and special interest groups, such as CASA, SACA, paediatric, trauma, cardiology, and regional anaesthesia. Whilst this trend was laudable and desirable, it did tend to dilute financial and manpower resources. Dr. Brown recommended that the AARS, with WFSA help, encourage the involvement of these other groups with the AARS, particularly in the area of joint meetings. This would present economies of scale, cost savings, and maintenance of the support of the medical industry. It was agreed that these proposals be considered for the 12th AACA in Singapore in 2006.

Following bids by two member societies, a secret ballot was held during the 2nd regional assembly. The 13th AACA will be hosted by the Japan Society of

Anesthesiology in the new International Congress Centre in Fukuoka in 2010.

The treasurer, Dr. Kuzuo Hanaoka, reported on the high level of accumulated finances and that they should be used effectively for educational activities and the development of standards in the region. Following the ensuing discussions it was agreed to allocate the sum of U.S. $ 15,000 over the next 4 years to items such as improving lines of communication, better liaison with and between members societies and the special interest groups, incident monitoring surveys, and the development of Asian and Australasian standards of anaesthetic practice.

The bylaws were amended to enable a member of the board, who had not served as chairman during his/her 8-year term, to be so nominated and elected. AARS and WFSA affairs are increasing in complexity and this change would allow an experienced board member to further contribute to regional affairs.

The new regional board was elected as: chairman Dr. Florian Nuevo (Philippines), vice-chairman Dr. Sylvian Das (Malaysia), secretary Dr. Alan Merry (New Zealand), treasurer Dr. Kazuo Hanaoka (Japan), and board members Dr. Rebecca Jacob (India), Dr. Jung-un Lee (Korea), Dr. Robert McDougall (Australia) (assistant secretary), and co-opted members Dr. John Richards (Australia) and Dr. Tat-Leang Lee (Singapore). Representatives of the WFSA Executive Committee were Dr. Deepthi Attygalle (Sri Lanka), Dr. Kester Brown (Australia), Dr. Peter Kempthorne (New Zealand), and Dr. Richard Walsh (Australia).

Hence, from those early beginnings, just over 40 years ago, at the 1st AACA in Manila, in November 1962, with an attendance of 177 delegates representing nine societies from the region, this Regional Section of the WFSA has grown to now include 22 member societies with over 17,500 members, as follows:

- Australian Society of Anaesthetists (established 1934) 2,300 members
- Bangladesh Society of Anaesthesiologists 50 members
- Chinese Society of Anesthesiology 245 members
- The Chinese Society of Anesthesiologists Taipei (established 1956) 580 members
- The Society of Anaesthetists of Hong Kong (established 1954) 80 members
- Indian Society of Anaesthestists (established 1947) 1,001 members
- Indonesian Society of Anesthesiologists 244 members
- Japan Society of Anesthesiology (established 1954) 8.568 members
- Korean Society of Anesthesiologists (established 1956) 2,010 members
- Malaysian Society of Anaesthesiologists (established 1965) 252 members
- Association of Anaesthesiologists of Mauritius (established 1989) 40 members
- Anaesthetists' Society of Myanmar Medical Association 14 members
- Society of Anaesthesiologists of Nepal 54 members

- New Zealand Society of Anaesthetists (established 1948) 250 members
- Pacific Society of Anaesthetists (established 1989) 21 members
- Pakistan Society of Anaesthesiologists 116 members
- Society of Anaesthetists of Papua New Guinea 10 members
- Philippine Society of Anaesthesiologists (established 1951) 1.012 members
- Singapore Society of Anaesthesiologists (established 1971) 155 members
- College of Anaesthesiologists of Sri Lanka (established 1972) 90 members
- Royal College of Anaesthesiologists of Thailand (established 1973) 575 members
- Vietnamese Society of Anaesthesiologists (established 1978) 100 members

(From WFSA Directory of Member Societies, November 2001)

This factual record outlines the progress of the AARS of the WFSA over 40 years. Hopefully, it places on record the tireless efforts of many dedicated anaesthetists who breathed life into the AARS and of those who continue this magnanimous act for the sake of the development of the profession of anaesthesia and the promotion of education in patient safety as they jointly work towards achievement of the basic purpose of the WFSA-making available the highest standards of anaesthesia and resuscitation to all people of the world and to disseminate the same amongst them.

I wish to record my sincere gratitude to the many people who have made this "history" possible. To Dr. Saywan Lim (past President, WFSA) who initially suggested and encouraged the proposal of writing this historical record. To Dr. Kenichi Iwatsuki (Sendai City, Japan) for making available his history of the AARS as published in the souvenir booklet for the 5th AACA in New Delhi. To Dr. Quintin Gomez (Manila, Philippines), Dr. Hideo Yamamura (Tokyo, Japan), the late Dr. Douglas Joseph (Sydney, Australia), and Dr. Robert Hare (Melbourne, Australia) for photographs and access to congress and assembly records. To Dr. John Richards (Adelaide, Australia) and the current secretary of the AARS, Dr. Alan Merry (Auckland, New Zealand), for contemporary records. The assistance of the present chairman of the AARS, Dr. Florian Nuevo (Philippines) is valued. To Mr. Patrick Sim (Wood Library/Museum of Anesthesiology) my gratitude for his archival assistance.

Whilst every endeavor has been made to verify the material of this history, I apologise for any errors and omissions. My appreciation to Dr. Donatella Rizza, Senior Editor, Springer-Verlag Italia, for the special effort made to ensure that this "History" is a full and complete record.

Note: this chapter is based on the publication in Seoul, Korea, by the Board of the AARS, of the book "History of the Asian and Australasian Regional Section" (author Cedric Hoskins) for distribution at the 8th AACA, September 1990.

11 WFSA AND EUROPE. A LONG BUT COMPLICATED RELATIONSHIP

D.J. Wilkinson

Introduction

Europe has always been a strong supporter of the World Federation of Societies of Anaesthesiologists (WFSA) and indeed they were instrumental in the original creation of the organisation. Much of that early contribution has been detailed elsewhere. Europe has always had a strong regional voice in anaesthesia and there has been a myriad of European general and specialist societies over the years that have contributed to or ignored the activities of the WFSA. This chapter will attempt to outline how some of these societies came into being and how they now contribute to European and world affairs.

National or regional?

Well before the creation of the WFSA there was a variety of strong national societies who, as part of their activities, ran scientific meetings. The Association of Anaesthetists of Great Britain and Ireland (AAGBI) had been founded in 1932, yet did not start running meetings until the early 1950s. The French started their meetings in 1946 and the Swedish society (founded in 1946) started to hold Scandinavian congresses from 1950 onwards.

In 1952 the Austrian society started the Central European Meetings of Anaesthetists, which rotated with the German and Swiss societies as organisers. In 1959 this meeting was held in Düsseldorf and was attended by Professor Cecil Gray who suggested that there should be a Europe-wide society and that it should hold its first meeting in Vienna. 1962 was mooted as an acceptable date as it fell between two World Congresses. At the next World Congress in 1960 in Toronto, Gray was appointed chairman of a WFSA Regionalisation Committee and the concept of a European region was officially adopted by the WFSA.

First moves

Professor Otto Mayrhofer was selected to be chairman of the Organising Committee for this meeting in his home city of Vienna. The Austrian society at this time had about 100 members. This 1st European Congress was held, in September 1962, under the auspices of the WFSA in the former Imperial Palace and was very successful. There were five lecture halls used simultaneously for the 3.5 days of the meeting. The main topics were "recovery and special care units", "anaesthesia for the aged", and "problems with anaesthesia for emergency surgery". Following on from the congress was a postgraduate course for a further 1.5 days using three lecture halls (one in English, one German, and one French). It is interesting to note that no speaker asked for expenses or a fee for their services. About 1,500 delegates attended from 48 countries around the world.

One of the useful contacts for the promotion of this meeting was made through the Council for International Organisation of Medical Societies (CIOMS), which was a sub-division of the United Nations Educational, Scientific, and Cultural Organisation and the World Health Organisation (UNESCO and WHO). CIOMS had already been instrumental in the setting up of the WFSA in 1955 and close liaison was maintained between officers of the WFSA and CIOMS through Dr. Boureau (France), as the organisation was based in Paris. He had been able to attend general assemblies of CIOMS in 1955, 1958, and 1961, and had secured some funding for the European meeting in Vienna in the form of travelling bursaries for young researchers. CIOMS was unable due to its constitution to directly fund anything other than World Congresses, and so this generosity was both unexpected and unique. Eight young researchers benefited from this award (U.S. $ 1,200) and attended Vienna from all over Europe.

The WFSA Executive Committee and the committee on regionalisation both held meetings during the conference and it was also decided to hold the next European Congress in Denmark in 4 years time.

By the time of the 3rd World Congress in Sao Paulo in 1964, Gray was able to report that three regions, "Europe, Australasia, and Latin America" had held regional congresses and that more were being planned.

Official creation of European Regional Section

During and following the initial European meeting in Vienna, and after widespread discussion with various other European protagonists, it was decided to set up a formal European Regional Section (ERS) of the WFSA. This was done using as a guideline the bylaws of the WFSA and a set of rules were put together so that the new organisation could be created at the 2nd European Congress that took place in Copenhagen in August 1966.

The Danish Society who hosted this meeting was aided by the societies from Norway, Sweden, and Finland. Ole Secher was congress President and

Henning Poulson secretary of the Organising Committee. This meeting was opened by His Majesty King Frederick IX.

All aspects of clinical anaesthesia were covered in the symposia, group discussions, or free paper sessions. In addition, 16 films relating to anaesthesia were screened. Twenty-five founder member countries were present and included Austria, Belgium, Bulgaria, Czechoslovakia, Denmark, Finland, France, East Germany, West Germany, Greece, Hungary, Israel, Italy, Yugoslavia, The Netherlands, Norway, Poland, Portugal, Rumania, Spain, Sweden, Switzerland, Turkey, United Kingdom, and USSR.

At a General Assembly of delegates from these European societies of the WFSA a set of rules were accepted that included the following:

1. The European section will consist of the European member societies of the WFSA with the addition of Israel.
2. Its activities will be consistent with the aims and objects of the World Federation.
3. A regional assembly will usually be held in connection with each European Congress of Anaesthesiology.
4. Each member society shall be represented by the same number of delegates as in the General Assembly of the WFSA.
5. The board of the European section shall be composed of the chairman, two vice-chairmen, the secretary, and the treasurer. Representatives of Europe within the Executive Committee of the WFSA are ex officio members without a vote.

The first board was elected at the General Assembly and comprised: chairman Dr. Steven Couremenos (Greece), first vice-chairman Professor Louis Lareng (France), second vice-chairman Dr. Borivoj Dvoracek (Czechoslovakia), treasurer Dr. Henning Poulsen (Denmark), and secretary Professor Otto Mayrhofer (Austria). Besides agreeing to hold further European congresses on a 4-yearly basis, the ERS set up a Standing Committee on professional affairs. This was chaired by Professor Lareng (France) and was composed of a single delegate from each member society of the ERS and it was planned that they would deal with financial, organisational, social, and departmental problems. In the WFSA Newsletter Number 3 of June 1967 it is stated that this new committee would continue "the efforts and accomplishments of the Association of European Anaesthesiologists during past years". I can find no record of this latter organisation and even Professor Lareng who chaired the Standing Committee has no recollection of its existence! Nevertheless the ERS had been created.

Other regional meetings

In Eastern Europe there were some barriers to free exchange of information with colleagues in the west. A symposium in anaesthesiology was organised in East Berlin in September 1959 by Professors Barth and Meyer. Although this was successful, there was then a 4-year gap before a 1st International Symposium of Anaesthesiology (ISA) was organised by the Hungarian Society in Budapest in September 1963. The President then was Dr. Harkanyi. As well as 150 delegates and speakers from Eastern Europe, there were five speakers from England, Sweden, and Austria. The meeting had an extensive scientific agenda, as well as discussing potential future meetings. It was agreed to hold such meetings on a regular 2-yearly basis.

The 2nd ISA took place in Prague in 1965, Dr. Hoder was in charge of the meeting, and intensive care appeared on the programme for the first time. Poland arranged the 3rd ISA in Poznan in 1967 with Professor Jurik as President. This meeting gathered some of the truly great names of anaesthesia together, including Robert Macintosh from Oxford, Henry Beecher from Boston, Torsten Gordh from Stockholm, and Rudolf Frey from Mainz. Otto Mayrhofer, then secretary of the WFSA, was also present and encouraged many Eastern European countries to consider attending the forthcoming World Congress in London.

However, many other meetings were taking place throughout Europe. For example, in 1965 the 8th Central European Meeting was held in September in Zurich and there was a Spanish/Portuguese meeting in Barcelona in October of that same year. Similar meetings continued on an annual basis, with a Central European meeting being held in Salzburg in 1967 with some 1,500 delegates and a Spanish/Portuguese meeting in Santiago de Compostella in the same year with some 400 delegates. Europe was becoming more and more active.

Consolidation

With the 4th World Congress being held in London in 1968 there was an opportunity for the European community to meet a wider group of colleagues "on their doorstep". Some 2,800 anaesthetists convened at the Royal Festival Hall on the South Bank of the River Thames. The meeting was a resounding success. A report was made at the General Assembly about the ERS, relating mainly to the meeting held in Copenhagen 2 years previously. Professor Henning Poulson was able to report another successful outcome and the formation of the official structure. It is interesting to note that this is the last reference to the ERS in the World Congress General Assembly minutes. The WFSA continued to take an interest in the developing regional meetings and often held Executive Committee and other Standing Committee meetings during the ERS congresses, but the ERS became self sufficient and continued to organise very successful 4-yearly meetings.

The WFSA also continued to send an officer to the Scandinavian and Central European meetings, as well as to the International Anaesthesia Symposia, indicating its support for and interest in the region.

The 3rd European Congress was held in Prague in 1970. The President of the meeting was Dr. Josef Hoder and his committee organised a 5-day meeting with 72 scientific sessions. Almost 1,600 attended what for many from "the west" was the first experience of Eastern Europe. This was a particularly memorable experience for all of those who attended and many heard stories of a lifestyle and professional life that was at great variance from that with which they were familiar. In the scientific sessions there were papers on neuroleptanalgesia, hyperbaric oxygen, muscle relaxants and their antidotes, toxicity of inhaled agents, ketamine, propanadid, regional anaesthesia, monitoring, and metabolic changes during resuscitation.

A new regional board was appointed at this time: Douglas Howat (Great Britain and Ireland) was made chairman, Emil Stojanov (Bulgaria) first vice-chairman, Alfredo Arias Alvarez (Spain) second vice-chairman, Otto Mayrhofer (Austria) secretary, and August Colding (Denmark) was made treasurer.

During these years, member societies paid U.S. $ 0.50 per member to the ERS and a different subscription to the WFSA. This payment started to cause huge problems as countries were unwilling to or had great logistical difficulties in paying two sets of subscription to two organisations. This would come to a head at the next European Congress in Spain in 1974.

In 1971 there were the usual Scandinavian, Central European, and Spanish/Portuguese meetings. With the World Congress taking place in Kyoto in 1972 the only other major European meeting that year was the International Anaesthesia Symposium held in Dresden in June. There had been good communication between the WFSA and the organisers of the congress and as it was felt that few delegates from this region would be able to travel to Kyoto this symposium was again supported by the WFSA in the form of their secretary Professor Mayrhofer who spoke at the Opening Ceremony. Some 300 delegates attended. Europe was strongly supportive of the Kyoto congress and many delegates found themselves elected to the executive and other committees.

In Madrid in 1974 the 4th European Congress took place. A new Board was elected with Alfredo Arias Alvarez (Spain) as chairman, Jean Lassner (France) secretary, Augustus Haxholdt (Denmark) treasurer, and John Zorab (Great Britain and Ireland) vice-President. Concern was re-iterated about the problem of payment of subscriptions to the organisation, with several societies refusing to pay both WFSA and its European section. The income generated by this subscription was not considerable and was used to fund the board's expenses. It was agreed that this was not really required, as most expenses could be met from the surpluses of European congresses.

The various national societies began to organise more and more local meetings and there started to be considerable overlap. The WFSA had acted as a "clearing house" for these and regional meetings, with a congress programme being published in the WFSA Newsletter, but the costs of publishing this leaflet had proved too much and it had stopped production in 1974.

A new society formed; The European Academy

The new secretary, Professor Lassner, attempted to record when meetings were taking place, but societies proved to be reluctant to co-operate and no true co-ordination was possible. As a result there were often multiple anaesthesia meetings taking place at the same time. Very little extra activity was generated by each of the European boards, their only function being to run a 4-yearly congress and act as a point of reference between the WFSA and the local societies.

With the World Congress in Japan in 1972 and Mexico in 1976 and the ERS meetings only every 4 years, some in Europe began to feel there was no opportunity for more regular cross-European anaesthesia discussion. In March 1977, after some preliminary discussions, Lassner convened a meeting in Paris to which the societies of Austria, Belgium, Finland, France, Germany, Greece, Great Britain and Ireland, Italy, The Netherlands, Norway, Poland, Spain, Switzerland, Turkey, and Yugoslavia sent representatives. At this meeting the goals of a European Academy were proposed and discussed. After another meeting in Dublin that September and a third in Paris in April 1978, the bylaws and structure of the organisation, as worked out predominantly by Professors Rosen and Vickers, were confirmed.

The 5th European Congress was held in Paris in September 1978 and for the first time a single topic was adopted for the whole meeting. This was haemodynamic variations in anaesthesiology. Lassner was made President of this ERS meeting. At this same meeting, the European Academy of Anaesthesiologists (EAA) was created and the first General Assembly approved its constitution and elected the first senate, as well as Lassner as its first President. Its main aim was to foster European scientific co-operation in anaesthesia and it existed as a non-profit making non-governmental organisation registered under French law in Paris. At the first ERS General Assembly the then President of the WFSA, Quentin Gomez (Philippines), gave an address that expressed his concern that the setting up of this new body (EAA) could potentially be harmful to the WFSA and doubted its value. Lassner who had invited him to the meeting was naturally disappointed with this approach and resigned from the WFSA Executive Committee.

The new academy was a relatively small organisation that was regarded by some as an elitist body. Its impact on European anaesthesia was soon to become highly significant with the setting up of an European examination in anaesthesia. Gomez's reservations proved unfounded, as the academy published the abstracts of the Paris 1978 ERS meeting within a year and Lassner wrote in the preface "this publication also marks the beginning of interaction between the Federation and the Academy which both bodies can legitimately expect to be productive." This proved to be true and the Academy and ERS maintained cordial relations throughout the next decade, with a full exchange of views, ideas, and personnel. Many "senior figures" in European anaesthesia were officials in both organisations.

The Academy created a series of innovative additions to European anaesthesia in addition to its meetings and the diploma examination. The *European Journal of Anaesthesia* was published and still continues today. There was the introduction of an accreditation programme for departments of anaesthesia across Europe and a series of awards made to trainees for research.

Further ERS development

The 6th Congress took place in London in 1982. Dr. Wylie was President of the congress and the meeting was opened by HRH the Princess Margaret, Countess of Snowdon, who was the Patron of the Association of Anaesthetists of Great Britain and Ireland. She was able to present every President of every European society with a special commemorative scroll at the Opening Ceremony and it was interesting to note the standing ovation awarded to Professor Marek Sych (Poland) as he crossed the stage to receive his. This was at the time when the Gdansk dock workers under Lech Walesa were striving to achieve a democracy in Poland and was a particularly poignant moment. A new board was elected with Professor Steinbereither (Austria) as chairman.

In Vienna in 1986 at the 7th ECA, a new board of the ERS was elected and comprised Dr. Baskett (Great Britain and Ireland) chairman, Professor Viby-Morgensen (Denmark) secretary/treasurer and Professors Pelosi (Italy), Peter (Germany), Rondio (Poland), and Noviant (France) This board started to take greater notice of educational opportunities within Europe and agreed to fund some of these. There was an understanding that ERS activity in this area should be co-ordinated through the WFSA Education Committee. Further European sub-groups were starting to emerge at this time, including the European Resuscitation Council.

In 1990 in Warsaw, at the 8th European Congress, Jorgen Viby-Morgensen (Denmark) was appointed chairman. His new board comprised Professors Rondio (Poland) and Peter (Germany) as vice-chairmen, Dr. Baird (Great Britain and Ireland) as secretary, and Professor Pelosi (Italy) as treasurer. Professor Gassner (Israel) was a further board member. The ERS, apart from organising this 4-yearly congress, was not very active, however, and meanwhile a new European organisation was emerging.

Another new society the European Society of Anaesthesiologists (ESA)

There was increasing dissatisfaction amongst younger specialists and trainees that there was no pan-European congress of anaesthesia where free papers could be presented and the academic quality of presentation was rigorously maintained. It was felt that too often people were selected to speak at meetings because of geographical considerations, i.e., seeking representation right across Europe, rather than by their ability to lecture or because of the quality of the science they were presenting. There were also very few meetings at which trainees could present free papers and detrimental analogies began to be drawn between European and American meetings.

It was certainly true that the ERS did little else but organise a meeting every 4 years and that it deliberately tried to provide opportunities for lecturers from all countries within its remit. The Academy meetings meanwhile were considered by many as elitist and difficult for trainees to access. An image of a "senior club" was the perception constantly referenced.

In 1987 a fledgling European Society of Anaesthesiologists (ESA) was set up in Brussels. In their introduction to their bylaws at that time it was stated that "Responsibility to the patient imposes special obligations in view of the freedom to provide services which will take effect in 1992 within the European community, and having regard to the variety of situations in which doctors, and especially anaesthetists, are working in the countries of the Community and to the conditions under which they are trained and exercise their profession." It appeared therefore to be focussing its interest particularly at that time within the European Community.

A more-detailed ESA constitution published in 1991 introduced itself as an international scientific society with the following aims:
1. To provide homogenous continuous education to advance the organisation of training and the improvement of the qualifications of anaesthesiologists in Europe.
2. To encourage and promote fundamental and applied research pursuant to scientific developments and to help publish the results in Europe.
3. To give due recognition to the work and authority of anaesthesiologists in relation to other medical disciplines and to the patients in Europe.
4. To encourage exchanges between European anaesthesiologists.
5. To make clinical recommendations for improvement of standards of clinical practice in anaesthesiology in Europe.

The first ESA meeting took place in Brussels in May 1993 and as stated in its advertising flyers modelled itself on the ASA meeting. The Steering Committee comprised: Dr. Andreen (Sweden) President, Dr. d'Hollander (Belgium) secretary, Dr. Gribomont (Belgium) treasurer, Dr. Aitkenhead (England) editor, and Dr. Reiz (Sweden) scientific organiser. There were 15 subcommittees to the Scientific Committee, each organised by an individual with a specific interest and "track record" in that area of specialisation. They created a scientific programme based on the ability of the lecturer to speak as well as the scientific content. Invited lecturers had their expenses paid by the organisation, but they were also expected to take on other tasks such as chairing sessions. The meeting was a resounding success with a huge trade sponsorship programme. This programme funded the attendance of a large number of delegates and ensured that the meeting was a financial success. The standard of the scientific programme was high and the meeting had a large free paper session. Whatever anyone said, the meeting was popular and proved to be a continuing success in the following years.

This innovative addition to European anaesthesia proved to be an unsettling influence to the longer-established organisations. It was soon apparent that there might be a limited "pot" of trade money available, and this would tend to go towards the most-popular and successful meetings. The ERS viewed these developments with alarm, especially as the ESA planned to hold "rival" meetings in the same years as the ERS was organising its own European Congress of Anaesthesiologists. Many societies, and particularly the national societies in Germany, Austria, and Switzerland, expressed their concern over the appearance of a new organisation that might not have the best interests of all of Europe at its heart. However, the ESA was here to stay as it was filling a void left by the Academy and ERS.

The ERS contacted the ESA and asked if discussions might be initiated to determine how the potential financial strain of running two major European meetings in 1998, the date of the next ERS Congress, might be mitigated. This debate was welcomed by the ESA board and an informal meeting was convened in Copenhagen in November 1992 to explore possible solutions. At this meeting the ERS representatives suggested that the ESA might defer their 1998 meeting or alternatively hold a joint congress that year. The ESA board meeting in 1993 was unable to accept the former proposal and was unenthusiastic over the idea of a joint meeting with the ERS. A willingness to maintain lines of communication was stressed, with a view to determining what might or might not take place in 1998. Discussions continued in early 1994 and these looked very promising with an outline proposal for a joint meeting gaining general support. However, by the time of the ERS Congress in Jerusalem, the mood appeared to have changed and the proposal for a joint meeting was not welcomed by the General Assembly of the ERS.

ERS developments

Viby-Morgensen, chairman of the ERS, described to the General Assembly of the ERS in Jerusalem in 1994 how there had been two informal meetings with representatives from the ESA. He reported that the interim ESA board had rejected a proposal that they should not hold a major meeting every 4th year coinciding with the ERS Congress. He highlighted the increasing level of confusion created by the multiple European societies that all claimed to "represent" European anaesthesia. Many anaesthetists, and perhaps more importantly, many people in trade organisations, felt unsure which organisation they should support.

During widespread debate during the assembly, the overall frustration appeared to be the lack of co-ordination in Europe that would in the long term be detrimental to anaesthesia on the continent. Some suggested that the ERS should consider holding more-frequent meetings. There was no support for joint meetings with the ESA.

At this 9th European Congress a new board was convened. Leslie Baird (Great Britain and Ireland) was made chairman; Dietrich Kettler (Germany) secretary; Gaby Gurman (Israel) treasurer; Gunter Hempelmann (Germany) vice-President and Elena Damir (Russia) the other vice-President. The meeting was a resounding success, with a gratifying number of delegates being undeterred by the threat of terrorist activity. For the first time in several congresses there was a positive budget and the ERS benefited proportionally. It soon became apparent, however, that the increasing activity of the ERS would need an increase in funding. This was discussed with the WFSA executive, but no clear answer emerged at this time.

Following this congress, further attempts were made to find an equitable way to unite the various European organisations. Prior to the EAA meeting in 1995 in Bern, a meeting was convened between representatives of all these organisations. Following initial discussions it was agreed that co-operation was crucial and that there was a need to set up a Steering Committee to be chaired by Leslie Baird, the ERS chairman. This committee was able to meet in London in November 1995. All were unanimous in their support of the ideals of the FEEA, as outlined by Philippe Scherpereel. The ESA affirmed their constitutional inability to miss a meeting in the 4-yearly intervals when the ERS was holding its European Congress. It was, however, prepared to consider holding a joint meeting on such an occasion and the EAA agreed to discuss this further. The UEMS, represented by Professor Scherpereel, was very supportive of this initiative.

There appear to have been many missed opportunities to finalise an agreement between the ERS and the ESA around this time due to poor communications, busy working schedules, and the constraints of European travel. It is very difficult to determine whether these were useful excuses or genuine missed opportunities, but time went by and no closer rapport developed.

During the later part of this decade the ERS also investigated the possibility of publishing a regular newsletter. This initiative was led by Gaby Gurman and a great deal of time and effort was spent on the project. In the end it was considered that the expense outweighed the benefits and the ERS contributed to the WFSA Newsletter instead. Throughout this period the EAA had been publishing a very effective newsletter and this often carried ERS news and views. Following the Frankfurt Congress in 1998, there was a regular CENSA (Confederation of European National Societies of Anaesthesia) page written by the secretary.

Another unofficial organisation becomes official

Dr. MacRae (Great Britain and Ireland) and Dr. Tekeres (Hungary) convened an unofficial meeting of Presidents of the European societies in the early 1990s at which a wide variety of topics were discussed. The meeting, called a President's collegium (or just college), appointed Professor Rolly (Belgium) as the chairman of the group, which talked about matters of mutual concern. They convened again on several occasions; in 1996 the German society sponsored the meeting in conjunction with its national meeting in Nuremburg. At this meeting, following a presentation from Dr. Baird the Presidents College agreed to meet under the auspices of the ERS, and would do so next in January 1997 in London on the occasion of the 150th anniversary of the introduction of anaesthesia. At the European Congress in Frankfurt this group proposed that they be considered part of the ERS organisation. This was readily agreed and they were incorporated into the statutes and bylaws of CENSA at the Florence Congress in 2001as an Advisory Committee to the CENSA board. Annual meetings have been hosted by the CENSA board for this renamed Committee of Presidents since 1998, and a pattern of concerns across European anaesthesia continues to emerge and solutions suggested. It is fascinating to learn of similar problems in many countries and gratifying when others are able to suggest effective solutions. The problems of manpower, training, lack of resources, and poor public relations continue to defeat universal solutions.

More negotiations

In 1997 the ESA again approached the ERS with a view to re-opening discussions on greater co-operation within Europe, and in particular the challenge of conflicting meetings. The problem was acute with the ERS Frankfurt meeting scheduled for 1998. A meeting took place in May of 1997 in Lausanne between representatives of the ERS, ESA, EAA, FEAA, and UEMS. There appeared to be an agreement to run a joint ESA/ERS meeting every 4 years if the financial aspects could be clarified, for the Academy to contribute a day of lectures at the ESA Congress on an annual basis, and perhaps to join with the ESA and ERS every 4 years in their congress.

By November things had taken a turn for the worse again. Many individuals made public statements about the various organisations that were uncomplimentary and did little to enhance productive co-operation. The Academy decided to reverse its decision to join with the ESA at its 1998 Barcelona meeting because of perceived problems with relation to the ESA's negotiations with the Academy with respect to the *European Journal of Anaesthesia*. Essentially the ESA board made a commercial decision not to take up an offer made by the EAA at that time regarding the journal, but still wished to keep lines of communication open.

The ESA board was still happy to run a joint meeting with the ERS, starting possibly in Lisbon in 2002. However, it tempered this offer by stating that any decision by the ERS to increase the frequency of its meetings would be regarded as a hostile act against the ESA and would negate any such co-operation. There was still a desire to find some method of creating greater unification and the concept of some overall umbrella organisation, to which all the current European anaesthesia groups could belong, began to be considered.

The creation of Confederation of European National Societies of Anaesthesia

In Frankfurt in 1998 at the 10th ECA there was a major re-organisation of the ERS. Dr. Baird had circulated a series of documents, each of which took sometime to consider. A significant change was to consider and adopt a revised edition of the statutes and bylaws. The General Assembly was reminded that the work of the ERS had increased dramatically in recent years, partly due to the integration of a large number of Eastern European countries into the organisation. In addition, there was a need to relate to an ever-increasing number of European anaesthesia groups. These included the ESA, the EAA, the FEEA, and the UEMS. The assembly accepted this extensive revision and also voted their approval of a change of the name of the organisation to the Confederation of European National Societies of Anaesthesia (CENSA).

The future of CENSA congresses was the subject of another discussion paper considered by the assembly. The majority favoured the holding of a meeting every 2 years in conjunction with a national society meeting, these meetings to be held in odd years so as not to clash with the World Congresses. The meeting was informed about recent meetings with the EAA board when collaborative measures had been discussed, including the *European Journal of Anaesthesia* becoming the official journal of CENSA, and perhaps other collaborations might be possible in the future. It was also announced that there were problems with the organisation of the 11th meeting in Lisbon due to a lack of the necessary infrastructure. The decision to hold this meeting in Lisbon had been made in Warsaw in 1990. It was decided that offers to hold future meetings in 2001 and 2003 would be invited in the near future.

To help alleviate the financial pressures of CENSA the delegates agreed to pay an extra levy of U.S. $ 0.50 per member to the WFSA, who would in turn pay this sum to CENSA. This was a re-introduction of the levy abandoned in 1978 in Paris.

The CENSA board was enlarged at this time to help deal with the increasing workload. Dietrich Kettler (Germany) became chairman, David Wilkinson (Great Britain and Ireland) secretary, Olav Sellevold (Norway) treasurer, Gunter Hempelmann (Germany) and Gaby Gurman (Israel) were made vice-Presidents, and Maria Janecsko (Hungary), Giampaolo Novelli (Italy), Thomas Pasch (Switzerland), and Philippe Scherpereel (France) were elected to the board. This new board determined to take the newly named CENSA further forward within Europe. It decided to cement its relationship with the national society members by hosting CENSA symposia within national meetings. This was offered to all member societies and proved to be particularly welcome in Eastern Europe and with societies that held meetings on a less-frequent basis.

Sadly from a financial viewpoint, despite a good level of registration at the Frankfurt meeting, there was a deficit in the overall budget. CENSA was therefore very dependent on the new subscription it had introduced.

Further European congresses

Following the consideration of a series of applications, the CENSA board awarded the 2001 congress to Florence, to be run jointly with SIAARTI, and the 2003 congress to Birmingham to be run jointly with the AAGBI. The time scale for the Florence meeting was recognised to be extremely challenging, 3 years instead of the usual 8 years, but Professor Novelli and his team were confident that a joint CENSA/SIAARTI meeting was feasible and would be a huge success.

The ESA regarded the changes in congress timing to be a direct competitive challenge and the concept of a joint congress for 2002 could no longer exist due to the change in dates for the CENSA meetings.

However, there appeared to be a renewed enthusiasm for more talks between the various protagonists within Europe to find a new way forward, and CENSA certainly wished to be involved in that process.

The Florence Congress of 2001 was a huge success culturally, socially, scientifically, and financially. Professor Novelli and his team created a truly memorable congress made more poignant by the death shortly after the Congress of Professor Novelli much to the sadness of all of his European colleagues. The board changed its composition again with Dr. Wilkinson (Great Britain and Ireland) becoming President (a change in title to bring CENSA in line with other European organisations), Professor Scherpereel (France), President-elect and Honorary Secretary, Professor Sellevold (Norway) honorary treasurer, Professor Janecsko (Hungary) vice-President, and Drs. Ward (Great Britain and Ireland), de Sousa (Portugal), Trenkler (Slovak Republic), and Conti (Italy) together with Professors Gurman and Hempelmann were elected as board members. By this stage CENSA symposia were established in a wide variety of national meetings. In addition, CENSA had adopted a much more-robust stance to educational matters and thanks to outstanding work buy Gaby Gurman a comprehensive pattern of educational aid was created in a West meets East document approved in Florence. This set up a series of educational initiatives funded by CENSA, the WFSA, and by wealthier societies in Europe that could benefit the less-affluent societies in the region. One example of this was that the educational projects that had been running for years in Beer-Sheva, Israel were duplicated in Romania and Italy for the benefit of Moldavia and Albania. Maria Janecsko chaired the educational subcommittee of CENSA that co-ordinated this activity.

The European Federation of Anaesthesia

In October 1998 the Academy hosted a meeting in London to try to take anaesthetic co-operation in Europe a step further. Representatives from the EAA, ESA, CENSA, and the UEMS had productive talks. A proposal was made that a European Federation of Anaesthesiology be formed as an umbrella organisation encompassing the EAA, ESA, and CENSA. It was further suggested that the *European Journal of Anaesthesia* become the approved journal of the three organisations, and that some method of organising joint meetings be determined. A working group took the concept further and the EFA board met again in January 1999 in Brussels. Here, after detailed discussion, it was agreed to work towards the creation of a single European entity. A further meeting would take place at the ESA Congress in Amsterdam in May and that meeting's programme would carry the logos of the ESA, EAA, and CENSA. No representative from CENSA attended that meeting following some confusion relating to the timing of statements concerning CENSA European Congresses. The ESA board withheld the CENSA logo from the meeting. The EFA board met again in Budapest in August of 1999 when CENSA again attended. Here the opportunity for a truly joint congress in 2003 in the United Kingdom was confirmed. A decision would be dependent on agreement with the AAGBI who had been awarded the congress on behalf of CENSA. The ESA agreed to open negotiations with AAGBI on this topic. Agreement was reached that the *European Journal of Anaesthesia* would be the official journal of all the EFA organisations and their logos would be appended to the front cover.

A further meeting of the EFA in January 2000 in London confirmed a mission statement and regulations of the new organisation. These were published in the EAA and ESA Newsletters. It was noted that in 2001 CENSA would hold a meeting in Florence and that the ESA and EAA would hold another conference at a separate venue several months away. (This was subsequently confirmed for Gothenburg.) In 2002 it was hoped to hold a collaborative meeting with all three organisations, leading up to a truly joint meeting in 2003. This proved to be the case with 2002 running in Nice and 2003 taking place in Glasgow instead of the original choice of Birmingham for commercial reasons. This latter meeting, although hosted by AAGBI, was essentially a ESA meeting. The term Euroanaesthesia was applied to the Nice and Glasgow meetings and would be the name for future congresses.

Board meetings for the EFA continued at regular intervals throughout 2000, 2001, and 2002. Step by step a greater confidence in the process was developed and this was greatly enhanced by a very productive EFA task force meeting held in Munster in June 2002. This was an attempt to create a binding form of statutes and bylaws to enable true amalgamation to take place by January 2005. However, in recent months legal constraints and a variety of decisions by individuals and boards have yet again caused a ripple of dissatisfaction to run through the EFA organisation.

Whether these problems can be resolved satisfactorily is unclear at this time of writing and the future of a fully unified single European anaesthesia organisation remains unconfirmed.

Latest congress

The most-recent congress to have taken place was that in Glasgow in 2003. Here for the first time the ESA, the Academy, and CENSA ran a joint meeting hosted by the AAGBI. It was an excellent meeting enjoyed by most and showed what might yet be achieved in the future with sufficient good will from all involved. The scientific, social, and financial success of the meeting was encouraging. The current CENSA board includes David Wilkinson (Great Britain and Ireland) President, Philippe Scherpereel (France) President-elect, Michael Ward (Great Britain and Ireland) Honorary Secretary, Olav Sellevold (Norway) honorary treasurer (co-opted), Maria Janecsko (Hungary) chairman of the Education Committee (co-opted), Stefan Trenkler (Slovak Republic), Carlos Couceiro de Sousa (Portugal), Giorgio Conti (Italy), Zeev Goldik (Israel), and Laslo Vimlati (Hungary).

The future

CENSA remains the European "arm" of the WFSA. It has over many decades struggled hard to promote and enhance anaesthesia across the whole of the continent. Its aims, like those of its parent body, the WFSA, are sound and achievable. There are few if any other voices in Europe that truly represent the whole of anaesthesia in this manner, and CENSA is bound to continue its endeavours in the future. It is hoped that these will be in some formal collaboration with other bodies within Europe, but this cannot be to the detriment of CENSA's basic aims. There is great enthusiasm within European anaesthesia and CENSA and the WFSA will continue to harness this together for the benefit of our profession.

Acknowledgements. I am very grateful to Michael Vickers and John Zorab for their efforts to provide me with accurate information on which to write this essay. I am particularly grateful to Professor Otto Mayrhofer for allowing me to read and use considerable portions of a draft paper he wrote, but never published, on the early development of the WFSA. Judy Robbins, of the Wood Library Museum of Anesthesiology in Chicago that holds the WFSA archive, has again provided invaluable assistance. My thanks also go to Ruth Hooper in the WFSA office in London who was able to unearth further relevant papers.

12 A HISTORY OF INTERNATIONAL CONTACTS OF RUSSIAN ANAESTHESIOLOGY

E.A. Damir

Introduction

Modern anaesthesia-early history in the USSR

The political situation in the USSR after World War II made international contacts difficult, with the Communist Party and the KGB controlling all personal contacts and correspondence. However, there were good medical libraries in the main cities (Moscow, Leningrad, capitals of republics), which were financed by the government. Moreover, in order to keep abreast with medical and research advances worldwide, it became important for Russian doctors to learn foreign languages. Leading surgeons started to realise the necessity of improving anaesthesia.

Early period of international surgical contacts

In the early period of modern anaesthesiology the most-important work was initiated by leading surgeons, who were the teachers and supporters of the first anaesthesiologists in the USSR. Leading surgeons were also very important for initiating international contacts in anaesthesiology.

The first visits of distinguished Russian surgeons and scientists to departments of anaesthesia in West European countries for training were organised in the early 1950s by Professor Alexander N. Bakulev, Professor Petr A. Kuprianov, Professor Eugeni N. Meshalkin, Professor Vladimir A. Negovski (Physiology), Professor Boris V. Petrovski, Professor Aleksander V.Vishnevski, Professor Sergei S.Yudin, and Professor Isaak S. Zhorov.

Professor Isaak S. Zhorov

Professor Isaak S. Zhorov was a surgeon and the author of the textbooks *Noninhalation Anaesthesia* (1936) and *General Anaesthesia* (1959). He was head of one of the first schools of anaesthesiology, and he organised the section of anaesthesiology of Moscow's Society of Surgeons. He initiated extensive contacts with British and German anaesthesiologists. He was elected a fellow of the Royal College of Surgeons (UK) for his work in anaesthesiology, and he invited Professor Rudolf Frey of Germany to Moscow to lecture on anaesthesiology.

Professor Boris V. Petrovski

Professor Boris V. Petrovski was a surgeon and academic. He was a Minister of Health who helped to establish anaesthesiology as an independent specialty. He organised one of the first schools of anaesthesiology, an independent department of anaesthesiology in his clinic (1959) and the first chair of anaesthesiolgy at a Russian medical school (1963) (Professor Olga D. Koliutskaja was its first occupant).

Professor B. Petrovski initiated extensive international contacts. He organised 6 months training in the United Kingdom for his pupil Armen Bunatian (at Dr. John Nunn's Department of Anaesthesiology). He was elected fellow of the Royal College of Surgeons (UK).

As Minister of Health he organised for Russian specialists to attend the 1-year WHO training courses in anaesthesia in Copenhagen (Elena Damir 1958, Victor Strashnov 1959, Stepan Zolnikov 1960).

Professor Alexander N. Bakulev

Professor Alexander N. Bakulev was a pioneer of pulmonary (1946) and cardiovascular (1948) surgery in the USSR. He was also an academic and former President of the Medical Academy of the USSR.

His clinic was the first in Russia to appoint two full-time anaesthesiologists-Dr. Gennadii Ryabov (1953), later an academic and distinguished scientist, and Dr. Juri Savinov. In 1956 Professor A. Bakulev organised an independent department of anaesthesiology and invited as a director Dr. Victor Smolnikov, who returned to the USSR after many years in China.

Professor Eugeni N. Meshalkin

Professor Eugeni N. Meshalkin, surgeon, professor, and academic, was a pupil of A. Bakulev and a pioneer of cardiovascular surgery. He introduced endotracheal anaesthesia into clinical pratice in Russia (1946) and was the author of a textbook *Intubation (endotracheal) Anaesthesia* (1953).

He was occupant of the first USSR Chair of Thoracic Surgery and Anaesthesiology (1956) at the Institute for Postgraduate Training of Physicians. In 1956 he first organised regular 4- to 5-month courses of anaesthesiology for surgeons, and in 1959 an independent Chair of Anaesthesiology (Dr. Elena Damir) in the Institute for Postgraduate Training of Physicians.

Professor Petr A. Kuprianov

Professor Petr A. Kuprianov, a surgeon and academic, was for many years Chief Consultant for Military Surgery at the Ministry of Defence and Director of the Clinic of Military Surgery at the Military Medical Academy in Leningrad (St. Peterburg). In 1947 he organised 3 months training in Sweden for his pupil Dr. M. Anichkov (at Professor Bjork's clinic). Dr. Anichkov introduced the use of endotracheal anaesthesia in thoracic surgery and published the book *Endotracheal Anaesthesia in Thoracic Surgery* (1948). Professor Kuprianov organised 2 months training in the Czechoslovakian Socialist Republic for two pupils - Dr. B.Uvarov (later, 1963, Professor of Anaesthesiology) and Dr. Ju. Shanin (later distinguished researcher in the field of controlled ventilation). Professor P. Kuprianov established the first Chair of Anaesthesiology (1958) at the Military Academy and remained its occupant until 1963.

Professor A.V. Vishnevski and his son A.A. Vishnevski

Professor A.V. Vishnevski and his son A.A. Vishnevski were the founders of local anaesthesia in the USSR (1930). Professor Vishenvski suggested the method of *"Tight crawling infiltration anaesthesia"* (the textbook published in 1932). He established the Research Institute for Surgery in Moscow (1948). In 1959 he established within the institute one of the first independent departments of anaesthesiology (chief Dr. T. Darbinian, later distinguished researcher). Professor T. Darbinian was elected as the first President of the independent Society of Anaesthesiology of the USSR (1957). He introduced neuroleptanalgesia into Russia. Due to his initiative the Society of Anaesthesiology became a member of WFSA (1972).

Professor Vladimir A. Negovski

The emergence of reanimatology (intensive therapy) as an independent specialty and an important part of anaesthesiology is connected with the work of Dr V. Negovski, academic, founder of the Experimental Research Laboratory (1936) and Research Institute (1985). Research into clinical death and resuscitation was started during World War II in 1942, and continued after the war in the clinic of Professor A. Bakulev (1948-1956) and in the Botkin Hospital, where the first independent department of reanimatology (intensive therapy) was established in 1959. V. Negovski initiated extensive international contacts and co-operation. Research, exchange of specialists, and collaboration in disaster medicine were carried out with P. Safar's institute (USA), Dr. R. Frey (West Germany), Dr. V. Kvetan (USA), and Dr S. Saev (Bulgaria), amongst others.

Early period of international anaesthesia contacts

Again it is necessary to remember the political situation in the USSR at that time. Russian doctors and scientists had to overcome enormous difficulties to achieve personal contact with our colleagues abroad, to participate in international congresses, and to invite guests from other countries. For any foreign contact we were required to obtain the permission of the Ministry of Health through its Foreign Department. The local Communist Party cell needed to give preliminary approval for each foreign initiative.

At that time all Soviet specialists were divided into "drive-out permitted" and "drive-out forbidden". This meant that some of us were not able to accept invitations from foreign colleagues even if all necessary arrangements had been made. The reasons for being "drive-out forbidden" were in most cases not known. I would mention that difficulties of this sort were even worse in some other socialist countries (e.g., the GDR).

In the early period of the development of modern anaesthesiology the WHO suggested that the Ministry of Health of the USSR send young doctors to a 1-year WHO Course of Anaesthesiology in Copenhagen, Denmark. The teachers were leading Danish anaesthesiologists. During the period, 1958-1960, three specialists were trained. The Danish teachers were Drs. W. Andersen, W. Dam, J. Jorgensen, Kirhoff, H. Ruben, and O. Seko, and Professor Churchill-Davidson (UK) and Professor H. Livingston (USA) were invited lecturers. The Russian trainees included Dr. Elena A.Damir (1958), later Professor of Anaesthesiology (1959), Institute for Postgraduate Training of Physicians; Dr. Victor Strashnov (1959), later Professor of Anaesthesiology (1966), Leningrad Medical School; and Dr. Stepan M. Zolnikov (1960), later director of the Research Institute of Reflexotherapy (1970).

WFSA and its European Regional Section (ERS, later CENSA)

WFSA and its European Regional Section (ERS, later CENSA) accepted as a member the All-Union Society of Anaesthesiologists and Reanimatologists in 1972. Since then we have had the continuing support of WFSA for our educational programme. Past and present WFSA Presidents have visited our country (Moscow, St. Peterburg, Tashkent, Kiev). These have included Professor F. Foldes (1970), Professor O. Mayrhofer (1974), Professor Q.Gomez (1978), Professor J. Bonica (1982), Dr. C. Parsloe (1986), Dr. J. Zorab (1988, 1990), Professor M. Vickers (1996), and Dr. K. Brown (1996). All participated in our congresses, gave lectures, visited hospitals, and discussed training programmes.

WFSA involvement in the Russian Society (Federation of Anaesthesiologists and Reanimatologists) since 1972

Since 1972 the following Russian doctors have held positions within WFSA: Professor T. Darbinian, vice-President (1976-1980); Professor A. Bunatian, member of Committee on Education (1992-2000); Professor E. Damir, member of Executive Committee (1988-1996), member of committee on resuscitation (1984-1988); Professor I. Molchanov, member of Committee on Statutes and Vylaws (2000-2004); Professor B.Gelfand, vice-chairman of committee on resuscitation, trauma and intensive care (2000-2004); Dr. M. Cherednichenko, member of committee on quality of practice (1996-2004).

WFSA Committee on Education supported refresher courses in Russia

With financial support from WFSA and societies of anaesthesiology of the United States, Japan and several Western European countries, our society was able to organise short-term international refresher courses in Moscow, St. Peterburg, Khabarovsk, Ekaterinburg, Yerevan, Tbilisi, Tashkent, and the Baltic Republics. The number of participants of some courses was as many as 150-200. Unfortunately severe financial problems made travel through our huge distances very limited. However, due to above-mentioned financial support we were able to have a visiting teaching programme organised by groups of distinguished specialists from many countries in the USSR and Russia.

Particularly important international contacts and teaching programmes were organised with the inestimable help of Professor George De Castro (Belgium), Professor Rudolf Frey (Germany), Dr. Richard Jack (UK), Professor Joachim Nadstawek (Germany), Professor Ellison (Jeep) Pierce (USA), Dr. Svetlana Rutter (Tchernikhovskaja) (UK), Professor Peter Safar (USA), Dr. Frank Walters (UK), Professor Vladimir Zelman (USA), and Dr. John Zorab (UK).

European Academy of Anaesthesiology

The Society of Anaesthesiologists of the USSR and Russia have had contact with the European Academy of Anaesthesiology (EAA) since 1978, when Professor Tigran Darbinian and Elena Damir were elected to the membership. We were sorry not to be able to participate regularly in the meetings. The reason was at first political and later financial. There was great interest in the European Diploma Examination in Anaesthesiology, especially when the Russian language was accepted and part I and part II examinations were organised in Moscow. Unfortunately the Academy discontinued this after 3 years. We consider that this might not bode well for the acceptance of our country into the European Union.

13 WFSA AND THE LAND OF THE RISING SUN

K. Shimoji

It was a truly memorable day, 19 September 1972, when the 5th World Congress of Anaesthesiologists (WCA), sponsored by the World Federation of Anaesthesiologists (WFSA) and organised by the Japanese Society of Anaesthesiologists (JSA), took place in the beautiful city of Kyoto, an ancient capital of Japan. This congress was presided over by Professor Hideo Yamamura, University of Tokyo, and chaired by the late Professor Akira Inamoto, Kyoto University. The Opening Ceremony of the 1st day of this meeting was attended by the "Kohtaishi" (Prince of Japan, now the "Tennoh", the Emperor) and his wife, Princess Michiko, and many other cabinet and local government representatives. Now, I think it is time that second - and third-generation members of JSA should host the WCA in Japan in the near future, welcoming as many WFSA members as possible from all over the world.

Since the establishment of the WFSA, the JSA has been supporting the Federation in various ways, such as sending many scholars to attend the WFSA meetings, serving as committee members of the WFSA, and donating to the anaesthetic societies of developing countries when necessary. WFSA committee members from Japan have actively served during the last 50 years and are listed in chronological order for the last 30 years in Table 1.

As most anaesthesiologists know, Dr. Seishu Hanaoka carried out general anaesthesia using Mafutsusan successfully for surgical extirpation of breast cancer in 1806, almost 40 years before Drs. Wells, Morton, Simpson, and Snow successfully used nitrous oxide, ether, and chloroform in 1845, 1846, and 1847, respectively [1]. Unfortunately, however, there have been few Japanese successors during the Edo era (during which Japan was isolated from the rest of the world) and even later eras that have developed and promoted Dr. Hanaoka's outstanding methods. Nevertheless, some of his students used the same methods for various forms of surgery during the Edo era by obtaining informed consent [2].

As soon as the Meiji era began, which marked the end of 300 years of Edo isolation in 1868, knowledge and techniques of western medicine, includ-

Table 1. *WFSA committee members from Japan in the last 30 years*

Years	Committee	Name (Professor)
1973-1980	Vice-President	Inamoto A*, Iwatsuki K
	Membership	Yamamura H (Chairman)
	Finance	Fujita T
1984-1991	Vice-President	Miyazaki M, Nishimura N, Iwai S*
	Executive	Nishimura N, Mori K
	Education	Fujimori M
	Statutes and Bylaws	Fujita M*
	Resuscitation	Fujita T
	Obstetric Anaesthesia and Analgesia	Fujimori M
	Safety in Anaesthesia	Oyama T
	Paediatric Anaesthesia	Iwai S*
1992-2000	Vice-President	Mori K
	Education	Fujimori M (Chairman)
	Statutes & Bylaws	Fujita M*
	Publication	Ogawa R
	Resuscitation	Yoshiya I
	Obstetric Anaesthesia and Analgesia	Kosaka Y, Aoki M*
	Safety, Equipment and Technology	Sato T, Fukushima K
	Paediatric Anaesthesia	Sankawa H
	Pain	Shimoji K (Chairman)
2001-	Executive	Hanaoka K
	Obstetric Anaesthesia and Analgesia	(Aoki M)*
	Resuscitation	Sakabe T
	Paediatric Anaesthesia	Obara H
	Safety, Equipment, and Technology	Kugimiya T

*Deceased

ing anaesthesia, flowed into Japan until the so-called second period of isolation during the Second World War.

Modern techniques and knowledge of anaesthesia were introduced into Japan by Dr. Meyer Saklad from America after the Second World War. Thus, modern anaesthesiology is a relatively new medical field in Japan. It used to be one of the subunits of general surgery like other surgical fields such as neurosurgery or orthopaedic surgery until the end of the Second World War [3]. During the occupation of Japan by GHQ (General Headquarters, American Army), Dr. Saklad was invited to Japan to introduce modern anaesthesia practice by the Japan-America Association of Medical Education. Dr. Saklad's lecture had a strong impact on surgeons who were involved in post-war medical education in Japan.

Due to the importance of anaesthesia for vital physiological processes and intensive medical care, the JSA introduced a board examination system (written, oral, and practical) in 1962, which has been held once a year. At the same time, the Japanese Ministry of Health and Welfare (JMH) introduced a license for practising general anaesthesia for medical doctors who had trained for 2 years under the supervision of the JSA board holders (category I) or those with experience of more than 300 cases of general anaesthesia evenly distributed throughout the surgical fields (category II). The number of the JSA board holders has increased from considerably in the last 4 decades [4]. Surprisingly, however, the number of JMH license holders practising clinical anaesthesia exceeds those of JSA members [4], which indicates that there are many practising clinical anaesthesia who are not members of the JSA.

This might be because JMH license holders are legally permitted to practise clinical anaesthesia in Japan, excluding dentists who are allowed to administer general anaesthesia only for dental treatment. In other words, some JMH license holders are practising general anaesthesia as a part of their own surgical specialties because of a shortage of anaesthesia specialists or to save costs on general anaesthesia.

Despite the rapid increase in the numbers of JSA board holders in Japan, the total number of specialists is still far behind those in the United States, England, and Europe (Table 2) [5–7].

Another characteristic feature of anaesthesiologists in Japan is the uneven distribution of JSA members among the prefectures [8, 9]. Although it is conceivable that anaesthesiologists like other medical specialties tend to concentrate in large cities such as Tokyo and Osaka, where there are many large hospitals, large variations in distribution are noted by regions. In general, numbers of JSA members are low in the eastern part of Japan compared with western Japan, excluding Hokkaido (the furthest outreach of eastern Japan): west high, east low (the phrase spoken frequently to express a wintry pressure pattern over the Japanese islands).

The inadequate number of anaesthesiologists in Japan seems to arise from four factors. Firstly, the independence of anaesthesia from general surgery was delayed until the end of the Second World War. This still results in a lack of familiarity among the general public, as demonstrated by the fact that approximately 50% of patients in our university hospital were unaware of the role

Table 2. *Comparison of anaesthesiologist numbers in Japan with those in other countries*

	Japan	**USA**[b]	**England**	**EU**
A Numbers of anaesthesiologists per population (10^5)[a]	3.7	9.0	4.6	9.2
B Numbers of all medical doctors per population (10^3)	1.8	2.6	1.6	3.5
C A/B (10^2)	2.05	3.46	2.87	2.63

[a]Grossly calculated through the data in (1) the Japanese Ministry of Health and Welfare: a white paper on health and welfare, 2001, (2) Japan Society of Anaesthesiologists: Directory of Members, 2002, (3) American Society of Anaesthesiologists: Directory of Members, 2002, and (4) Rolly G (1996) Eur J Anaesthsiol 13:325–335
[b]Besides anaesthesiologists, nurse anaesthetists provide much of the care (modified from reference 3)

of anaesthesiologists at the pre-anaesthetic interview (unpublished personal data). Secondly, medical school departments in Japan still adhere to a bureaucracy that prevents radical and open treatment of patients under a medical team that includes anaesthesiologists. Thirdly, all payments and claims by national and private sector medical insurance must be made through one doctor (a front desk doctor) in the main department where the patients is treated, not by each specialist in different departments, such as anaesthesiologists, radiologists, or pathologists. This system makes it difficult for anaesthesiologists to claim payment for their own surgical anaesthesia practice from an insurance organisation or directly from the patients. Fourthly, payment from medical insurance organisations in Japan is based upon the total costs of the treatment for each patient. This system again tends to favour staff without a JSA board license or private hospital owners who pay the anaesthesia specialist. Thus, surgical anaesthesia is inclined to be administered by a JMH license holder or other surgical staff without a JSA board license. However, the high prefectural variability in numbers of JSA members seems to be due to regional differences in the first and second factors rather than the third or fourth.

Although it is difficult to define the anaesthesia workforce in different countries simply, due to their different medical insurance systems, this gross comparison might allow anaesthesiologists, particularly those in developing countries, to educate the public.

References

1. Matsuki A (2000) New studies on the history of anesthesiology - a new study on Seishu Hanaoka's "Nyugan Chiken Roku" (a surgical experience with breast cancer) (in Japanese with an English abstract). Masui 49:1038-1043

2. Yamauchi K, Fuwa H (1996) Analysis of old surgical operations of the Drs Ishin Fuwa who graduated from Hanaoka School of Medicine (in Japanese with an English abstract). Nippon Ishigaku Zasshi 42:61-76

3. Taga K, Fujihara H, Baba H, Yamakura T, Shimoji K (2002) Workforce and regional distribution of anaesthesiologists in Japan. Eur J Anaesthesiol 19:530-532

4. Japan Society of Anesthesiologists (2002) Annual report (in Japanese) 32, pp 172-73

5. The Japanese Ministry of Health and Welfare (2001) A White Paper of Health and Welfare (in Japanese), pp 162-179

6. American Society of Anesthesiologists (2001) Directory of Members

7. Rolly G (1996) Anaesthesiological manpower in Europe. Eur J Anaeshtesiol 13:325-335

8. Japan Society of Anesthesiologists (2002) Directory of Members (in Japanese)

9. Saito T (1996) Sogo Chireki Shinchizu (General Historical New Map) (in Japanese). Teikoku-Shoin, Tokyo, pp 117-118

14 THE SOUTH AFRICAN SOCIETY OF ANAESTHESIOLOGISTS AND ITS ROLE IN THE WFSA

N. Parbhoo

he foundation of the South African Society of Anaesthetists (SASA) on 1 August 1943 was an event of major significance in the development of South African medicine. It was the result of a historical chain of events and the tireless service and selfless devotion of a few dedicated individuals. It is thus to the lasting credit of those that came after the "masters" that the ideals of the society were perpetuated.

Although Dr. William Thomas Green Morton is acknowledged as the father of anaesthesia for having successfully demonstrated ether anaesthesia at the Ether Dome at Massachussetts General Hospital, Boston, on 16 October 1846, South African doctors were not far behind in experimenting and successfully using this agent.

Dr. Ebden at the Old Somerset Hospital, during early trials with ether in Cape Town in April 1847, used an ordinary bullock's bladder fitted with a mouthpiece with a sponge in it. On 20 April 1847, it was reported in *De Verzamelaar* (The Gleaner) that Mr. Raymond, a dental surgeon of Cape Town, had successfully used ether vapour to extract teeth from two men. In June 1847 Dr. William Guybon Atherstone recorded in detail his success in amputating a leg using ether vapour as an anaesthetic.

In 1862, the rebuilt New Somerset Hospital became the first teaching hospital in South Africa. In the north, when the discovery of gold in 1886 caused Johannesburg to grow into a large city of 50,000 inhabitants, a need arose for the building of Johannesburg General Hospital. In 1907 Dr. G.W. Bampfylde Daniell was appointed its anaesthetist, the first such appointment in the country. He was a prolific writer and a very keen lecturer. Credit is due for establishing the specialty in South Africa. Ralph Waters once wrote: "The foundation of any specialty is dependent, I suppose, first upon men, second upon publications and third upon organisations through which men meet for mutual development by exchange of ideas".

As in the United States and the United Kingdom, general practitioners and dentists gave the anaesthetics. Among those were men dedicated to advancing this sphere of practice. In Cape Town, Drs. Harry Berelowitz, Royden Muir, and Eric van Hoogstraten, and in Johannesburg Drs. Benjamin Weinbren and Frank B Mudd, were the senior anaesthetists involved in the teaching of techniques in anaesthesia.

With the advent of World War II, there was an acute shortage of anaesthetists and many doctors joined the Royal Army Medical Corps and South African Medical Corps and offered their services. At the end of the war, anaesthetists returned from overseas and were able to teach local staff new techniques. South African doctors with their brief exposure to anaesthesia expressed a keen desire to improve their skills and knowledge. They often used to meet informally at each other's homes and listen to lectures by experts in their field. It was at one of these informal meetings that Dr. R.A. Moore-Dyke proposed the formation of a South African Society of Anaesthetists (SASA). SASA was inaugurated on 1 August 1943 on a Sunday afternoon at the Johannesburg General Hospital (later known as the Hillbrow Hospital). Dr. Moore-Dyke was proposed as President but he declined in favour of his senior, Dr. Benjamin Weinbren. Dr. Weinbren had been a part-time anaesthetist to the Johannesburg General Hospital since 1916. Born in Lithuania in 1889, he came to South Africa at a very early age, received his education in Johannesburg, and obtained his MBChB in Edinburgh in 1912. He continued with postgraduate studies for a further 2 years and then returned to South Africa to general practice. From 1920 he devoted his practice solely to anaesthesia.

"Pom" Dyke was elected secretary/treasurer. Invitations to attend the meeting were sent to all practising anaesthetists in the Union of South Africa (most of whom were in the Transvaal), as well as to the volunteer anaesthetists in the South African Medical Corps stationed at the various military hospitals in the Union.

The South African Medical and Dental Council Register in 1943 recorded that there were 26 anaesthetists, 48 ear, nose, and throat surgeons, 40 obstetricians and gynaecologists, 53 ophthalmologists, 9 orthopaedic surgeons, 73 general surgeons, and 12 urologists. Those present at the meeting were Benjamin Weinbren, Harry Grant-Whyte, David Crawford, Sam Hoffman, David Feldman, Sam Lipron, Blumy Segal, Miriam Barlow, Cyril Becker, Ronald Moore-Dyke, Duff Scott, Hymie Samson, John Duffield, and Charles Arkles.

Weinbren stated that the chief aims of the society would be to safeguard the economic status of anaesthetists (looking back we must commend him on his foresight), to educate so that the specialty might be recognised, and to encourage self criticism, lest local anaesthetists fell behind in the scientific advances in anaesthesia.

A constitution was drawn up and apart from the addition of various bylaws and some amendments, it remains essentially the same today. One of the first decisions taken was to approach the Federal Council of the Medical Association to form this society under the auspices of the association. The next was to approach the International Anaesthesia Research Society for affiliation. This research society was formed in 1925 as an extension of the National Anaesthesia Society, with Dr. Francis Hoeffer McMechan as executive secretary/editor. The third item for discussion was the registration of anaesthetists by the South African Medical and Dental Council and the question of minimum requirements for such registration. At that time all that was required was a medical qualification plus proof of having spent 1 year in training at a hospital in that specialty under the supervision of an anaesthetic specialist.

By the end of the 1st year, of 31 practising anaesthetists, 30 had become members of SASA. Already in its formative year the council of SASA had successfully negotiated an improvement in the emoluments of recent appointments and there had been an advance in the status of anaesthesia per se. The executive now took up the task of convincing authorities that independent departments of anaesthesia should be set up at the medical schools of Witwatersrand and Cape Town.

By 1946 SASA was a recognised body and at the 34th South African Medical Congress, anaesthetists were for the very first time accorded the privilege of a section devoted solely to anaesthesia; this was in addition to the plenary session to commemorate the centenary of ether anaesthesia. It was at this congress that a resolution was passed to request the establishment of chairs in anaesthesia at the existing medical schools. It was also at this meeting that the idea of a SASA "newsletter" was born. Drs. C.S. Jones and J.T. Hayward-Butt as editors brought out the first issue in February 1947.

Most of 1948 was spent in correspondence with the dean of the Faculty of Medicine, University of Witwatersrand regarding the possible introduction of a diploma in anaesthesia. This came to fruition in 1949 when the DA in anaesthesia was offered by the University. In 1950, after the tabling of a report on postgraduate education that a body akin to the colleges in the United Kingdom should be established in South Africa, SASA was the first specialty society to ask for separate faculties, each having the right to examine under the aegis of the college.

The 2nd decade of SASA

Highlights of the 2nd decade included SASA becoming a founder member of the World Federation of the Societies of Anaesthesiologists (WFSA) in Holland in 1955. SASA also liaised with the South African Nursing Council to formulate a syllabus for the training of nurses in the care of the unconscious patient - just one facet of such meetings. A firm stand was also taken by SASA to convince the South African Medical and Dental Council to institute compulsory training in anaesthesia for interns. On the medico-legal side, the speed with which the Inquest Act was being altered was a matter of concern to the society and negotiations with the Department of Justice continued for many years, ultimately with success in November 1972 with the arrival of form H471.01.06 - the forerunner of paper inquests.

The quest of the society to have chairs in anaesthesia established finally succeeded when Professor O.V.S. Kok was appointed to the University of Pretoria in 1959, Professor J.C. Nicholson at the University of Witwatersrand in 1962, Professor H. Grant-Whyte in Natal in 1964, and Professor A.B. Bull at the University of Cape Town in 1965.

In 1960, as part of its role in ongoing education, SASA started a visiting lecturer's fund, based on a proposal put forward by Dr. Jack Abelsohn in August 1950. This fund still enables SASA to invite overseas lecturers to various congresses. Tariff determination, remuneration for sessional appointments on the South African Railway and Harbour Fund, and salaries for full-timers occupied the major portion of the SASA council's deliberation.

In September 1962, Dr. Dennis T. Glauber, acting for the tariff subcommittee, proposed a unit value schedule for tariff determination. This tariff has stood the test of time for 40 years and is presently in 2003 an issue of copyright for the South African Medical Association.

The 3ʳᵈ decade of SASA

In the 3rd decade, the SASA's endeavours shifted more towards the business sphere; prolonged negotiations with medical aid schemes took place in an attempt to improve the economic status of its members. SASA also held its first congress, separate from that of the Medical Association of South Africa. A group of academic anaesthetists felt that SASA was not devoting sufficient attention to academia and as result the Association of University Anaesthetists (AUA) was formed in September 1972. In later years their role overlapped in continuing medical education, both with SASA and the College of Medicine of South Africa and the society was disbanded.

During this period SASA also dealt at length with the controversial issue of nurse anaesthetists. Medico-legal implications finally, years later, did away with this. The first human heart transplant in December 1969 was the outstanding event of this decade, indicating to the world the interdependence of the anaesthetist, surgeon, and transplant team.

The 4ᵗʰ decade of SASA

Over the next 10 years, the public health aspects of anaesthesia came to the fore, with SASA playing a leading role in setting the standards for the safety of theatre equipment and the control of in-theatre pollution. Congresses were a regular feature of the society's activities. SASA continued to promote education with the award of the Diploma in Anaesthesia medal (renamed the SASA John Couper Medal). These efforts continued into the next decade, which saw the publication of *Guidelines for Practice* and subsequently *Guidelines for Intensive Care*.

Like all established bodies, SASA now felt that there was a need for an easily recognisable corporate identity. This led to the registration of the society's crest and coat of arms. For his role in first administering ether anaesthesia for a major operation, the amputation of a limb, in Grahamstown, South Africa on 12 June 1847, the family coat of arms of Dr. W.G. Atherstone was chosen, modified, and registered.

As a result of an unforeseen profit from the first SASA congress, separate from that of MASA, the Council of SASA voted in favour of setting up a research fund with this money. This was named the Jan Pretorius Research Fund in honour of the congress organiser Dr. Jan Pretorius who was killed tragically soon after.

The 5ᵗʰ decade of SASA

As the years went by, the outstanding efforts of certain members in enhancing the reputation of SASA and that of anaesthesia per se did not go unrecognised. Periodically in recognition thereof, honorary life vice-presidencies were awarded, the highest award SASA is constitutionally able to award. Since 1954, nine members have been recipients: Drs. Benjamin Weinbren, Jack Abelsohn, and Don Fisher Jeffes and Professors O.V.S. Kok, Hilde Ginsberg, Drs. Dennis Glauber, Jimmy Durham, Oscar Rosenzweig, and Professor John Couper.

The quest to raise the standard of anaesthetic training to equal that anywhere in the developed world was achieved by the Joint Conference of Boards and Faculties of Anaesthetists, represented initially by the English speaking countries - the United Kingdom, Ireland, Australia, South Africa, Canada, and the United States, in 1980.

To commemorate the first 50 years of the society, the official history of SASA-"*Five Decades - The South African Society of Anaesthetists 1943-1993*", by Nagin Parbhoo was launched at the society's Jubilee Congress held in Cape Town in March 1993.

For decades, SASA members have been clamouring for a publication of their very own. Apart from the *South African Medical Journal* and the MASA branch newsletters, there was no other conduit for the dissemination of anaesthetic matters to members throughout the land. This was remedied by the publication *Pipeline/Pyplyn*, a quarterly newsletter. In September 2001, *The South African Journal of Anaesthesia and Analgesia* - the official journal of the South Africa Society of Anaesthesiologists was launched at the 2ⁿᵈ All Africa Congress in Durban (ISSN-1027-9148).

WFSA and SASA

WFSA was established in Scheveningen, the Netherlands on 9 September 1955. The 26 founder member societies included the South African Society of Anaesthetists. Their official WFSA delegate was Dr. F.W. (Bobby) Roberts who was also the signatory for Zuid Afrika approving the statutes of WFSA. SASA was the 9th anaesthetic society to be established in the world and the very first in Africa. Nine SASA members attended this 1st WFSA Congress, making South Africans the largest group representing a country. From the rest of Africa two other countries were represented, with Egypt sending three delegates and Kenya one.

Since foundation, SASA members have continued to play an important role in the WFSA, the highest council in anaesthesia. Professor O.V.S. Kok was first elected to the executive, finance, and Regional Committees and was then regional director for Africa (1960-1964), then chairman of both the finance and Nomination Committees (1964-1968), and later elected a vice-President of WFSA (1968-1972). For this latter period Professor H. Grant-Whyte was elected to the committee on membership. During 1972-1976, Professor A.B. Bull was on the WFSA foundation board of trustees, Professor H. Grant-Whyte on the committee on obstetric anaesthesia, and Dr. Dennis Glauber chaired a scientific session at the 5th World Congress in Kyoto, Japan. Professor J.L. Couper served on the Membership Committee (1980-1984) and Professor J. Downing on the Obstetric Committee for the same years. For 1984-1988, Dr J. Danchin was elected to the Finance and Nomination Committees and Professor P. Foster to the Executive, Scientific Committee of congress and the Committee on Education and Scientific Affairs.

For 1988-1992, Dr. B. Murray served on the Safety Committee, Dr. J. Danchin on the Finance Committee, Professor P. Foster on the Executive Committee, and Professor J.L. Couper on the Education Committee. The years 1992-1996 saw B. Murray on the Safety Committee, Professor D.F. Morrell on quality of Practice Committee, Professor P. Foster as honorary vice-President and editor of the WFSA newsletter, Publications Committee. Both Professors D.F. Morrell and D.A. Rocke chaired scientific meetings and served on the trauma and obstetric scientific Session Committees, respectively.

The period 1996-2000 saw the first edition of *World Anaesthesia,* the joint adventure of *World Anaesthesia Newsletter* (Bill Case) and *Anaesthesia Worldwide* (editors Patrick Foster and Bosseau Murray), which appeared in April 1997. April 1997 also saw the first All-Africa Anaesthesia Congress in Harare, Zimbabwe. This event was sponsored by the Zimbabwe Anaesthesia Association and WFSA and assisted by the South African Society of Anaesthesiologists (President Leon du Preez). Professor D.F. Morrell arranged the academic programme and Professor D.A. Rocke was involved with obtaining sponsorship and the sale of exhibition space to the trade. During this congress the Africa Regional Section of the WFSA was established, with chairperson Professor D. Ffoulkes-Crabbe of Nigeria and Dr. Hannes Loots of SASA as treasurer and Professor D.F. Morrell elected to the Executive Committee board. The South African Society of Anaesthesiologists was requested to host the next All-Africa congress in 2001. Professor D.A. Rocke continued to serve on the committee on obstetrics, Professor Adrian Bösenberg was elected to the committee on paediatric anaesthesia, and Professor D.F. Morrell on the committee for quality practice.

At the 11th WFSA Congress in Sydney, Australia in 1996, the SASA bid committee successfully convinced the venue committee of WFSA of South Africa's suitability to host the 14th WFSA World Congress for the year 2008. Other contenders were Japan, Singapore, India, and Brazil.

During September 2001, SASA, under the convenorship of Professor D.A. Rocke, successfully hosted the 2nd All-Africa Anaesthesia Congress of the Africa Regional Section of WFSA at the International Convention Centre, Durban.

We now look forward to welcoming the world to the 14th WFSA World Congress in 2008. In the words of Dr. Anneke E.E. Meursing, secretary to WFSA, "Some national member societies feel and are more involved with WFSA than others. The national societies of Australia, Canada, France, Great Britain and Ireland, Israel, Japan, the Netherlands, South Africa, and the United States of America deserve a special mention for their contributions to the world of anaesthesia beyond the call of duty."

15 CONTRIBUTION OF WFSA TO THE DEVELOPMENT OF PRACTICE OF ANAESTHESIA IN AFRICA

M. Chobli

The marvellous developments in the practice of anaesthesia during the last 3 decades have permitted very safe anaesthesia for most patients undergoing surgery in Europe and America, but have had no benefit for the population of the developing world. In Africa, despite real progress in the past few years, the situation is one of the worst in the world. However, there has been a positive evolution in several areas: the training of physician anaesthetists, the acquisition of better materials and drugs, and the better organization of departments of anaesthesiology.

The role of WFSA in these advances has been very important and due to the actions of its Dynamic Committee of education, it is possible to envisage a bright future for our specialty.

African anaesthetists from English-speaking areas took early advantage of this co-operation, mainly in Ghana with Professor Koffi Oduro and in Nigeria with Professor Foulkes-Crabe. Several refresher courses have been organized in Accra, Lagos, and Ibadan since the 1970s.

East African colleges also benefited from the help of WFSA in Kenya, Uganda, and Tanzania. WFSA activities in African French-speaking countries began later, due to the tireless efforts of Professor Philippe Scherpereel. He contributed to the foundation of the Society of Anaesthesia and Intensive Care of Sub-Saharan Africa (SARANF) in 1984 and helped it to become full member of WFSA 4 years later.

Year after year, thanks to the very good relationship between Professor Scherpereel and these young colleagues from Africa, the standard of anaesthesia practice has become better and safer in Cameroon, Cote d'Ivoire, Congo, Benin, Burkina Faso, Senegal, and Guinea. Today, we can be proud of the increased number of physician anaesthetists (from 22 in 1984 to 148 in 2000) in our geographical area. We can also be proud of the organization of our departments, which now use new anaesthetic drugs that are safer for patients undergoing surgery. From 1993 this programme was implemented by the late Professor Pascal Adnet, Professor Scherpereel's pupil, who gave to the young anaesthetists of Africa a beautiful lesson in co-operation and friendship. The fact that he died in Africa during WFSA training in Benin in October 2000 has further elevated his status among African anaesthetists.

Unity of all anaesthetists in Africa is a great goal for the development of the specialty. WFSA has again been important for fostering the development of unity. The WFSA African Regional Section (ARS) was set up in Harare, Zimbabwe in April 1997. This was very important for the history of anaesthesia in Africa. Dorothy Ffoulkes-Crabbe, the first President of ARS, and her board members worked to develop standards of anaesthesia practice and to inform most anaesthetists about new modalities. The ARS board regularly emphasises to all practitioners the need to train more physicians in anaesthesiology and to use simple but safe materials and drugs. In 2001, more than 3,000 anaesthetists attended the second all-Africa anaesthesia congress in Durban, South Africa.

This meeting showed that we are progressing in different areas: manpower, equipment, and organiszation. Improvement of the quality of the practice of anaesthesia throughout the continent was noticed through the number but also mainly through the quality of papers presented during the congress. Dr. Angela Enright, chairman of the WFSA Education Committee, was present in Durban to encourage us. The role played by WFSA in the positive changes occurring in developing countries is well known today, and is appreciated by established anaesthetists and students.

The WFSA Special Assistance Programme to help training of physician anaesthetists is a success. It is true that nurse anaesthetists are more numerous today than physicians, but it is an important objective to train primarily doctors in anaesthesia. However, while waiting for this, it is important to improve the practice of our nurse-anaesthetists. The great success of Professor Michael Dobson's book *(Anaesthesia in the District Hospital)* shows the educational demand from the nurses. African anaesthetists have appreciated the effort of WFSA to provide books and newspapers for continued training and we thank especially Dr. Eltringham and his team. A new generation of anaesthetists soon understood the great need to work with the Executive Committee of WFSA and particularly the Committee of Education, to quickly change the practice of anaesthesia in Africa.

Tony Roche in South Africa, Henry Burkiwirwa of East Africa, Fidele Binam in Central Africa, Laïtan Soyananwo in West Anglo-Africa, and Martin Chobli in West Francophone Africa form today a solid group able to improve the practice of anaesthesia in Africa.

Kester Brown, Anneke Meursing, and Angela Enright can rely on this new team.

16 WFSA: EDUCATIONAL ACHIEVEMENTS

T.C.K. Brown, R. Eltringham

In 1964, at the World Congress in Sao Paulo, Brazil, Robert Hingson of Cleveland Ohio reported his ideas of a "brother to brother foundation" to provide assistance for anaesthesia in developing countries. The WFSA executive supported the concept and established an "Anaesthesia Education and Relief Foundation". Its members included John Bonica, Francis Foldes, and E.M. Papper of the United States, Luis Cabrera of Chile, and two or three others. The aim was to raise funds for educational projects. At the same congress in 1964 the Executive Committee decided to produce a newsletter. The first edition, edited by the Secretary, Otto Mayrhofer, was published in four languages in 1965.

The official decision to create a WFSA Committee on Education in Anaesthesiology was made by the Executive Committee at the European Congress in Prague in 1970. This committee was renamed the "Committee on Education and Scientific Affairs" during the 5th World Congress in Kyoto in 1972, to be assisted and controlled by a board of trustees. Jack Moyers (USA) was the first chairman. The other members were Barry Fairley (USA), D.D.C. Howat (UK), Douglas Joseph (Australia), Carlos Parsloe (Brazil), and Ole Secher (Denmark). The board had representatives from 20 countries and was chaired by J. Beard from the United Kingdom.

Jack Moyers, who organised the World Congress in Washington in 1988, remained on the Education Committee between 1972 and 1984. His personal CV indicates that he was chairman for the whole of that period. He initiated the idea of voluntary educational teams (VETS) to visit countries that requested help.

VETs were formed by two or three anaesthesiologists who went to one or several countries. They gave lectures and conducted teaching in the operating room. Ty and Penelope Smith were the first team. They went to South America. Their trip was organised by Carlos Parsloe (Brazil), Carlos Castaneo (Bolivia), Francisco Lopez and Virgilio Paez in Ecuador, the three countries that they visited. They gave over 30 lectures and visited 16 hospitals, performing anaesthesia in many of them. In 1981, Professors Nalde and Duarte visited South America and Professor Rosen led an obstetric anaesthesia team to Malaysia. Funding, or lack of it, limited the amount of activity that could be undertaken. In 1983 the secretary, John Zorab, indicated that the Federation could afford to send two or three VETs a year. In 1986, when Howard Zauder from New York was chairman, the VET programme was changed to a visiting professor programme where one or two people would visit somewhere for a week. These visits are supposed to include some hands on teaching.

Training centres were initiated by the World Health Organisation in *Copenhagen* where Ole Secher played a major role as the director. People came from all over the world to attend this course. Later WFSA opened further centres in *Caracas, Venezuela* (1969) and *Manila*, Philippines (1971). These served the purpose of providing basic training for 1 year in anaesthesia to people from countries in the region that did not have their own training programmes. They gradually ceased functioning as more and more countries established their own training and the need declined. In recent years several other centres have been established to cater for similar needs in other regions where anaesthesia is less developed.

The *WFSA Lectures in Anesthesia* were produced twice a year from 1984 to 1988, mainly due to the drive of John Zorab, former secretary and then President. Committees of the Federation also produced *manuals* on obstetric anaesthesia (edited by John Bonica) and resuscitation (edited by Peter Safar), prepared by the Relevant Committees. Around 1992 the Paediatric Committee produced one on paediatric anaesthesia (edited by Anneke Meursing).

Catalysts for activity

The vital components for generating educational activity were enthusiasm of the chairman, active support from committee members, funds, and communication. The period between 1984 and 1988 was disappointing. Funding was very limited and the committee was small, not proactive and communication was difficult. One member in East Germany, for example, never made contact, another had a wife who developed cancer and was not able to contribute much, and yet another did not receive his mail very often because of war in his country. The committee only responded to requests from national societies and these were few. The chairman resigned in 1987 because of other major responsibilities. Kester Brown became chairman and continued through the following 4-year term. He travelled through South America on his way to the World Congress lecturing and finding out about that region. The most-important lesson learned on that trip was the value of using speakers from the region who spoke the language, understood the nature of practice and the problems of the region so that they could teach what was relevant. These lessons were used during the next 4 years and this principle has been encouraged since.

Refresher courses

John Zorab was a very active secretary at the time. As well as editing the lecture series, he also advocated the idea of refresher courses, particularly for Africa. The first attempt was a 1-day paediatric anesthesia course at the end of the East African meeting in Arusha in 1985. The idea evolved further during a social gathering over a few Tusker beers between John Zorab, Roger Eltringham, Hatibo Lueno (Dar es Salaam), and Phares Huma (Nairobi) at the conclusion of the Society of Anaesthetists annual meeting held in Arusha, Tanzania in 1986. It was decided that a refresher course would be run in conjunction with their annual meeting the next year, 1987. This was organised and eight lecturers came, although one who had hoped to come from South Africa was not allowed to enter the country by the Kenya government. It was also disorganised as the venue was changed at the last minute. Several participants finding no one at the original venue went home, although many managed to find the new venue. The transport failed to arrive to take the lecturers to the venue and finally the official certificates of attendance for the participants did not arrive. To the credit of Phares Huma, new copies were made at short notice and, much to everyone's surprise, arrived in time for the meeting. Sadly, a few years later Phares Huma, a man of great promise, died.

These refresher courses gradually evolved over the following 4 years (1988-1992) and were run in many countries, particularly in Africa, the South Pacific, and later in other regions. They became a successful component of the WFSA education programme, but their success was largely due to those active members on the committee, particularly Roger Eltringham and Philippe Scherpereel. They were members of the new, expanded committee elected at the Washington World Congress in 1988 (Fig. 1).

The organization of the Education Committee was modified at that time so that each member had an area of responsibility, was given some autonomy to organise courses, and was allocated the necessary funding. The com-

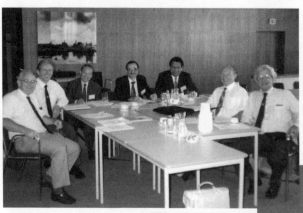

Fig. 1. *Education Committee meeting in The Hague, 1992. From left: Kester Brown (chairman, Australia), Philippe Scherpereel (France), Mitsugi Fujimori (Japan), Jamal Shariff el Shenablah (Jordan), Virgilio Paez (Ecuador), Roger Eltringham (UK), John Cooper (South Africa)*

mittee became much more proactive, not merely waiting for requests to arrive, but actively sending people to different countries. This increased the role of the Federation and made education a major component of its activity. These were exciting times with new developments.

English-speaking courses in Africa were organised over the next decade by Roger Eltringham (Gloucester, UK) and subsequently continued by Bill Casey (Cheltenham, UK) in 1996. They followed the success of the initial course held in Nairobi in 1987. The aim now is for these courses to be arranged by the African members with the others acting as a resource for finding appropriate visiting lecturers.

In response to a request from a national society, the WFSA would select a team of three to four visiting lecturers, who would combine with local speakers to give lectures, tutorials, and demonstrations over a period of 3-5 days, covering subjects selected by the hosts. Key factors in a successful course included local input, audience participation, and adequate time for questions and panel discussions. Each course ended with a quiz with prizes for the winners and distribution of WFSA certificates of attendance. As the pattern of courses was established and their popularity grew, so the demand for them increased, eventually exceeding the budget available from WFSA. Fortunately, several member societies gave valuable assistance by sponsoring speakers. In particular these included the Association of Anaesthetists of Great Britain and Ireland, the Dutch and German Societies, and several regional and specialist societies in the United Kingdom.

Valuable help also came from individuals who were willing to pay their own expenses. This enabled five or six courses to be run each year in countries throughout east, west, and central Africa, including Kenya, Tanzania, Uganda, Sudan, Nigeria, Ghana, Botswana, Malawi, Zambia, Zimbabwe, Mauritius, and Ethiopia.

Francophone courses in Africa were run by the French Society of Anaesthesia and Resuscitation (SFAR) and the West African Society of French-Speaking Countries (SARANF). During the same period Philippe Scherpereel moulded the WFSA contribution into the existing programmes. By contributing financial help, the WFSA was able to support the parallel French activities, serving 15 countries in West and Central Africa including Mauritania, Senegal, Mali, Burkina Faso, Niger, Chad, Guinea, Ivory Coast, Benin, Togo, Cameroon, Gabon, and both Congos.

The Australian Society of Anaesthetists (ASA) Overseas Aid Committee, with help from New Zealand, established a course in Fiji for the South Pacific anaesthetists as a collaborative project with WFSA in the late 1980s. Some Australian and New Zealand anaesthetists went to the other Pacific islands to provide locums on a voluntary basis, having only their fares paid, so that the island anaesthetists could attend the course. After about 4 years the Australian government Aid agency (AIDAB) donated significant support, as they could see that it was already a successful aid project. This aid increased and eventually provided a visiting lecturer (Steve Kinnear) for 2 years. During his time he established a diploma training programme, which eventually led to the first postgraduate medical diploma in the South Pacific - an impressive first for anaesthesia.

The ASA began to encourage the process of self sufficiency whereby the local anaesthetists gradually took more responsibility for themselves. Unfortunately, in the late 1990s the formula for the provision of government aid changed so that the ASA became less directly involved. The programme has been extended so that there is now also a masters programme run under the auspices of the Fiji School of Medicine. Unfortunately the political upheavals in Fiji have had an adverse effect on the training programme, but it is continuing.

In Asia the support has been mainly in South and South East Asian countries in the form of lecturers, some of whom have also done some theatre work. The use of lecturers from other countries in the region has had the benefit of building bridges in the region.

In 1991 John Zorab, in collaboration with Elena Damir, the President of the Russian Society and a member of the WFSA executive, organised the first refresher course in Europe, which was held in Moscow. Other lecturers included Professors Clergue (Paris), Kettler (Gottingen), Viby Mogensen (Copenhagen), Drs. Monk and Jack (UK) and Krassner (New York).

Study travel grants was another idea promoted by John Zorab. Each Eastern Bloc country was invited to send a promising young anaesthetist, who was considered to be a potential leader of the future, to a western department for a month. In 1989 this was a significant development as it preceded perestroyka in the USSR. Some of the anaesthetists selected, such as Maria Janecsko (Hungary) and Ivan Smilov (Bulgaria), have gone on to hold leading

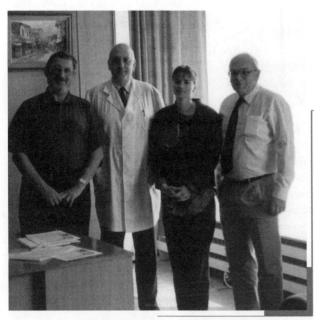

Fig. 2. *Sofia, Bulgaria, 1997. From left: Gabriel Gurman (Israel), Ivan Smilov (Bulgaria), Dessislava Shonperlieva (Bulgaria), Kester Brown (chairman, Executive Committee, Australia)*

positions in their country and in WFSA. Israel took responsibility for Romania, taking three people and adding some funding of their own to support the project. This programme with Israel continued, and WFSA support was increased to allow participation of several other countries in that region, such as Bulgaria and Moldavia. Gabriel Gurman (Education Committee 1996-2004) has coordinated this effort, going to teach in these countries and selecting appropriate anaesthetists to attend for 1- or 2-month courses. It has been an important and much valued help to people in those countries emerging from communist dominance (Fig. 2).

In the early 1990s the WFSA began to send representatives to speak at annual conferences of the Russian Society of Anaesthetists. The contacts forged at these meetings have led to a series of subsequent refresher courses supported by WFSA in the Baltic states, Ukraine, and Archangel. Elena Damir requested the inclusion of the Russian Far East in the WFSA programmes. In 1994 Professor Fujimori (chairman of the Education Committee at that time) arranged Japanese speakers and financial support for the first WFSA course in Siberia in the city of Khabarovsk. Further courses continue to be organised by Japan.

Stopover visits

An important development was the establishment of a number of different categories of help in addition to the visiting lecturers for courses. One of these was to provide a limited grant to anaesthetists travelling through a region to enable them to stop off to lecture and teach for 2 or 3 days. This has been used to a limited extent but effectively, particularly in 1988, when 11 paediatric anaesthetists on their way to meetings in Australia stopped over to teach in six major South East Asian cities - Singapore, Kuala Lumpur, Bangkok, Manila, Hong Kong, and Colombo. Unfortunately a typhoon struck Manila and civil unrest made it necessary for Anneke Meursing to leave Colombo in a hurry.

The budget in the 1988-1992 period was U.S. $ 50,000 per year but, by collaborating with some national and other societies, it became possible to send lecturers to 50 countries, with some others benefiting by attendance at regional courses. In addition, the teachers came from 25 countries, so that the whole programme had become truly international. Outside agencies such as national societies, pharmaceutical and equipment companies, and government agencies have also been able to make helpful contributions to worthwhile projects that they probably would not have done on their own.

The Education Committee has been the main beneficiary of the surpluses generated at subsequent World Congresses making it possible to increase the annual budget and thus support more ventures. The committee has continued with the members each having individual areas of responsibility and funds, so that the wide range of courses continues but has spread to include other parts of Asia, Eastern Europe, South and Central America and, through the Australian Society, Micronesia. The chair of the committee between 1992 and 1996 was Professor Mitsugi Fujimori (Osaka, Japan). It continued with the active promotion of the refresher courses. In 1996, Haydn Perndt, from Hobart, Australia, became chairman and pushed the boundaries of education further. He had had wide experience working in many of the Pacific Island countries, as well as with the Red Cross in several areas of conflict. This gave him an understanding of the needs of less-affluent countries, which he was able to convey to others on the committee, thus inspiring them to participate more actively. The same overall strategy has continued since Angela Enright (Canada) took over the chair in 2000.

Training centers

Training centres have been a major development since 1996 to provide for specific regional anaesthetic manpower needs. Bangkok formed a group from the various university departments with the support of the Thai College of Anaesthesiologists to train some anaesthesiologists from Indo-China, particularly Cambodia and Laos. The initiative spread to include Vietnam, Myanmar, and Mongolia. The aim was to take people with some experience and train them so that they could return to contribute as teachers in their own countries. Three or four trainees come each year and rotate through Bangkok training hospitals and attend the teaching programme. Professor Thara Tritrakarn, a member of the Education Committee, has been active in developing and supporting this programme, ably assisted by others representing the departments involved (Fig. 3).

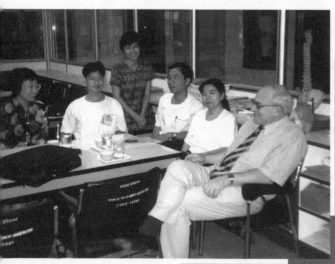

Fig. 3. *Teaching at the Bangkok Training Centre course, May 1997. From left: Jariya Lertakyamanee (course supervisor, Bangkok), Sinongkham Phanmany (Laos), Sirilak (instructor, Bangkok), Traycheth Chanthisiri (Laos), Vanphong Norasingh (Laos), Kester Brown (chairman, Executive Committee, visiting lecturer)*

The American Society, stimulated initially by Nick Greene following his visit to Kenya in 1987, has contributed to programmes in Africa, such as that at KCMC in Arusha, and more recently to a joint venture with WFSA and the Ghanian government to train anaesthesiologists in that country. Most of the trainees are from Ghana but one of the conditions of WFSA support has been that at least one should be from one of the neighbouring English-speaking countries where training facilities are inadequate. The Americans are responsible for sending volunteer lecturers, usually for a month at a time.

Similar centres have been developed independently by the French Society in Senegal and a Belgium group from the University of Louvain (B. De Poulin, P. Baele, and F. Veckyemanns) in Benin, with some support from their government.

Specialist training in obstetrics for Africa was set up to take a candidate for 3-6 months at a time in Durban. In Santiago, Chile there is a training position in paediatric anaesthesia for someone from a less-affluent country in South America. So far participants have attended from Ecuador and Guatamala. These are all beneficial to the individuals and, hopefully, also to their home country when they return. It is hoped that more of these centres will develop when funds become available. Unsuccessful attempts have been made to give some form of recognition to hospitals that train people from other countries. There are many of these such as the Royal Children's Hospital in Melbourne, which has trained people from 39 countries, Gottingen in Germany, University of Louvain in Belgium, several in France, Gloucester in England, Hamilton in New Zealand for the Pacific, and many others. There has to be someone in the hospital department who is prepared to organise and administer these programmes and look after the trainees.

Difficulties in deciding which departments should be recognised have prevented this concept coming to fruition. The standard of the programme has to be assured but how should it be monitored? Another major problem is that of avoiding the feeling that a centre is selected merely because the person in charge is closely involved with WFSA. This may be justifiable because those people may, through their involvement, know where there is a need and have the necessary contacts in these places. The problem of recognition has not been resolved, but the satisfaction of knowing that one's department is contributing to helping other countries is often all the reward that is needed, especially when the people returning to their country are able to improve conditions and participate in teaching programmes. Teaching the trainees how to teach and to organise meetings and training programmes can make these people even more effective.

Primary trauma care courses were developed initially by Douglas Wilkinson in Oxford and Marcus Skinner in Tasmania, following encouragement from Haydn Perndt and Michael Dobson. Stephen Swallow and Rob McDougall in Australia joined them later to help with the further development of the courses and manuals. The aim has been to provide basic training in primary trauma care for less-affluent countries that might not have all the facilities that are available in many more-affluent countries. The course is delivered initially to doctors, then healthcare workers. Potential trainers are selected from those attending and given further instruction so that they can train others. These people then help the outside trainers at subsequent courses and then take over running the courses in their country themselves. This has been successfully achieved in several countries. In 2000 these courses became the responsibility of the Education Committee, which funds some of the courses.

Challenges when teaching

Flexibility is essential when lecturing on such courses. In 1988, Kester Brown ran a 1-day paediatric anaesthetic course in Quito, Ecuador. The official who was to open it failed to arrive. During the waiting period the projector was checked. No light, so a new bulb was obtained. Then the carousel went backwards when the forward button was pressed! It also went backwards with the reverse button! Another projector was obtained. Dud bulb! Once the good bulb was inserted all was well. But then the video projector did not focus. Another video player was obtained and VHS videos were collected so proceedings could begin. Elsewhere, on other occasions the video jammed and could not be shown, there was a power cut preventing slides from being projected, or the speaker was suddenly asked to cut the lecture short because the programme was running late. Flexibility and adaptability are essential.

Publications

The Publications Committee was established in 1992, with the hope that it would become another important arm of the educational activity of the Federation. About the same time, the journal *Update in Anaesthesia*, edited by Iain Wilson, was introduced by World Anaesthesia, a philanthropic group of anaesthetists from many countries, whose aims were similar to WFSA. Unlike the WFSA, the membership of World Anaesthesia is open to individual anaesthetists and provides the opportunity for them to channel their energies into international programmes such as those run by WFSA. They run on a relatively small budget derived from annual subscriptions of those who can pay.

Initially WFSA gave meagre support to *Update in Anaesthesia,* but in 1996 when Roger Eltringham became chairman of the Publications Committee and more funds became available to WFSA, support for the production and distribution of this publication became a priority and an excellent example of collaboration between WFSA and World Anaesthesia.

The aim of *Update in Anaethesia* is to provide concise, easily readable, and up-to-date advice on practical problems for dissemination to anaesthetists who have difficulty obtaining anaesthesia literature. It is produced twice a year, in English, Spanish, Russian, Mandarin, and French. It has proved extremely popular with anaesthetists all over the world. The total distribution of the printed editions in the various languages during 2001 was 14,000 distributed to over a hundred countries. The increasing cost of printing and distribution has led to greater emphasis being put on its dissemination via the Internet. English, French, and Russian versions are available on the Internet, being widely accessed in 134 countries. It is hoped that the Spanish and Mandarin versions will soon become available on the Internet. There has been a request for its translation into Indonesian, and other languages may follow. All that is necessary is to have someone who will reliably translate it and organise its distribution. This could be done through society web sites if they exist.

During the period 1996-2000 the WFSA and World Anaesthesia newsletters were combined to become an interesting and informative journal attracting contributions from all over the world. Unfortunately the rising costs and the need for the Federation to have its own newsletter in a more-concise format led to separation of the two in 2001.

The literature Distribution Committee was introduced in 1994, following a recommendation by Bernie Wetchler, then chair of the Executive Committee. The distribution of packages of books has gradually been replaced by donations of particular textbooks in response to specific requests made to the WFSA office from departments that lack books. Unfortunately this programme is the first to be cut in times of financial stringency and economic difficulty. One of the books distributed has been the French edition of *Safe Anaesthesia* by Lucille Bartholomew, an anaesthetist who worked for many years in Africa. The French translation, printing, and distribution was organised by Lois Gibson who has been working in West Africa.

The distribution of journals was another scheme launched in 1999 by the Publications Committee. Individuals were invited to send their current journals, once they had read them, direct to anaesthetists in the less-affluent world who were unable to afford the subscription. Within 12 months of launching the scheme, over 100 donors had volunteered to send their journals. Lists of those willing to send their journals and also those wishing to receive them are held by the WFSA. Those wishing to join the scheme as donor or recipient can do so by contacting the WFSA office.

The aims of the Federation are to promote the highest standards of anaesthesia that can be achieved in the various parts of the world. The work of the education and Publications Committees is the most-effective way to achieve this along with the four-yearly World Congresses, which enable many people from all over the world to meet, exchange information, and hear about the latest developments. In recent World Congresses, great emphasis has been placed on trying to make them effective update and continuing education meetings for all the specialty and special areas of anaesthesia, thus enabling anesthesiologists to attend meetings on their special interest within the wider congress. This was achieved by having well-organised and integrated programmes. Having speakers from all parts of the world has also been encouraged to make them really international. The teachers and contributors to the publications come from many countries.

Many anaesthesiologists have given generously of their time to participate in the courses and educational activities of the WFSA. Some have gone to places that have not always been safe-coups, civil unrest, and political upheavals have sometimes occurred. They travel economy class, and while the hosts are usually expected to look after their accommodation and living needs, occasionally this is not economically feasible. Flights may be erratic, and problems with customs, immigration, and other similar trials can add to the difficulties of travelling in some of the countries. On several occasions, examination of baggage found that a suspicious object on the X-ray scanner was the WFSA President's Medallion! On another occasion a teaching film was looked on with great suspicion by the customs officer because it was in a blue box-a blue movie! Despite all this, many anaesthetists have had great satisfaction and made many friends from being involved in this educational work - the gratitude of the recipients and their kindness makes one feel that the effort is all worthwhile and appreciated.

17 WFSA FINANCES: WHERE DOES THE MONEY COME FROM AND WHERE DOES IT GO?

M. Rosen

The treasurer, with the Finance Committee, and financial advisers, proposes to the Executive Committee financial and budget plans, to implement the aims of the WFSA, advises on changing circumstances; and supervises the implementation of the plans and budgets.

The WFSA was founded at the 1ˢᵗ World Congress in the Netherlands in 1955. Finance was required to fund a secretariat to integrate the involved countries, their aims for WFSA, and to organise the location and requests to hold the World Congress every 4 years. The financial requirements were therefore modest. These were met by agreement with each national society to pay an annual subscription to WFSA that was based upon the number of their members. Societies varied in size, and, at that time, particularly in their ability to transfer cash because of currency regulations. There were differences in definition of "members" (full member, part-time, associate, or trainee) that gave rise to underestimates. The power to influence WFSA was related approximately to the number of members, upon which was based the number of delegates to the General Assembly. Later during Dr. Henning Poulsen's (Fig. 1) term (1964-1968) currency transfer problems were met, to some extent, by setting up bank accounts in-country (but not transferable) that were then used for educational visits and training in that country or bloc. Salary differences (low salaries) and "member" definitions led to membership under-reporting (which exists to this day), sometimes due to lack of exchangeable currency, which has been largely

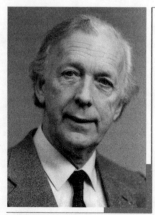

Fig. 1.
Henning Poulsen, first separate Treasurer of WFSA

overlooked by treasurers and the Executive Committee in the higher interest of ensuring the widest representation for WFSA.

These policies and arrangements were developed mainly in the period of the first separate treasurer (The office of secretary/treasurer was held by Sir Geoffrey Organe from 1955 to 1964), Dr. Henning Poulsen, and continued under Professor Quinton Gomez (1968-1976), and Professor Carlos Rivas Larazabal (1976-1984). In addition, there were always difficulties in collecting the annual dues on time, and in communicating with the officers of some societies because of frequent changes of address. In 1980, Dr. (Professor) Richard Ament was appointed deputy treasurer, specifically, and particularly, to improve communications with societies and to speed up collection of the annual dues. The success of this Rivas/Ament team is attested to by the financial results. Capital assets of WFSA in 1976 amounted to U.S. $ 73,725 and by 1984 had risen to U.S. $ 243,374 - a threefold increase! In that period, too, the WFSA bank accounts were reduced from eight to two, with great improvement in efficiency.

Particular problems exist in operating any international organisation; there are widespread administrative difficulties - high costs of communication, very high costs of transfers of funds, and, sometimes, substantial losses due to exchange rate variations. Communication problems have somewhat diminished with the arrival of the Internet; but to date there is no solution to the high cost of money transfers coupled with extensive delays and exchange rate fluctuations.

In 1976 after the 6th World Congress in Mexico, informal discussions between the officers led to the conclusion that a World Congress belonged to the WFSA together with any surplus. It became clear, too, that there should be such surpluses if each congress was properly organized, mainly arising from the technical exhibitors. Therefore to encourage good management it was eventually agreed at the 7th World Congress (1980) that any surplus would be shared with the organising country. It was agreed that the WFSA share would be used to support the educational aims of the WFSA, particularly in developing countries.

In 1984, Dr. Richard Ament (Fig. 2) became treasurer and implemented major changes in the organisation of WFSA. He registered the WFSA as a Not-for-Profit (NFP) charity in New York State, United States. This had financial implications, which enabled WFSA to be untaxed, and any donations to WFSA also to be untaxed, which were great advantages, but also required audited accounts, which had costs, and a necessity to comply with NFP rules. These rules were, mainly, to ensure that the

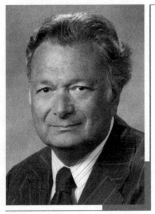

Fig. 2.
Richard Ament became Treasurer in 1984

major part of the income was used each year for the charitable aims of WFSA. In 1992, I became treasurer and was able to recommend greatly expanded expenditure for the education and Publications Committees.

Financial advisers

Mr. Ernest Warburton, lately treasurer of Guy's Hospital and adviser to AAGBI, was honorary adviser from 1992 to 1999. Mr. Francis Wirgman (also adviser to AAGBI) became adviser to WFSA in 1999.

Investment brokers

Smith Barney (Buffalo) were appointed by Dr. Ament in 1984. In 1992 the appointment was thrown open. The Finance Committee recommended the re-appointment of Smith Barney and Couriers, the funds being divided almost equally. In 2000 Tirschwell and Loewy (who had been considered in 1992) were appointed, in place of Smith Barney with Courier. Mr. Warburton had found Smith Barney records unsatisfactory.

Auditors

Dr. Ament in 1984, appointed Deloitte and Touche (in Buffalo) (previously Touche Ross) who have continued as auditors since.

WFSA funding (years indicate "year ending")

Expenditure
Education. In 1984, the Education Committee budget supported projects totaling U.S. $ 39,167; in 1992 this expenditure was U.S. $ 18,537, it was expanded in 1996 to U.S. $ 67,208, and in 2000 to U.S. $ 156,061. These budgets paid for courses, lectures, and lecturers, as well as the WFSA regional training centres in Ghana, Israel, Chile, and Thailand.

Publications. In 1984-1996 publication expenditure was solely for the newsletter and cost between U.S. $ 500 and U.S. $ 2,000. The Publication Committee expanded its important work distributing literature and also the journal *Update* in five languages, with an expenditure of U.S. $ 4,558 in 1996, increasing greatly by 2000 to U.S. $ 49,720.

Administrative expenses. (These include all the WFSA expenses, less education and Publication Committee expenditures and grants for future congresses.) In 1984 the administrative expenditure was U.S. $ 53,846; in 1988 it rose to U.S. $ 74,002, and in 1992 to U.S. $ 110,474. In 1994, a central office (shared with the European Academy) was opened in London at the Royal College of Anaesthetists and expenditure increased, a little, to U.S. $ 117,140. In 1996, with a separate office in London, expenditure rose steeply to U.S. $ 311,655. In 2000 it rose further to U.S. $ 444,931. The costs in that year were exceptionally increased because of major secretarial staffing difficulties, many changes in procedures, and because of World Congress expenditure. These expenditures also reflected substantial increases in activities of the WFSA.

WFSA assets

The earliest accounts available to me (1976) showed WFSA assets of U.S. $ 73,725, which grew in 1984 to U.S. $ 499,133 (about 7 times). In 1988 the assets were U.S. $ 1,241,246 (U.S. $ 15,000 from the European Congress in 1986 and U.S. $ 500,000 from the 9th World Congress in the USA in 1984) (about 17 times). In 1992 the total had risen to U.S. $ 1,780,129 (U.S. $ 609,296 from the 10th World Congress in The Netherlands) (about 24 times). In 1996 the total assets were U.S. $ 2,605,921 (U.S. $ 742,207 from the 11th World Congress in Australia (about 36 times). In 2000 the total assets were U.S. $ 2,997,427 (U.S. $ 248,102 from the 12th World Congress in Canada (about 40 times from 1976). Accounts for 2001 show assets of U.S. $ 2,624,920, reflecting the fall in stock markets.

Income

Dues are U.S. $ 1.25 per member per society. These have increased the following total income: 1984 U.S. $ 56,776; 1988 U.S. $ 66,220; 1992 U.S. $ 87,868; 1996 U.S. $ 85,778; 2000 U.S. $ 94,029.

These dues have not altered since 1984. It is difficult to persuade national societies to agree to any increase based upon this method. It might therefore be more acceptable to focus on a fixed proportion (e.g., 5%) of the annual subscription of the society instead of an increase based on per capita. Reliance on voluntary contributions may be another possible option.

World Congresses, since 1988, have been the major source of WFSA income as follows: 1988 (USA) U.S. $ 500,000; 1992 (The Netherlands) U.S. $ 609,296; 1996 (Australia) U.S. $ 742,207; 2000 (Canada) U.S. $ 248,102.

Other funds. The WFSA Foundation. At the 12th World Congress it was agreed by the Executive Committee to explore an organisation (charitable NFP) to raise funds for the WFSA aims, with Professor Michael Rosen as chairman. In April 2001, it was agreed that such an organisation should be known as the WFSA Foundation, and should be a subcommittee of the WFSA.

The Association of Anaesthetists of Great Britain and Ireland agreed jointly with WFSA to raise in the United Kingdom in 2002-2003 U.S. $ 150,000. This, it is hoped, will act as a model for other national societies to similarly raise funds. These funds come from the United Kingdom anaesthetic organizations (AAGBI donated U.S. $ 15,000), British members, and British business-es active in the developing countries. At the time of writing (July 2002), the total stands at more than U.S. $ 50,000, before the appeal being sent to all British members. In 2004, a decision will be taken on the future activities of this organisation. If successful it could be an opportunity to raise substantial funds to improve the woeful anaesthetic services in developing countries.

Other funds. In 1998, the United Kingdom government was approached by a group of British anaesthetists, including the treasurer, for help to devel-op a distance learning postgraduate educational system that could be used by technicians, nurses, and physicians in developing countries using CD Roms, the Internet, telephone advice, and personal visits. This was super-vised by Dr. Michael Dobson and was successfully completed in 2002 in Zim-babwe. It cost U.S. $ 200,000 and was paid for by the British government. Fur-ther testing is proposed in Africa. After that the programmes will then be made available worldwide at low cost.

In 1998, Dr. Roger Eltringham received a grant of U.S. $ 300,000 from the British government to test the Glostavent anaesthetic apparatus (an oxygen con-centrator, a draw-over vaporiser, and a gas pressure-operated ventilator with a back-up battery) in Mozambique, Zambia, and Tanzania. Tests are ongoing and will be completed during 2003. If successful this will represent an impor-tant development of a low-cost, locally repairable anaesthetic apparatus and ventilator for use in the operating theatre and intensive care unit. In addition, development is being sought, in collaboration with industry, of a low-cost, sturdy oximeter that could have important implications for safety.

Conclusion

In summary, it is noteworthy that the WFSA treasurers have been clinical anaesthetists, albeit distinguished and leaders in their countries, but without special financial training. Nevertheless, their records in international finance, and as officers of the WFSA, can be looked upon with pride.

I feel sure that the WFSA and its present treasurer, Dr. Richard Walsh (2000 to present), and each future treasurer will continue to ensure that the finances enable progress to be maintained, with due economic rigour, in achieving the important aims of WFSA, which can undoubtedly benefit mil-lions worldwide.

I wish them well in their important quests. The data used in this paper have been taken from the accounts of 1976-2000 and from my memories.

18 WFSA: ACHIEVEMENTS AND CHALLENGES

C. Parsloe

he World Federation of Societies of Anaesthesiologists (WFSA) was founded in 1955 at the 1st World Congress of Anaesthesiologists (WCA) with a clearly stated and noble objective: "to make available the highest standards of anaesthesia to all peoples of the world" [1]. The 1996 statutes re-stated that objective as "anaesthesia and resuscitation". To that end several pursuits are listed, including: (1) to assist and encourage the formation of national societies of anaesthesiologists; (2) to promote education and the dissemination of scientific information; (3) to arrange at regular intervals a WCA and sponsor regional congresses; (4) to recommend desirable standards for the training of anaesthesiologists; (5) to encourage the establishment of safety measures, including the standardisation of equipment; (6) to advise, upon request, national and international organisations [2]. In this chapter it will become evident that all those pursuits were ably and extensively achieved, but it will also become evident that the WFSA still faces considerable challenges, over which it has no control.

World globalisation was not a common concept in 1955, but without any question at its inception the WFSA looked at the world in a global fashion, attempting to promote safe anaesthesia worldwide. Professor J.J. Bonica entitled his 1984 presidential address "Achievements of the past and challenges of the future" [3]. That report offered an overall view of the development of the WFSA over its first quarter of a century. As it approaches its 50th anniversary it is a good time to ponder the challenges it still faces in trying to fully accomplish its objectives.

Membership growth has been gratifying since the original 26 founding national societies, plus observers from 14 other national societies [1], have now increased to 108 [4]. Similarly, the number of anaesthesiologists has increased from the original estimated 4,500 to approximately 100,000. This can be considered a very positive achievement. WCAs were held every 4 years, covering most continents: 1st, 1955, in Scheveningen, The Netherlands; 2nd, 1960, in Toronto, Canada; 3rd, 1964, in São Paulo, Brasil; 4th, 1968, in London, United Kingdom; 5th, 1972, in Kyoto, Japan; 6th, 1976, in Mexico City, Mexico; 7th, 1980, in Hamburg, Germany; 8th, 1984, in Manila, the Philippines; 9th, 1988, in Washington, D.C., United States; 10th, 1992, in The Hague, The Netherlands; 11th, 1996, in Sydney, Australia; 12th, 2000, in Montreal, Canada. Thus Europe had 5, North America 3, Asia 2, South America 1, and Australia 1 World Congresses. The 13th World Congress will be held in 2004 in Paris, France, and the 14th World Congress in 2008 in Cape Town, South Africa, including the one continent so far still without a World Congress.

There are now four Regional Sections within the WFSA: the Confederation of European National Societies of Anaesthesiology (CENSA), formerly called the European Regional Section (ERS), the Confederation of Latin-American Societies of Anesthesiology (CLASA), the Asian and Australasian Regional Section (AARS), and the African Regional Section (ARS) [4]. All Regional Sections hold periodic congresses.

The growth of anaesthesiology

Anaesthesiology has rapidly progressed to a highly scientific and well-structured branch of medicine, with its field of action clearly delineated and expanding to areas outside the traditional operating room environment. The increasing field of activities of anaesthesiologists is matched by the changing names of the original departments of anaesthesiology to departments of anaesthesiology and critical care medicine, pain medicine, resuscitation, and ultimately to perioperative medicine. It could be argued that the name is less important than the capacity to well fulfill the wide scope of duties. Anaesthesiology *lato sensu* has always been involved with those several aspects of medical care as they evolved, without the need for added denominations. The increasing demand for surgical anaesthesia plus what has become known as perioperative medicine, both in the operating room environment and the ambulatory setting, requires additional manpower, additional training, and additional funds to well accomplish the whole spectrum of duties. The treatment of acute and chronic pain has placed an added but welcome burden that now constitutes an important part of the anaesthesiologist's daily activities. Additionally, interventional procedures in the cardiology, radiology, computed tomography, magnetic resonance, endoscopy, and nuclear medicine units require either anaesthesia or analgesia and sedation, adding to the anaesthesiologist's traditional operating room role. Technology has invaded the operating room, the ambulatory settings, and indeed permeates all areas where anaesthesiologists work. We now live in a technologically dense environment. Endoscopic operations are increasingly using robotic arms that can be commanded by the surgeon's voice and advances are continuing in remote control surgery. Anaesthesia must accompany and adapt to such innovations. It is only a matter of time before autonomous robots are used in the perioperative areas for patient transport and for assistance with anaesthesia. Anaesthesiologists must be prepared for the operating room of the future, which is already being delineated. The future holds challenges beyond the imagination of the founding member societies. We must look into the future. Therefore, in this essay I have given equal emphasis to the WFSA achievements in its first half century of existence and to the challenges that it still faces.

WFSA Committees

The deliberative body in the WFSA is the Executive Committee, but it also has a number of committees that look at specific aspects of improving anaesthesia care, particularly in the less-fortunate areas of the world. These are divided into two categories: (1) Standing Committees, comprising the education, finance, publications, and the Statutes and Bylaws Committees; (2) Specialty Committees, comprising the obstetrics, pediatric, pain relief, resuscitation, trauma and intensive care medicine, safety and quality of practice, and the technology, information, and Equipment Committees. A WFSA Foundation, which superseded the original Anaesthesia Educational and Relief Foundation, ably chaired by the late Dr. Robert A. Hingson, is in charge of raising necessary funds for the diverse educational projects. Respective chairpersons and committee members are in charge of overseeing the many and increasing activities. There are two special WFSA representatives: Dr. Michael Dobson, from the Nuffield Department of Anaesthetics in Oxford (UK) for the World Health Organisation (WHO) and Dr. Joseph Rupreht, from the Department of Anaesthesia, Erasmus University in Rotterdam, The Netherlands, as honorary archivist [4].

Publications

The WFSA prepares annual reports and the WFSA Newsletter, edited by John Moyers [5], and sponsors two publications [6] particularly aimed at the developing world: *Update in Anaesthesia*, edited by Iain Wilson [7] and *World Anaesthesia*, edited by W.F. Casey [8]. Dr. Michael Dobson of Oxford founded in 1987 an organisation called *World Anaesthesia* with the aim of advancing anaesthesia throughout the developing world. Its main activity has been the preparation and distribution of the above-mentioned two publications [9]. These publications have proved their value in providing a means for the exchange of opinions among members from national societies in less-developed countries. *Update* is distributed to 134 countries and is published in five editions: English, French, Mandarin, Russian, and Spanish [5, 6]. This impressive achievement speaks for itself. In 1965 the secretary, Professor O. Mayrhofer, started publishing the well-printed *WFSA Newsletter* [10] in four languages (English, German, French, and Spanish) with support from Springer-Verlag. Due to loss of financial support, this comprehensive newsletter had to be discontinued with number 9, in 1973. Subsequent newsletters were distributed in a simpler fashion, mainly in English.

Manpower

From the beginning the field of anaesthesiology has been plagued with a shortage of physicians interested in full-time specialisation, with the consequent intrusion of non-medical personnel in such medical activities. Some countries have succeeded in maintaining the administration of anaesthesia by physicians only, even in the so-called developing world. However, in many countries the high demand, coupled with insufficient numbers of properly qualified physicians, have resulted in dentists, nurses, and paramedical personnel administering surgical anaesthesia. Developed countries have the economic means to sustain several different categories of medical and non-medical personnel in many fields. Some societies developed what became known as "The anaesthesia care team" comprising medical and para-medical personnel. With the increasing demands for monitoring, critical care, pain relief, and analgesia and sedation outside the operating rooms, anaesthesiologists should benefit from the help of qualified assistants, allowing them to fulfill their many activities without relinquishing their main duties to provide qualified medical care.

However, in underdeveloped countries social and economic factors create significant problems for medical care, including surgery and anaesthesia, as well as for public health. Inadequate budgets, wrong priorities, the lure of the developed world, and the dissatisfaction with having to work under considerably less than ideal circumstances are not conducive to training the required number of full-time physician anaesthesiologists or even sufficient numbers of physicians with the ability to administer safe anaesthesia on a part-time basis. Such circumstances, where minor surgery can be practiced by non-physicians, have led to the training of non-physicians in the administration of surgical anaesthesia. It is impossible to dissociate anaesthesia from the overall surgical and medical care and the existing local infrastructure. Such inadequate conditions need to be overcome before anaesthesia can be practiced in a consistently safe manner in less-developed regions. There is one hidden danger in training non-physicians in anaesthesia that needs to be well understood. In attempting to cover present needs, it may discourage physicians from entering a field with practicing non-physicians. Therefore, this approach generates a vicious circle: a lack of physician anaesthesiologists-non-physicians administering surgical anesthesia - a lack of interest among physicians in practicing anaesthesiology - no present and future provision of additional physician anaesthesiologists. In the long term it is a self-defeating situation.

General versus local anaesthesia

A major drawback in the administration of safe anaesthesia under less than ideal circumstances is the emphasis on general anaesthesia rather than on local anaesthesia. The types of surgical operations performed in underdeveloped regions are suitable for local infiltration anaesthesia or simple regional blocks. Intrinsically these procedures are safer than poorly managed general anaesthesia. Some regions do not always have adequate supplies of equipment to ensure safe general anaesthesia, such as suction equipment, medicinal oxygen, and airway devices such as working laryngoscopes and tracheal tubes or laryngeal masks. Knowledge of the essential basic principles for the safe administration of anaesthesia is also sometimes lacking. Oral airways are not consistently obtained in many operating areas. Over the years surgeons have lost their ability to use local anaesthesia, but they should be taught this simple art, which is useful for the great majority, if not all, surgical operations performed in the underdeveloped world [11]. Regretfully, this simple and sound approach has not met with much enthusiasm. There is a wide scope for regional anaesthesia societies (American Society of Regional Anesthesia, ASRA, European Society of Regional Anesthesia, ESRA, and particularly the Latin-American Society of Regional Anesthesia, LASRA, and the Asian and Oceanic Society of Regional Anesthesia, AOSRA) to become involved in collaborative projects with the WFSA.

Anaesthesiology training centres

The most-significant step towards training anaesthesiologists from Europe and other countries was the "Anaesthesiology Centre Copenhagen" which was set up by the World Health Organization (WHO). It started in 1950 and over its 23 years' existence trained 220 anaesthesiologists from Denmark and 453 anaesthesiologists from 71 other countries, who became, in turn, active in the dissemination of the specialty in their countries of origin [12]. This centre was immensely successful at a crucial time for the development of anaesthesiology, when the WFSA did not exist. Subsequently, the WFSA in collaboration with the WHO sponsored two WFSA/WHO training centres, the Ibero American Anaesthesiology Training Centre, in Caracas, Venezuela, officially dedicated in October 1966, and the Anaesthesiology Centre Western Pacific in Manila, the Philippines in 1970. Both centres were essentially maintained by the local universities [3, 11]. Professor Carlos Rivas-Larrazabal conceived and was the *primum movens* for the Caracas centre, which he directed from the Anaesthesia Department, University Hospital, Central University of Venezuela. Professor Juan A. Nesi, on the invitation of Carlos Rivas, directed the post-graduate course, founded at the Central University Hospital in 1958, until 1985. His teaching for a number of years at the Ibero American Centre became a major factor in the training of generations of anaesthesiologists in Venezuela and in Latin America [13, 14].

Professor Quintin J. Gomez, was responsible for the creation of the Anaesthesiology Centre Western Pacific at the University of the Philippines College of Medicine as a joint activity of the Regional Office for the Western Pacific, WHO, the Department of National Defense, Republic of the Philippines, the China Medical Board of New York, and the WFSA [15]. Both centres served their adjoining geographic areas well and successfully trained hundreds of anaesthesiologists. The WFSA sent visiting professors to both centres, but that was the extent of its financial help. Some of the professors for the Caracas centre were paid by the WFSA relief foundation committee.

Yearly detailed reports were prepared and sent to the WFSA. The work of those centres in the early years of the WFSA was of lasting benefit. Regretfully, they were eventually closed for lack of continuing financial support.

Another training centre was started in 1996, the Bangkok Anaesthesia Regional Training Centre, in collaboration with The Royal College of Anaesthetists of Thailand [16, 17]. Professor Thara Tritrakarn from the Department of Anaesthesiology, Faculty of Medicine, Siriraj Hospital, Mahidol University, has had a major input into this centre. Its seventh group of trainees started in January 2003.

The Paediatric Anaesthesia Training Centre, started in 1997 and run by Dr. Silvana Cavallieri, at Luis Calvo McKeena Hospital in Santiago, Chile, provides excellent training to young anaesthesiologists from Latin America [17, 18].

A training Centre in Accra, Ghana, started in 1999, is a project of the American Society of Anaesthesiologists overseas teaching programme, which offers support and sends teachers. WFSA pays the expenses of the trainees [17].

. During 2002 other WFSA-supported training centres were initiated. These include The Soroka Medical Centre at Beer Sheva, Israel, Department of Anaesthesia, Professor Gabriel Gurman; Milan, Italy, Professor Bruno Turchetta; Cluj-Napoca, Romania, Spitalul Clinic, Professor Iurie Acalovsichi, with help from CENSA, and Basingstoke, UK, Dr. David Robins at the North Hampshire Hospital [17].

A cardiovascular training center was officially opened on September 2003, at the Catholic University Medical School Hospital in Santiago, Chile, with Professor Jorge Urzua as Program co-ordinator [18].

Such remarkable achievements require leadership and adequate budgets for their inception and maintenance, and are definitely beneficial towards raising the overall standards of anaesthesia practice.

Educational activities and refresher courses

During the 3rd WCA, in 1964, the Executive Committee approved the formation of a new Standing Committee, the Committee on Education and Scientific Affairs (CESA), ably chaired by the late Professor Jack Moyers. It created a visiting educational team programme and succeeded in organising a series of 1- to 2-week-long visits to different countries. It was soon realised that a few professorial lectures were quite inadequate to sustain the interest and to effectively raise the standards of anaesthesia care in the less-developed regions. The observed tendency was for the national societies to request visiting professors to attend their anaesthesia meetings rather than to work for any length of time under prevailing local conditions and to offer effective suggestions for improvement. In 1986 this project was changed to a "visiting professor programme", which gave more emphasis to clinical work [11]. It must be stated that in certain circumstances, given the different agents and equipment, and even of diseases, unknown to the visiting professors, they had to admit that they were probably learning as much as they were teaching.

Two courses in "anaesthesia for the developing world" are given annually at the Department of Anaesthesia, John Radcliffe Hospital, Oxford and at the Department of Anaesthesia, Frenchay Hospital, Bristol, directed respectively by Dr. M. Dobson and Dr. C. Jukes [19]. They offer basic instruction and suggestions for simple and reliable anaesthetic techniques and equipment applicable to developing regions. These courses can also serve as orientation for First World colleagues desiring to improve anaesthesia in less-developed regions. The courses have been well attended and proved their worth on both instances.

The WFSA sponsors primary trauma courses adapted to developing countries and courses on the maintenance and repair of essential anaesthesia equipment in Africa [20]. These new developments are proving to be of significant benefit to less-developed regions.

The education and pain committees worked together to provide the first pain seminars in 2003. Dr. Dilip Pawar, from India, Dr. R. Vijayan, from Malaysia, and Dr. R. Goucke, from Australia taught seminars in Bangkok (Thailand), Colombo (Sri Lanka), Dhaka (Bangladesh), and Surabaya (Indonesia) [17].

The Education Committee is engaged in organising and supporting a number of refresher courses and visiting teachers to many countries. A complete report on the educational achievements can be found in the specific chapter in this book.

WFSA-WHO collaboration

The WFSA collaborated in 1983 with the WHO in the revision of the anaesthetics/analgesics section of the "Model List of Essential Drugs". The objective of this document was to provide source material for adaptation by national authorities, particularly in developing countries [21]. Dr. Michael B. Dobson wrote a clear and concise book entitled *"Anaesthesia at the District Hospital"* specifically oriented to anaesthesia in developing countries, which was published in 1988 by WHO in co-operation with the WFSA [22]. A second revised edition has just been published. Details on this extended collaboration can be found in the specific chapter: WFSA and WHO.

WFSA manuals

The WFSA has sponsored the publication of several monographs mainly intended for the lesser-developed regions. These include *Manual on Cardiopulmonary Resuscitation* by Peter Safar, 1968 [23], *Cardiopulmonary Cerebral Resuscitation*, a considerably enlarged 3rd edition, written by P. Safar and N. Bircher, 1987 [24], *Cardiopulmonary Resuscitation for Lay Persons* by N. Caroline, subsidized by the International League of the Red Cross with joint sponsorship of the WFSA [3, 25], *Obstetric Analgesia and Anaesthesia* by John Bonica, 1972 [26], with a 2nd revised edition published in 1980 [27], *Handbook of Obstetric Analgesia and Anaesthesia*, edited by Graham H. McMorland and Gertie Marx, 1992 [28], *Basic Techniques of Nerve Blockade* by D. Bruce Scott, 1992 [29], and *Basic Considerations of Paediatric Anaesthesia*, written by Anneke E.E. Meursing and David Steward, 1992 [30]. Some of these manuals were revised and reprinted, as well as translated into several languages. The authors deserve special recognition for the time and effort they donated to those highly successful endeavours.

In 1984, the secretary, Dr. John Zorab, started a series originally entitled *"WFSA Lectures"*, which, in 1985, changed its name to *"Lectures in Anaesthesiology"* [11, 31]. It consisted of two issues per year. Due to lack of continued financial support this worthwhile project was discontinued, with the publication of volume 5 in 1988.

In 1984, upon being elected President of the WFSA, I chose two key words as representative for the quadrennium: *communication and co-operation* [11]. There is a strong need to establish proper communication in order to understand each other's positions, essential needs, and aspirations. It is only after proper communication is attained that any kind of co-operation can hope to prosper. No project leading to common goals can evolve successfully without adequate understanding between human beings.

Monitoring standards

In 1992 an International Task Force for the Safe Practice of Anaesthesia met in The Hague, during the 12th WCA, to prepare a document defining basic standards for all national societies [32]. These standards were adopted by the WFSA on 13 June 1992. It must be recognised that at present it is impossible to impose worldwide standards, however meritorious, such is the asymmetry in knowledge, manpower, and technology between countries. Compliance with the standards is a desirable goal, but represents a present and future challenge.

Clinical competence and technology

When considering the quality of medical and anaesthesia care it could be argued that technology should take second place to proficient knowledge and personal empathy. Dedicated physicians can offer comfort and psychological support even when lacking proper equipment. From the patient's point of view trust in a person is considerably more important than a paraphernalia of non-communicating and fearsome equipment. High tech does not necessarily imply high quality of medical care and low tech need not be equated with low quality of medical care [33]. It could be stated that in developing regions even no tech is far better than wrong tech [33, 34]. In other words, developed regions need not necessarily be assumed as the overall paradigm for medical practice and, on the other hand, developing regions should not be considered as stereotypes of inadequate medical care. The diversity is large and there are enclaves of different degrees of development in most countries. The quest for extended clinical competence is essential. Electronic instruments are useful, provided they are complemented by a supporting infrastructure. Otherwise they are useless and may even be dangerous. *A technology dependent anaesthesiologist is an anathema in the undeveloped world.*

Donated equipment

Ill-guided attempts have been made to try to "improve" anaesthesia simply by sending modern or discarded equipment to underdeveloped regions without providing instructions for its proper use and maintenance. Under such conditions equipment may last 1 year, 1 month, 1 day, 1 h, or 1 s. There are cemeteries of unused and unsuitable equipment lying idle in the underdeveloped world without any benefit to patients [34]. Most donations stem from good will. However, it seems that they may only create a warm and complacent feeling in the donors rather than helping the receivers. A common mistake is to send equipment with wrong connections or with fittings for a nonexisting gas supply. Another common error is to send electrical equipment with the wrong voltage. Such mistakes reflect the degree of ignorance in relation to prevailing local conditions, and obviously render the equipment useless. To be effective, donated equipment must be adapted to local needs.

Offering equipment and technology to unprepared minds and introducing it to an unprepared milieu is an exercise in futility and waste. D. Mackenzie well describes the scenario of wasting assets: "Another way technologies lose their potency is by disconnection from the infrastructure that supports them. The Third World is littered with real, rusting examples of disconnection: with the remains of technologies that work well enough under First World conditions but fail in the absence of supporting networks" [35]. Guidelines for the donation of anaesthesia equipment have been described for the information of donors and the optimisation of the deed. In order to obviate inadequate use and waste of limited resources, the WFSA offers training in Africa on the maintenance and repair of essential anaesthesia equipment. Such courses are invaluable for the proper and safe use of available equipment [20].

World asymmetry: the challenge facing the WFSA

It is regrettable that at the turn of the century and the beginning of the new millenium the world continues to show great social and economic asymmetry. Roughly three-quarters of the 6 billion human beings still suffer from inadequate living conditions. The three medical scourges of humanity as singled out by the WHO - malaria, tuberculosis, and AIDS - still afflict hundreds of millions of human beings in underdeveloped regions and are responsible for a large number of preventable deaths yearly. Consider malaria as an example: in any year, 10% of the global population suffers its debilitating chills and fevers, and more than 1 million die; 90% of these deaths occurs in sub-Saharan Africa; most are children under the age of 5 years. The link between malaria and underdevelopment is much more powerful than generally appreciated [36, 37]. Jeffrey Sachs concisely expresses its major impact on human suffering: "Where malaria prospers most, human societies have prospered least" [36]. The United Nations publishes yearly a United Nations Human Development Report (UNHDR). Chapter 1 of the UNHDR for 2001, "Human development - past, present, and future", reveals, in the section "New challenges and setbacks", the catastrophic impact of AIDS, especially in Africa: "At the end of 2000 about 36 million people were living with HIV/AIDS - 95% of them in developing countries and 70% in sub-Saharan Africa" [38]. Inadequate living environments prove to be a culture medium for the resurgence of tuberculosis.

The UNHDR for 2001 shows a technological map of the world dividing geographical areas according to the degree of available technology [39]. Descriptive terms such as technology leaders, potential adopters, and technology marginalised regions are self-explanatory, again showing the immense disparity in existing infrastructure. Jeffrey Sachs describes a new map of the world identifying world technological asymmetry in terms of technology innovators, technology receivers, and technology excluded regions [33]. In a similar vein Sachs' well-documented article "The geography of poverty and wealth" [40] delineates global distribution of economic output by means of a "world map showing GNP density - the product of population density and gross national product per capita".

The UNHDR for 1999, "Globalization with a human face", states the desirable aim: "Global markets, global technology, global ideas, and global solidarity can enrich the lives of people everywhere. The challenge is to ensure that the benefits are shared equitably and that this increasing interdependence works for people - not just for profits" [41]. Regrettably, the reality is quite different as the UNHDR for 2001 reveals: "Human development challenges remain large in the new millennium. Across the world we see unacceptable levels of deprivation in people's lives. Of the 4.6 billion people in developing countries, more than 850 million are illiterate, nearly a billion lack access to improved water sources, and 2.4 billion lack access to basic sanitation. Nearly 325 million boys and girls are out of school. And 11 million children under age 5 die each year from preventable causes - equivalent to more than 30,000 a day" [38].

A definition of underdevelopment implies regions where life and work are cheap, nutrition, health, and access to medical care are inadequate, poverty, illiteracy, and violence are abundant, constitutional rights are mere words, and hope for a better future is absent [33, 34]. A list of the essential needs of developing regions consists of any number of the following: food, potable water, sewage disposal, housing, clothing, education, work, transportation, leisure, access to medical care, eradication of endemic disease, and control of epidemic disease [33, 34]. The undeveloped world is best defined as any region lacking some or all of these essential needs, in other words, devoid of adequate infrastructure. Surgery and anaesthesia could be listed as the very last of the many basic needs. Under such dire living conditions the WFSA can hardly succeed in fully achieving its main objectives.

There exists an indisputable asymmetry in social and economic conditions throughout the world. Infrastructure and the basic tenets for adequate nutrition and health are regrettably extremely unequal. It can hardly be expected that all patients will uniformly receive safe and comfortable anaesthesia under such disparate living conditions.

The information age myth

It was thought that technology and the information age would decrease worldwide disparity and in a given time close the existing gap between rich and poor nations. However, it seems to have increased it. M. Dertouzos believes that "The gap between rich and poor can be closed but it will require concerted efforts, charity and more" [42, 43]. In plain words, unequal living conditions can not be corrected simply by injections of money and with technology transfer. It will require time to create the necessary infrastructure and a critical mass of capable and educated personnel to consistently and in a sustainable fashion increase living standards. Obviously, overcoming human poverty [44] remains outside the WFSA capacity. The UNHDR for 2001 describes the problem well: "Making new technologies work for human development" [38].

Many scientists have looked into the problem of world asymmetry and left us with more questions than solutions. Freeman Dyson asserted: "I am looking for ways in which technology may contribute to social justice, the alleviation of differences between rich and poor, to the preservation of the earth" [45]. WFSA's considerably smaller objective can not be achieved without adequate solutions for those larger overall problems.

Norman Borlaug, Nobel Peace Prize, 1970, wrote: "Don't think even for one minute that we will have permanent world peace on empty stomachs and human misery. It will not happen" [33]. Quite obviously, anaesthesia can only be improved after essential requirements for adequate living conditions, are implemented.

Amartya Sen, Nobel Economy Prize for 2000, makes a strong case for ethics in economics. "Progress is more plausibly judged by the reduction of deprivation than by the further enrichment of the opulent" [33, 46]. Indeed, technology is deaf/mute, non-communicating, and frightening to most patients; it is also morally neutral and by itself can do either good or evil. It requires proper use by intelligent, educated, and ethically oriented individuals.

In short, whereas the developed world has become technology dependent, the undeveloped world remains devoid of proper technology. As long as such disparities persist, the challenges facing the WFSA and similar international organisations will impede required and desired achievements. Worldwide anaesthesia care with safety and comfort depends ultimately on the overall symmetrical improvement of the dire social and economic conditions under which the larger part of humanity still lives.

Paul Valéry, a French poet, left in 1932 the following harsh synthesis: "Humanity has never known so much power with so much disorder, so much leisure with so much anguish, so much wealth with so much poverty, and so much knowledge with so much uncertainty" [33]. It is a sad reflection of our times that 70 years later those words can be repeated in their full context. Despite a veritable revolution in technology and explosive increase in wealth, the overall majority of human beings are still living in conditions of abject poverty. This challenge is beyond the realms of the WFSA. Unfortunately, without its correction it is unrealistic to consider that the WFSA main objective, that of "offering safe anaesthesia to all peoples of the world", can be accomplished. The ugly question lurking ahead is: for how much longer will the terrible gap between rich and poor countries continue to exist? It is no consolation to those suffering that a comparable statement, made a few centuries ago by the French moralist La Bruyére (1645-1696) indicates that asymmetric living conditions have plagued our planet for a very long time indeed: "Il y a une espèce de honte d´être heureux à la vue de certaines misères" [33, 47] (There is a special kind of shame on being happy in view of such misery).

This long-standing incapacity to ameliorate widespread inhuman living conditions should make us pause to consider a sober sentence written by the neurobiologist and ethicist, Jean-Pierre Changeux: "Qu´a-t-il donc dans la téte, cet *Homo* qui s´attribue sans vergogne l´épithète *sapiens?*" [48] (What then, does he have in his head, this *Homo* who shamelessly calls himself *sapiens?*). Have science and technology become overly arrogant and dissociated from basic human values?

Conclusion

In conclusion, it is evident that the challenges facing the WFSA far surpass its ability to fully achieve its objectives. This should not serve as an excuse to despair of any solution. With its educational activities in developing regions leading to the possible effective and sustained transfer of knowledge and technology what little can be done signifies a step upwards from the inadequate medical care still prevailing in many parts of the world. In the face of millions of yearly deaths from violence, avoidable diseases, and deprivation, if anaesthesia can contribute to one life saved, one patient made comfortable, one painless delivery, no matter where, the effort will be worthwhile and represents positive achievements against seemingly insurmountable challenges. The WFSA looks ahead towards forthcoming years with the continuing commitment to achieve its now enlarged mission statement [20]: WFSA objectives are to make available the highest standards of anaesthesia, pain relief, and resuscitation to all peoples of the world and to disseminate the same amongst them".

References

1. Griffith HR (1963) History of the World Federation of Anesthesiologists. Anesth Analg 42:389-397

2. WFSA statutes and bylaws (1996)

3. Bonica JJ (1984) WFSA presidential address

4. WFSA annual report (2002)

5. WFSA Newsletter, May 2003

6. Eltringham R Chairman, WFSA Publications Committee (2003) Report, February 2003. WFSA Newsletter, May 2003

7. Update in Anaesthesia. WFSA. A Journal for Anaesthetists in Developing Countries

8. World Anaesthesia. WFSA

9. (1997) World Anaesthesia 1:2

10. WFSA Newsletter 1-9, 1965-1973. Springer-Verlag

11. Parsloe C (1988) WFSA presidential report

12. Secher O (1985) Anaesthesiology Centre Copenhagen. In: Rupreht J, van Lieburg HJ, Lee JA, Erdman W (eds). Anaesthesia essays on its history. Springer, Berlin Hlidelberg New York

13. Garcia LEH (1995) El Centro Latino-Americano de Anestesiologia. In: Carlos Rivas Larrazabal y la Anestesiologia Venezolana. Edited by the Cátedra de Anestesiologia de la Faculdad de Medicina, UCV. Caracas

14. Parsloe C (1998) An outstanding anaesthetist - Professor Juan Armando Nesi. World Anaesthesia 2:14

15. Anesthesiology Center Western Pacific. University of the Philippines College of Medicine. Folder, January 1973

16. WFSA annual report 1996/1997

17. WFSA Education Committee report. Angela Enright (Chair), February, 2003

18. Urzua J. Personal communication

19. (2003) Courses in anaesthesia for the developing world. World Anaesthesia 7:20

20. WFSA about us web site: http://www.anaesthesiologists.org/aboutus_mission.html

21. WHO Model Prescribing Information. Drugs used in anaesthesia. World Health Organisation. Geneva, 1989

22. Dobson MB (1988) Anaesthesia at the District Hospital. WHO. Prepared in collaboration with the World Federation of Societies of Anaesthesiologists.

23. Safar P (1968) Cardiopulmonary resuscitation. A manual for physicians and paramedical instructors. Prepared for the World Federation of Societies of Anaesthesiologists

24. Safar P, Bircher NG (1988) Cardiopulmonary cerebral resuscitation, 3rd edn. Prepared for the World Federation of Societies of Anaesthesiologists. Saunders

25. Caroline N. Manual on cardiopulmonary resuscitation for lay people

26. Bonica JJ (1972) Obstetric analgesia and anesthesia. A manual for physicians, nurses and other personnel. Prepared for the World Federation of Societies of Anaesthesiologists, Springer-Verlag

27. Bonica JJ (1989) Obstetric analgesia and anesthesia. A manual for medical students, physicians in training, midwives, nurses, and other health personnel. Prepared for the World Federation of Societies of Anaesthesiologists. Amsterdam

28. McMorland GH, Marx G (1992) Handbook of obstetric analgesia and anesthesia. Prepared for the World Federation of Societies of Anaesthesiologists, by the committee on obstetric anaesthesia and analgesia

29. Scott DB (1989) Basic techniques of nerve blockade. A WFSA manual. Mediglobe AS

30. Meursing AEE, Steward DJ (eds) (1992) Basic considerations of paediatric anaesthesia. A WFSA manual

31. Zorab JSM (ed) (1984-1988) Lectures in anaesthesiology. Published in Association with the World Federation of Societies of Anaesthesiologists. Blackwell Scientific Publications

32. International Standards for a Safe Practice of Anaesthesia. Eur J Anaesthesiol (1993) [Suppl 17]:12-15

33. Parsloe C (2003) Worlds apart? Healthcare technologies for lifelong disease management. IEEE Eng Med Biol 22:53-56

34. Parsloe C (1994) The introduction of technology in the Third World: problems and proposals. J Clin Monit 10:147-152

35. Mackenzie D (1997) Wasting assets. London Rev Books 19:24-25

36. Scientific American editors (2002) Perspectives. A death every 30 seconds. Sci Am 286:2

37. Dunavan CP. (2002) Men, money and malaria. Sci Am 286:86-87

38. United Nations Human Development Report 2001. Chapter 1. Human development-past, present and future

39. United Nations Human Development Report 2001. The geography of technological innovations and achievements

40. Sachs JD (2001) The geography of poverty and wealth. Sci Am 284:62-67

41. United Nations Human Development Report 1999. Globalization with a human face

42. Leutwyler K (1997) Profile: M.L. Dertouzos. Sci Am 277:28-29

43. Dertouzos ML (1998) What will be. Harper Edge, San Francisco

44. United Nations Human Development Report 2000. Overcoming human poverty

45. Dyson FJ (1998) The sun, the genome and the internet. Tools of Scientific Revolution. Oxford University Press, New York

46. Sen AK (1987) On ethics and economics. Cambridge University Press

47. La Bruyère J de (1688) Les caractères ou les moeurs de ce siècle, 1688. In: Encyclopaedia Brittanica, 15th edn. Micropaedia 1978, 5:971

48. Changeux JP (1983) L'homme neuronal. Librairie Arthème Fayard, Paris

19 THE FUTURE OF WFSA

T.C.K. Brown, A.E.E. Meursing

*M*uch has happened since it was decided at the International Anaesthesia Congress in Paris in 1951 that a world organisation should be set up. An Interim Committee was set up with Harold Griffith as chairman. The other members were Alexandre Goldblatt (Belgium), John Gillies (UK), Jacques Boureau (France), Torsten Gordh (Sweden), with Jean Francisque Delafresnaye from the Council for International Medical Organisations as a consultant. They met in 1953 with some others and again in 1954. It was decided to hold the First World Congress in the Netherlands in 1955. This was held at Scheveningen in September 1955 under the chairmanship of Ritsema van Eck.

This book reviews the history of the first 50 years of the organisation. It is appropriate that the 2004 World Congress is being held in Paris where the idea of the establishment of WFSA originated.

Anaesthesia organisations

The International Anaesthesia Research Society (IARS) was formed many years before the WFSA. The major difference between the organisations is that IARS has individual membership whereas WFSA takes physician anaesthesiology associations and societies (minimum 10 members) as their members. The number of anaesthesia societies in the WFSA and worldwide has quadrupled. New anaesthesia training institutions have developed in many countries and hence the number of anaesthesiologists has increased considerably - 15-20 times since the inauguration of the WFSA. Anaesthesia has expanded to include new branches such as intensive care and pain management. Many subspecialties such as obstetrics, paediatrics, cardio-thoracic, regional, and neuro-anaesthesia have arisen and organised themselves into specialty groups.

WFSA has regional groups in Europe, Latin America, Asia-Australasia, and Africa. In addition, there are smaller regional organisations such as the South Asian and ASEAN Confederations and the Pan Arab group.

Anaesthesia per se

Fifty years ago ether was still widely used even in affluent countries. Spinal anaesthesia was used. The methods were not totally dissimilar in affluent and poor countries. Progress came in the form of new drugs, which offered many advantages, but had their own inherent dangers and added complexity and costs.

The move towards total intravenous anaesthesia resulted from improved understanding of the pharmacokinetics, the availability of accurate and adjustable infusion pumps, and concern about environmental pollution. It is not yet universally applicable.

Monitoring was minimal - a blood pressure cuff, maybe electrocardiography and, for children, a precordial stethoscope. It improved slowly - it needed to progress to counter the problems created by newer, more-potent drugs, which sometimes had their own hazardous side-effects, particularly when used by inadequately trained people. Pulse oximetry led to an advance in safety because it provided an early warning of decreasing oxygen delivery to the tissues. Capnography provided a tool, which indicated ventilatory status but also warned of failed intubation and diminished cardiac output with decreased blood flow through the lungs following air embolism or other causes. Measurement of agent and gas concentrations and other forms of invasive and non-invasive monitoring have been introduced in more-affluent countries. Monitoring of the depth of anaesthesia is also becoming more widespread. How relevant are these if a country or hospital cannot afford them or does not have staff who know how to use them?

It is difficult to foresee major discoveries that will alter how anaesthesia is administered. Changes often occur gradually. The introduction of the laryngeal mask airway has reduced the need for intubation and the use of muscle relaxants. Total intravenous anaesthesia has many adherents, but will it become generally applicable in all countries?

In recent years major changes have taken place in the treatment of diseases that were previously treated with traditional surgery. Endoscopic surgery and interventional radiology avoid the complex surgical procedures of the past and their problems, including blood loss.

Will the work of the anaesthesiologist change and maybe become less demanding? Will new technology or drugs be developed that will simplify the process of anaesthesia and pain control? Electrical anaesthesia was used briefly years ago. Will some other completely new concept develop that will totally change what we do or will work stations develop so that they include computer control of the anaesthetic? Lampard et al. at Monash University, Melbourne, Australia developed computer control of halothane anaesthesia using a feed back loop with blood pressure in 1972. They also developed the use of computer-controlled muscle relaxation with elecromyography in about 1975. Similar means of drug administration could be developed for wider use. The limiting factors are the complexity of the equipment and the need to have adequately trained people to use and maintain it.

The knowledge base has expanded, new techniques, equipment, and drugs have become available, but there are still two problems that work against uniform progress - the world population continues to increase and the economic gap between rich and poor nations widens. In addition, progress is also halted in many countries by the disruption caused by economic instability or armed conflict.

Economics

The divergence between the wealthy and poor countries continues to increase. Costs increase with each step in improving equipment and the development of new drugs. While these increases may be small compared with the total surgical and hospital costs, they are still significant, sometimes increasing by a factor of 10 or more. Other fields in medicine have been expanding at the same time, many, such as radiology, to a much greater extent than anaesthesia. Healthcare costs have exploded as investigation and treatment possibilities have expanded. Governments have begun to restrict health budgets. However, affluent countries can still afford much more than poor countries who have health budgets of as little as U.S. $ 2-3 per head of population. Advances in poor countries have been slower and these countries have fallen further behind. Today wealthy countries provide aid, often for political reasons. Frequently, this aid comes in an inappropriate form because the poorer countries do not have regular supplies of basics such as electricity and gas. Less-affluent countries cannot afford the replaceable accessories. They may never learn how to use the equipment or may have nobody to maintain it. Helping to bridge this gap is one of the greatest challenges for the WFSA. One WFSA development was the establishment of the maintenance and repair of equipment workshop. This project was initiated in Uganda with the support of Penlon. It was designed to teach those giving anaesthetics, as well as technicians and engineers, how to repair and maintain their equipment. The project has now spread to surrounding countries. Hopefully this is the beginning of a process that will help to overcome this problem.

A major economic downturn can affect the funding of healthcare, but it can also influence the funding available to the WFSA for education, publications, and administration. A financial depression will inhibit creative development of new initiatives. Thus, the WFSA Foundation (a charity) has been developed to raise additional funds to enhance the WFSA programs. The credit for this initiative goes to the past Treasurer, Professor Michael Rosen.

Manpower

The inadequate number of physician anaesthetists has been a problem throughout the history of the specialty. Some countries have solved the shortage by training non-physicians: nurses, clinical officers, or medical assistants. The number of medical, and hence anaesthesia, graduates is inadequate to deal with the increasing population. This should be a matter of concern to our specialty, particularly as anaesthesia becomes more complex and the consequences of trauma become more serious.

There are several influencing factors. First, there must be enough trainee physician graduates. Deficiencies can be due to lack of interest in the specialty, poor remuneration and conditions, or lack of training positions. In addition, training time has been increasing in many countries to cater for the requirement for increased knowledge and the reduction in working hours. The latter was introduced because of economic factors and concern about the safety of long working hours. If funds and positions are limited, lengthening training time may result in decreasing the number of trainees, which is unacceptable in areas where there are already not enough anaesthesiologists. In addition, funds may not be available to train doctors in the specialty or governments may see reduced funding as a means of cutting costs, not realizing that quality of care and safety are jeopardized.

There is a body of opinion that the specialty should change its name to *Perioperative Medicine* to extend the anaesthesiologist's work to include preoperative assessment and preparation, anaesthesia, postoperative care, pain management, and intensive care. This may reflect the anaesthesiologist's work in some countries but, again, it requires an increase in manpower. To continue to ensure the highest standards of patient care during surgery is of paramount importance.

The *relief of pain* during surgery is the purpose of anaesthesia, but postoperative pain management, chronic pain, and palliative care attract the interest of an increasing number of anaesthesiologists. This is appropriate in view of the knowledge and skills of anaesthesiologists but it does demand a significant time commitment by more people. Other medical specialists, as well as nurses, physiotherapists, and psychologists, are also involved in these fields, which may, in more-advanced countries, gradually separate off as a new specialty, again with loss of anaesthesia manpower.

Intensive care in many centres was begun by anaesthesiologists and, particularly in Europe, remains largely under their control. As the work becomes more specialised so the tendency for a separate specialty evolves.

These are some of the changes that have been occurring at different rates in different countries, which affect not only manpower but also the workload of our specialty. The role of the anaesthesiologist is widening and needs to be redefined.

These developments create a dilemma. We can widen our role to become perioperative physicians. We have the broad training to do so. However, in countries where the specialty is advanced, there is increasing specialisation within this field and eventually people become dedicated to pain management or intensive care and stop contributing to anaesthesia. New specialities emerge and the anaesthesiologist's boundaries retract back to the more-immediate care of the patient before and during surgery. This has already occurred in a few countries.

However, if we demonstrate a level of clinical expertise that is recognised by other specialists, anaesthesiologists could become leaders of the perioperative team. If they do, in countries where there are inadequate numbers of anaesthesiologists, it may be appropriate that anaesthesiologists supervise adequately trained non-physicians giving routine anaesthetics. The key to success is dependent on the adequacy of the supervision. Anaesthesiologists have to supervise thoroughly if they are to be respected by their colleagues. Failure to do so will create the opportunity for non-physicians to become independent and so demean our medical specialty. This is already a threat in some countries. If leadership of the perioperative team can be achieved, it may enhance the specialty but surgeons may not want others to control the care of their patients. In countries where there are enough doctors, adequate numbers can be trained as anaesthesiologists so that the highest standards can be maintained. These standards are attained by physician anaesthesiologists. This is the situation in some countries, but the reality is that there are many countries where this is unlikely ever to be achieved. In those countries anaesthesiologists must set the standard and ensure that the best possible anaesthesia is achieved under the circumstances by training and properly supervising anyone else giving anaesthesia.

Education

The WFSA has been very active in continuing education and publications as a means to improve the standards of anaesthesia worldwide. These are areas where great changes are occurring. The explosion of information and advances in the means of communication presents a challenge to ensure that appropriate methods are used. There has already been a decline in the publication of books and journals as printed works with increasing availability on CDs and on the Internet. The rapid rise in the number of people from an increasing number of countries accessing *Update in Anaesthesia* from the Internet indicates that even relatively poor countries have Internet access. Update is already available in several languages and there is potential for more to follow.

Journals, groups of journals, and proceedings of congresses are available now on CD so that the cost of postage of the journals is eliminated. There is great potential for teaching and learning using the Internet, which will make it easier to provide anaesthesia education by distance learning. More anaesthesiologists will have access to all the information. The problem is that there will still be some people without Internet access. These people are already disadvantaged by lack of access to literature. Maximising the use of the latest accessible technology will be important for those in the WFSA responsible for the teaching programmes. Distance learning programmes are already being developed.

Improving safety needs constant attention. Reporting and analysing complications so that we learn how to manage them better would help anaesthesiologists to correct problems more readily. The International Patient Safety Foundation and the Australian Incident Monitoring Study promote such programmes. These need to be developed in more countries with the help of the WFSA Patient Safety and Quality of Practice Committee.

The introduction of simulators, whether they be complex set or simple computer-based programmes, and immediate access to comprehensive anaesthesia information online will help to improve our response to complications and thus reduce serious complications, morbidity, and mortality.

Training

Training in anaesthesia varies around the world. Methods and duration of training, assessment, and standards vary widely. The Federation can encourage the introduction of uniform training standards, but implementation would need to be done on a regional basis. The European Academy has already established a European standard, but the numbers sitting these examinations is still limited, many people opting only to have their national qualification.

Development of a common syllabus and assessment or examinations should begin regionally. Some moves to standardise training have already been made in regions outside Europe. CLASA and parts of Africa have been discussing this. Eventually regional diplomas might evolve, but more political co-operation is probably necessary to allow this to progress. National bodies often like to control their own standards and qualifications.

There are some regions where basic training of physician anaesthesiologists is still deficient. The Federation and several national societies or groups have supported the development of training centres to fill this need. These and similar programmes continue to be necessary. Some specialty anaesthesia training centres have been established and more are needed, especially in obstetric and paediatric anaesthesia. As finance becomes available, the number of these training centres should be increased.

Congresses

One of the prime reasons for the existence of the WFSA is to hold the 4-yearly World Congress where members of societies from all over the world can meet to discuss their problems, share their knowledge, become acquainted, and make friends. The increasing ability to transfer information through the Internet could threaten the survival of these large congresses because the information is so easily accessible. Even in 1996, sessions were relayed to Italy from the World Congress in Sydney. Travel, accommodation, and conference expenses can be saved as well as time. It is hoped that this will not happen. The opportunity to meet and talk to people from all over the world affords the chance for people with a common interest to become acquainted and develop mutual understanding. They are occasions to make friends from other parts of the world and possibly initiate exchanges, which would benefit both parties. Maybe these meetings can also help to reduce the prejudice and conflict, which arise so often when people of different races and creeds do not know and understand each other.

The Federation is made up of many societies, most of which belong to Regional Sections. These have developed for various reasons, often initially to hold a congress. They have had periods of activity and other periods of inactivity. It is hoped that these bodies can help to bring cohesion in their regions, developing standards and educational programmes, for instance, and that their member societies will continue to support and be involved with the activities of the World Federation.

An increasing number of specialty meetings are being held. They are often shorter but are held more frequently. They bring people with common special interests together, which has many advantages, but there is still a place to hold larger congresses involving all groups of anaesthesiologists so that cohesion is retained in the field. The idea, which has already been taken up in some centres, that anaesthesiologists are part of specialist surgical departments rather than an anaesthesiology department, should be discouraged if anaesthesia is to remain an important independent specialty.

Conclusion

In order for the Federation to perform to its full potential it is important that it has officers and committee members who will work together and contribute effectively towards the achievement of its goals. Efforts must continue to ensure that the committees are effective, functional units so that they can promote policies that improve the standards and safety of anaesthesia. The Federation needs the support of its member societies financially and help with its projects to ensure that it remains viable and can successfully pursue its aims and objectives.

Anaesthesia is now one of the largest medical specialties. WFSA should provide leadership in the field. The future of WFSA depends on the integrity of the specialty. The specialty needs a body that oversees all branches so that cohesion is retained. Anaesthesiologists must be competent in all aspects of their work and perform to a standard that will earn the respect of their colleagues, their patients, and the community.

20 WFSA STATUTES AND BYLAWS COMMITTEE: PROVIDING THE FRAMEWORK

D.J. Wilkinson

Introduction

Every organisation needs a legal existence, a structure, and a set of reference points. Its purpose and aspirations need to be carefully defined and regularly reviewed. There should be some clearly defined processes to encompass its day-to-day running, its overall management, and its planned development. Meetings, publications, and liaison with other organisations need to be carefully orchestrated and follow a repeatable and transparent process. Financial matters should be circumspect, with audited accounts being published and presented according to defined processes. The mechanisms whereby members join or leave need to be described and their roles within the organisation need to be spelt out. For an international body there are considerations relating to different cultures, languages, religions, and social mores. All of these subjects require regular review and development to ensure that the organisation does not become stagnant and ineffective in a changing world.

The statutes and bylaws of the WFSA provide this framework. It is the bedrock on which the organisation is founded. The framework is monitored by the Statutes and Bylaws Committee, one of the Standing Committees of the WFSA. They are a small group who meet infrequently but correspond regularly. This chapter will outline the development and processes of this crucial committee, together with the development of the "rules" that currently provide the framework in which the WFSA now functions.

In the beginning

The first sign of a constitution for an international anaesthesia society appears to have been that produced by Dr. Marcel Thalheimer, a French surgeon, who co-organised an annual anaesthesia congress in France entitled Société Française d'Anésthesiologie. In 1951 he attended a meeting held in

London jointly organised by the Association of Anaesthetists of Great Britain and Ireland and the International Anaesthesia Research Society (IARS), bringing a draft constitution for a new truly international anaesthesia group.

The constitution, and the concept of an international society, was considered by British, American, and Canadian anaesthetists, as well as practitioners from several other countries, both in London and then subsequently at a further meeting in Paris that same year. There was no enthusiasm for the proposed constitution as set out by these French surgeons, but the concept of a world-wide anaesthesia society gained much support.

In Paris at this time was Dr. Jean Delafresnaye, the Secretary General of the Council for International Organisation of Medical Societies (CIOMS), which was a sub-division of the United Nations Educational, Scientific, and Cultural Organisation and the World Health Organisation (UNESCO and WHO). He suggested the formation of a special Anaesthetic Committee to consider the formation of a world organisation further. Over the next few years a selected group of five anaesthetists collected information about the state of anaesthesia in the majority of countries across the world. These five were to become the first Bylaws Committee, although without that name. They were Dr. Alex Goldblat (Belgium), Dr. Ritsema van Eck (The Netherlands), Dr. Jean Delafresnaye (France), Dr. Harold Griffiths (Canada), and Dr. Geoffrey Organe (Great Britain and Ireland).

In 1953 they decided that they had enough information to consider at a formal meeting and they met in Brussels in June of that year with several further colleagues. Having made the decision to form a world organisation, a large portion of the 3-day meeting was devoted to the formulation of a constitution. Dr. Delafresnaye took a leading role in this work using his experience of other international groups gleaned while working with CIOMS.

It was agreed that the new organisation should be a federation of societies rather than a new membership organisation to prevent it "falling into the hands of any ambitious and possibly unscrupulous groups or individuals" [1]. The basic aim of the organisation was, at the suggestion of Dr. Delafresnaye, set in very simple terms namely "Better anaesthesia for more people throughout the world". (Harold Griffiths suggested that someone paraphrased this as "Better dope for more dopes"!)

Initial proposals in the constitution

The main power of the proposed federation was centred on the General Assembly, a group of anaesthetists (delegates) who would meet at a World Congress every 4-5 years. These delegates would be elected by their national societies, and it was felt crucial that no matter how small a society was it should still have a reasonable voice within this assembly. A plan was formulated so that every society had one member, and then depending on a simple formula more delegates were permitted depending on the size of the society (e.g.,

1-500 members=1 delegate, 501-1,000 members=1 further delegate, and then 1 more delegate for each further 1,000 members). A similar process was planned for the financial contribution of each society to this World Federation so that the larger the society the greater the contribution to the finances.

The assembly would elect an Executive Committee that would carry out the work of the Federation assisted by an elected President and secretary/treasurer. The Executive Committee would have representation from each geographical area, and it was felt important that those two countries with the majority of members must always have a place on the committee. The group also believed it would be important to hold a World Congress of Anaesthesia on a regular basis.

Preliminary committee

The group realised that the creation of an effective constitution was vital for the new federation and set up the first named constitution committee. The members were Dr. Alex Goldblat (Belgium), Dr. Ritsema van Eck (The Netherlands), Dr. Jean Delafresnaye (France and CIOMS), and Dr. Geoffrey Organe (UK and Ireland). This group sent out the proposed constitution to every national society and invited their comments.

These comments were then reviewed and a new constitution and bylaws were created at a meeting held in Scheveningen, The Netherlands, in June 1954. This was a meeting of the whole interim Organising Committee that had met in Brussels in June 1953 plus one or two others.

It was noted that the majority of societies had approved the preliminary constitution and the scene was set for the first World Congress of the WFSA held 5-10 September 1955 in Scheveningen, The Netherlands.

During this meeting the final version of the constitution and bylaws was created and nominations for the Executive Committee were made. On the last day of the congress, 9 September 1953, the first formal General Assembly was convened. At this meeting those member societies present were recognised together with the delegates they had nominated to be present at the General Assembly. The first item of business was the acceptance of the new constitution and bylaws as proposed by Dr. Goldblat the chairman of the preliminary Statutes Committee. The new articles and bylaws had been discussed at a preliminary meeting of delegates and had been translated into Dutch to conform with the legal requirements of a constitution under Dutch law. This translation was reviewed by Dr. van Eck and a public notary and the Minister of Justice, all of whom had been most helpful. Dr. van Eck then moved that the assembly accept this first constitution, and this was seconded by Dr. Mayrhofer and accepted unanimously by the delegates. This action heralded the official formation of the WFSA.

The new constitution was then resubmitted to the Minister of Justice and the Queen of The Netherlands to ensure full legal recognition and registration of the WFSA in The Netherlands. It is strange to read that the WFSA is referred to as an "association" with a fixed time existence, namely "for a period of about 29 years and this until the ult. of December 1984". This is presumably a legal requirement in The Netherlands. It is important to note that at this time the Dutch translation of this document was regarded as the authoritative document. This new constitution was then "published" in English as an annexe to the Netherlands Official Gazette of Friday 17 August 1956, no. 160.

Next developments

A new, elected, Bylaws Committee met to continue to develop the structure of the new Federation. It was chaired by Professor Ciocotto (Italy), and Professor Gordon (Canada), Professor Yamamura (Japan), Dr Boureau (France), and Dr Failing (USA) served on the committee. Dr Organe, the new secretary/treasurer, made the headquarters of the WFSA in his London home, even though the headquarters according to the constitution were "situated in Amsterdam where it has its domicile in the Burger Ziekenhuis (Hospital)", and effectively ran the organisation from there. The new organisation had limited finances and so there were no regular meetings of the various committees. In 1959 the United States finally agreed to join the Federation just in time to contribute to the 2nd World Congress held in Toronto in 1960. At the General Assembly of this congress a new chairman of the Committee on Bylaws was elected, Dr. Joseph Failing (USA), and a new member Dr. Suarez y Munoz-Ledo (Mexico) replaced Professor Ciocotto (Italy). The bylaws had been modified during this time, as experience determined different working patterns, but the next major review was presented at the 3rd congress in Sao Paulo, Brazil in 1964. This established a pattern of working for the General Assembly. The formal Standing Committees of the WFSA were now well established, credentials, nominations, membership, finance together with statutes and bylaws. This latter group was to be made up predominantly from the old Bylaws Committee.

In the General Assembly minutes there is confusion created by the use of two headings, one of bylaws and the other of statutes. Under bylaws the chairman of the committee, Dr. Failing (USA), announced that a variety of changes had been suggested and these were approved by the General Assembly. Then under statutes the secretary/treasurer announced that all delegates would need to sign a document recognising and agreeing changes to the statutes to bring them in line with the changes in the bylaws. These would then have to be taken to the Dutch authorities for official approval. The final circulated and published document is entitled *Bylaws of the WFSA* and that is what is contained. However there were separate statutes that did not seem to be circulated in the same manner. The initial bylaws essentially repeat the statutes and then go on to develop other matters. The statutes are written as numbered articles while the bylaws appear as chapters.

There were three further significant changes in the bylaws at this time. The first emphasised the importance of the role of the chairman of the Executive Committee who was stipulated to immediately take over the role of President of the WFSA should the elected President be unable or unwilling to adopt that role.

Next there was an increase in the number of delegates attending the General Assembly with the adoption of the following representation: societies with up to 250 members=1 delegate, 251-500 members=2 delegates, 501-1,000 members=3 delegates, and then 1 further delegate for each 1,000 members or fraction thereof.

The other major change was the separation of the roles of secretary and treasurer. Up to this time it had been a single post held by Geoffrey Organe, now two officers replaced Organe; Henning Poulsen (Denmark) became treasurer and Otto Mayrhofer (Austria) became secretary.

Subsequently the new bylaws document was apparently signed by all of the assembly delegates and the revised statutes/bylaws was resubmitted to the Dutch Ministry of Justice and subsequently approved by Queen Juliana of The Netherlands on 9 June 1965.

1964 objectives

It is worth reiterating the objectives of the WFSA at this time. "To make available the highest standards of the anaesthesia science to all peoples of the world and to try and disseminate the same amongst them and it shall in pursuit of that aim try:

a) to assist and encourage the formation of national societies of anesthesiologists;
b) to promote the dissemination of scientific information;
c) to recommend desirable standards for the training of anaesthesiologists;
d) to provide information regarding opportunities for post-graduate training and research;
e) to encourage research into all aspects of anaesthesiology;
f) to encourage the establishment of safety measures including the standardisation of equipment;
g) to advise on request national and international organisations;
h) apply all other lawful means which may be conducive to the object of the Federation."

These new 1964 bylaws of the WFSA were circulated in English to all member societies and responses and suggestions encouraged.

Time of consolidation

Over the next 4 years there was a time of consolidation. The General Assembly at the 4th World Congress in London made minimal changes to the bylaws. For the first time regional anaesthesiology societies came into the picture. These could be admitted as members if they existed in an area where no national societies had been convened. The only other major change was the recognition that some nations might be divided into two or more areas by political divisions, and if each of these divisions formed a national society then they could both be elected to membership and have delegates at a General Assembly. The committee membership was at this time Jan Crul (The Netherlands) {chairman}, John Beard (Great Britain and Ireland), Joseph Failing (USA), Rudolf Frey (West Germany), and R. Gordon (Canada).

In Kyoto in 1972 the General Assembly requested a complete revision of the bylaws and charged a new committee to do this. The members were now Professor Jan Crul (The Netherlands)(chairman), John Beard (UK), C. Castanos (Bolivia), D. Joseph (Australia), and E. Siker (USA). The committee adopted the policy of meeting during other major congresses and convened a meeting at the European Congress in Madrid in 1974. Unfortunately only two members of the committee were able to be present and the work of revision continued by letter. The essential changes brought to the Mexico City General Assembly in 1976 were the addition of the posts of deputy treasurer and deputy secretary, the abolition of an ad hoc pre-trial committee for the investigation of the terms of expulsion or suspension of a member society, the date at which the annual subscription is due, and most important of all for the future work of the Federation, the institution of a Committee on Education and Research Affairs.

It was proposed at this time that the Federation should recognise that it had three types of committee, Standing Committees (membership, statutes and bylaws, finance, and education and scientific affairs), Ad Hoc Committees (credentials, nominations and World Congress Venue Committee), and also Special Committees (set up as the need arose). Prior to this the credentials committee had been a Standing Committee and the Venue Committee was a new concept.

There were however some subtle small changes that were of importance. There were new aims for the Federation, the promotion of education was highlighted and more formally it was proposed "to organise at regular intervals a World Congress of anaesthesiology and sponsor regional congresses"; and also "To encourage meetings of special interest groups within the specialty and make provision for them to meet where appropriate at such congresses". A member society now needed 10 members rather than 5. The newly proposed deputy secretary and treasurer positions were not to be officers but would be members of the Executive Committee without a vote. It was also recognised that the Federation needed a World Congress Venue Committee, and this was established as an Ad Hoc Committee. Interestingly, the General Assembly approved the formation of a foundation within the Education Committee that would have a board of trustees, nominated by the Executive Committee, and this foundation would administer the financial aspects of education. Three thousand copies of the bylaws were then printed (in Manila where the WFSA President Quintin Gomez resided) and circulated to all member societies. The new Bylaws Committee was composed of Jan Crul (The Netherlands) (chairman), D. Joseph (Australia), John Zorab (Great Britain and Ireland), G. Converse (USA), and Luis Rodriguez Alves (Brazil).

In Paris in 1978 at the European Congress of Anaesthesiology, Jan Crul, who was still the chairman of the Statutes and Bylaws Committee, convened a meeting that noted very few further suggestions had been put forward. There were one or two financial matters that required clarification particularly the definition of "active members" of a society as it was this that the WFSA used as a basis for their subscription request. With the approach of the Hamburg Congress in 1980 a significant increase in the membership of the Executive Committee was proposed, from 13 to 16, to reflect the increase in member societies of the WFSA. In addition, it was thought that the period of time members of Special and Standing Committees served should be fixed, and there was the suggestion that societies that failed to respond to repeated communications from the secretary should be considered for expulsion. The exact remit of the foundation created in Mexico remained unclear and some even suggested that they might organise the scientific as well as the financial aspects of a World Congress. After much discussion by letter and at initial meetings in Hamburg, the statutes and bylaws were modified only slightly with a few minor textural changes. The expulsion of non-communicating societies, the fixing of membership of committees to "not normally more than two 4-year terms" and the abolition of the foundation and its board of trustees were the final major proposals that were accepted. The idea of increasing the size of the Executive did not find favour at this time. The amendments to the bylaws at this time took up three pages of the General Assembly minutes! There was much debate at the 2nd General Assembly in Hamburg over the composition of the Organising Committee for future World Congresses. The statutes and Bylaws Committee had suggested that two to three members of the Executive Committee should be seconded to the local Organising Committee. There was considerable discussion with some totally opposed to this and others suggesting that perhaps one or two Executive Committee members might be seconded. In the end it was agreed that the executive would "review the work of the national Organising Committee", although some in the assembly were unhappy that this was introduced without prior circulation and then passed without sufficient time for consideration.

A complete re-write

Several people had in the run-up to 1980 noted that the WFSA's constitution had been originally set for 29 years and thus would "run out" in 1984. There was the need for a major revision of the statutes and bylaws by this time and indeed the creation of a new legal constitution. A new chairman was appointed, Professor Michael Vickers (UK), and he immediately set about completely re-writing both the statutes and bylaws. His committee now included Jan Crul (The Netherlands), D. Joseph (Australia), G. Rolly (Belgium), and Gaby

Gurman (Israel). It was apparent to Vickers that the regular small changes that had taken place over the past decades had left various inconsistencies between the statutes and the bylaws. In addition there was a great deal of repetition between the two documents. He proposed to his committee in January 1981 that they take the opportunity to identify statutes that were the fundamental aspects of the WFSA and bylaws that would become the detailed operational document. By July 1981 he was able to circulate a formidable document that took this approach. It listed side-by-side the current text and his new suggestions and asked for their feedback. In a third column he indicated the nature of the change made and the reason for that change. By January 1983 this new document had been read, re-read, and modified by his committee and the Executive Committee. A new era was emerging as the WFSA considered these proposals at the General Assembly in Manila in 1984.

The statutes were divided into eight sections and were numbered as articles. These dealt with the name and objects of the Federation, membership, the General Assembly, the Executive Committee, finance, reports, dissolution, and the bylaws. These statutes were essentially modifications of the old ones, together with appropriate passages from the bylaws. The objects of the Federation were transferred from the bylaws unchanged into the statutes. There had been at this time some correspondence relating to the creation of a WFSA distinguished service award; this did not find favour and was abandoned.

The bylaws were divided into seven sections, membership, General Assembly, Executive Committee, committees, funds, and expenditure, secretariat, and amendment and interpretation of the bylaws. There was significant clarification and rationalisation created by this new document. In addition the major innovations were the constitution was amended to bring the Federation in line with tax law in the United States, the selection of chairmen of Standing Committees would be made by the Executive Committee, and a new membership category of associate member society was created for those for whom payment of membership subscription was not possible. This latter group would be made at the discretion of the Executive Committee. This new set of statutes and bylaws broke the link with Dutch law and for the first time the English version of the document became the authoritative one.

The Statutes and Bylaws Committee was restructured again at this time; Dr. Bill MacRae (Great Britain and Ireland) became chairman and was joined by A. Hare (Australia), G. Rolly (Belgium), G. Gurman (Israel), and R. McKechnie (USA).

All change but all the same

In the following 8 years there was a period of further consolidation, with some major changes in procedural matters. In Washington in 1988 the structure of the Nominations Committee was clarified. This is one of the most-powerful committees within the WFSA organisation and determines the nominations to the post of President and those nominated to the Executive Committee. It was therefore vital that its composition was diverse and yet that it retained the experience to ensure effective working of the executive and therefore of the WFSA. It was agreed that the executive would select 16 full societies 1 year prior to the General Assembly and then create a ballot from all of the membership to select 8 of these to form the committee. This was accepted by the General Assembly and is still the rule today. The other significant change was that the chairmen of the Standing Committees became members of executive; this permitted their input at a high level and did much to ensure the smooth running of the organisation. At this time Professor Benad (GDR) and Professor Fujita (Japan) replaced Dr. Rolly (Belgium) and Professor Gurman (Israel) on the committee.

In 1992 at The Hague Dr. MacRae presented five pages of amendments to the statutes and bylaws at the first General Assembly. The major amongst these were that the chairman of the Executive Committee became an officer of the WFSA, the size of the Finance Committee was increased, and there were a variety of financial amendments, and perhaps the most-significant addition to the WFSA, the formation of a Publications Committee as a new Standing Committee. The detailed amendments were published in 1993 and again sent out to all member societies. Professor Benad (Germany) became the new chairman of the Statutes and Bylaws Committee and was joined by Professor Fujita (Japan), Eli Brown (USA), John Richards (Australia), and Manuel Galindo (Columbia).

In Sydney in 1996 there were further minor changes, and again in Montreal in 2000. The committee was chaired by Manuel Gallindo from 1996 and was composed of John Richards (Australia), Eli Brown (USA), K.P. Inbasegaren (Malaysia), and David Wilkinson (Great Britain and Ireland). I took over the chairmanship in Montreal and have been helped by K.P. Inbasegaren (Malaysia), Alfredo Cattaneo (Argentina), Bill Owens (USA), and Igor Molchanov (Russia). Over these last 8 years meetings have been very infrequent and the committee has been fairly dormant.

It is likely that there needs to be a major revision at this time of the way the WFSA is both structured and the way it runs its business. What was right for the 1980s is not so relevant in a new millennium. It will be interesting to see in the future whether this can take place and the exact nature of these changes. Changes to the basic statutes and bylaws should not be rushed or undertaken lightly, as they have been carefully scripted and refined over the years to enhance the work of the WFSA.

Conclusions

The Statutes and Bylaws of the WFSA form the bedrock on which all of the activity of the organisation is based. The changes in those "rules" reflect the changing social, economic, and educational states and needs of its member countries, and provide a fascinating insight into the development of the Federation.

Change for change's sake is not useful and the old adage of "if it ain't broke don't try and fix it" holds true in this context. Many of the regulations that control the functioning of the Federation are sound but appear archaic to the present day individual members, and this reflects both a degree of truth and also a lack of understanding of the basic rules.

Communication is the essence of a good organisation and that communication needs to be of a very high standard in both directions. This is perhaps where greater emphasis needs to be placed in the future so that the work of the WFSA may continue to benefit patients world wide.

Statutes and bylaws will undoubtedly change but the basic aims of the WFSA should remain. Currently these are:

a) to assist and encourage the formation of national societies of anaesthesiologists;
b) to promote education and the dissemination of scientific information;
c) to arrange at regular intervals a World Congress of Anaesthesiologists and sponsor regional congresses, to encourage meetings of special groups within the specialty, and make provision for them to meet where appropriate at the above congresses;
d) to recommend desirable standards for the training of anaesthesiologists;
e) to provide information regarding opportunities for postgraduate training and research;
f) to encourage research into all aspects of anaesthesiology;
g) to encourage the establishment of safety measures including the standardisation of equipment:
h) to advise, upon request, national and international organisations;
i) to apply all other lawful means that may be conducive to the objects of the Federation.

References

1. Griffiths H (1963) History of the World Federation of Anesthesiologists. Anesth Analg 42:389-387

Acknowledgement. I would like to thank both Judy Robbins of the Wood Library Museum and Ruth Hooper at WFSA London headquarters for their archival help with the preparation of this chapter. This chapter is based on personal experience, interviews with many of the protagonists, and the published statutes and bylaws. Much detail has been gleaned from the General Assembly minutes from 1955 to the present day, together with the WFSA annual reports and considerable correspondence. This material is currently held at the Wood Library Museum (WLM) of Anaesthesiology in Park Ridge, Chicago, USA and at the offices of the WFSA in London, UK.

21 BIOGRAPHICAL NOTES ON WFSA PRESIDENTS

J.S.M. Zorab

Let us now praise famous men, and our fathers that begat us.
Ecclesiasticus 44.1

Founding President

Harold Randall Griffith (1894-1985). President 1955-1960

Harold Randall Griffith was born in Montreal and graduated from McGill University in 1922. Although he had no university affiliation, Griffith soon became an internationally respected leader. Perhaps his greatest claim to fame should be ascribed to the fact that he, together with Enid Johnson, on 23 January 1942, was the first to use curare to produce muscle relaxation, thereby revolutionising the practice of general anaesthesia. It was almost 10 years later when, stimulated by the activities of Francis Hoeffer McMechan, Griffith started to become involved in the preliminary meetings that subsequently led to the foundation of the World Federation of Societies of Anaesthesiologists (WFSA) on 9 September 1955, on which occasion he was elected the first President. At the 2nd World Congress in Toronto in 1960, he decided that the time had come to retire from office and also from the Executive Committee and withdrew his name from nomination. He was, however, given the formal title of Founding President which, he noted, "confers the privilege of continuing to take part in the activities of the Federation and is one which I value as a very high honour indeed". His successors also decided that some permanent recognition of his contribution was appropriate and, in the late 1980s, the Executive Committee agreed that the scientific programme of each WFSA World Congress should include a "Harold Griffith Symposium".

2ⁿᵈ President

Cornelis Robert Ritsema van Eck (1905-1979). President 1960-1964

Cornelis Ritsema van Eck was known to his friends as Kees (pronounced "case") and also as Rits. He was born on 23 May 1905 in Semarang, Java. He studied medicine at the University of Utrecht, graduated in 1930, gaining his MD in 1931. He trained first as a bacteriologist and then as a surgeon. He went back to the East Indies, to Sumatra, as a military surgeon. In 1942 he was taken prisoner by the Japanese. A ship he was on was torpedoed, but he survived and, with others who were wounded, was taken to a camp in Malaka. He was liberated in 1945 and re-united with his family. He returned home and, in 1947, was invited to set up an anaesthetic department in the University of Groningen. He then spent a few months in the Nuffield Department of Anaesthetics in Oxford, England. In 1948, he became one of the founders of the Netherlands Society of Anaesthetists. At the time of the 1ˢᵗ World Congress, he was President of the Netherlands Society of Anaesthetists and, as such, became chairman of the congress Organising Committee. He was also co-opted to the first Executive Committee of the newly formed WFSA. He was elected President of WFSA at the 2ⁿᵈ World Congress in Toronto, Canada in 1960.

3ʳᵈ President

Geoffrey Stephen William Organe (1908-1989). President 1964-1968

Geoffrey Organe was born in Madras on Christmas day 1908. After his initial schooling at Taunton School, he went to Cambridge where he demonstrated his prowess as an outstanding athlete and started to study medicine. His further medical education was at Westminster Hospital, London, and he graduated MRCS, LRCP in 1933. After joining Patrick Shackleton in general practice, he became "house anaesthetist" in Reading and, in 1937, took the Diploma in Anaesthetics. Following this, Dr. Ivan Magill took him on as house anaesthetist at Westminster Hospital. Later that year, he developed cancer of the colon and underwent numerous operations. He survived for another 50 years! However, he was deemed unfit to serve in the forces during the war. After a number of training posts in anaesthesia, he was appointed consultant anaesthetist at Westminster immediately after World War II. He was heavily involved in the foundation of WFSA and was elected its first secretary/treasurer at the 1ˢᵗ World Congress in Scheveningen in 1955. Although heavily involved in anaesthetic affairs in the United Kingdom, he worked unceasingly on behalf of WFSA, travelling to many countries at his own expense to recruit new member societies. At the 3ʳᵈ World Congress in São Paulo, Brazil in 1964, the combined post of secretary/treasurer was split into two and Organe was elected President of WFSA.

4th President

Francis Ferenc Foldes (1910-1997). President 1968-1972

Francis Foldes was born in Budapest on 13 June 1910. His early years were difficult and he lost three of his four brothers in the holocaust. Francis graduated in Budapest in 1934 from Pazmany Peter University of Budapest Medical School. In 1941, Francis escaped to the United States. He began his career in anaesthesiology at the Massachusetts General Hospital. Later he was appointed Clinical Professor of Anaesthesiology at the University of Pittsburgh School of Medicine. In 1964, he was appointed Professor of Anaesthesia at the Albert Einstein College of Medicine in New York. He was elected President of WFSA at the 4th World Congress in London, England in 1968.

5th President

Otto Mayrhofer-Krammel (1920). President 1972-1976

Otto Mayrhofer (known to his friends as Teddy) was born in Vienna on 2 November 1920. He graduated from the Medical School of the University of Vienna in 1944. He studied anaesthesiology in England and did postgraduate training in New York. In 1976, he was appointed Professor and Chairman of the Department of Anaesthesiology at the University of Vienna. He was elected secretary of WFSA in 1964 and was elected President at the 5th World Congress in Kyoto, Japan in 1972 - the youngest person to hold this post.

6th President

Quintin Juan Gomez (1919-2003). President 1976-1980

Quintin Juan Gomez was born in Manila on 12 April 1919. He obtained a BA at the University of the Philippines in 1939 and graduated as a doctor from the College of Medicine at the University of the Philippines in 1944. In 1946, he went to Chicago, where he trained in anaesthesia for 2 years. He met Joseph Artusio in 1946 and continued his interest in anaesthesia. In 1949, he was appointed to the faculty of the College of Medicine in the University of the Philippines and went on to become the first Professor of Anaesthesiology. He was responsible for establishing anaesthesia as an independent medical specialty in the Philippines. He was elected treasurer of WFSA in 1968 and went on to be elected as President at the World Congress in Mexico City in 1976.

7ᵗʰ President

John Joseph Bonica (1917-1994). President 1980-1984

John Bonica was born on the small island of Filicudi, one of the Isole Eolie group north of Sicily on 16 February 1917. His family emigrated to New York in 1928. He graduated from Marquette University Medical School in Milwaukee, Wisconsin. He trained in anaesthesiology in New York. In 1960, he founded and became the first chairman of the Department of Anaesthesiology of the Washington School of Medicine in Seattle. He was elected secretary of WFSA in 1972 and was elected President at the 7ᵗʰ World Congress in Hamburg in what was then the Federal Republic of Germany in 1980.

8ᵗʰ President

Carlos Pereira Parsloe (1919). President 1984-1988

Carlos Parsloe was born in Santos in the state of São Paulo, Brazil on 28 November 1919. His medical training was at the Faculdade Nacional de Medicina *(National Medical Faculty)* of the University of Brazil where he graduated in 1943. He did his internship in Chicago and this was followed in 1946-1948 by a 2-year residency in anaesthesia at Wisconsin General Hospital (University of Wisconsin, Madison) with Ralph Waters. He gained further experience in Santos and has been in clinical practice in Sao Paulo since 1955. He was on the WFSA Executive Committee from 1972 until 1980, becoming a vice-President of WFSA in 1980. He was elected President at the 8ᵗʰ World Congress in Manila in 1984.

9ᵗʰ President

John Stanley Mornington Zorab (1929). President 1988-1992

John Zorab was born on 16 January 1929 in Southampton, England. He trained at Guy's Hospital, London, graduating in 1956. His anaesthetic training included jobs in London and Southampton. He completed his training at Westminster Hospital from where he was appointed consultant anaesthetist to Frenchay Hospital in Bristol, England. Following a period as secretary of the European Regional Section, he was elected secretary of WFSA in 1980 and elected President at the 9ᵗʰ World Congress in Washington D.C. (USA) in 1988.

10ᵗʰ President

Saywan Lim (1939). President 1992-1996

Saywan Lim was born in what was, at the time, Malaya, on 7 June 1939. He graduated from the University of Malaya in Singapore in 1963. In 1966, he started his anaesthetic training in Liverpool, England. He returned to Malaysia and, in 1968, was appointed consultant anaesthesiologist at the University Hospital in Kuala Lumpur. In 1974 he became consultant anaesthesiologist at the Kuala Lumpur Pantai Medical Centre. He was chairman of the WFSA Executive Committee from 1984 to 1988, when he was elected WFSA secretary. He was elected President of WFSA at the 10th World Congress in The Hague, The Netherlands, in 1992.

11th President

Michael Douglas Allen Vickers (1929). President 1996-2000

Michael Vickers was born in London on 11 May 1929. He trained at Guy's Hospital, London, graduating in 1955. He also started his anaesthetic training at Guy's, moving via Newcastle, Hammersmith, and Birmingham to Cardiff, where he succeeded William Mushin as Professor of Anaesthesia. He was heavily involved with national anaesthetic affairs and was first Honorary Secretary and then President of the Association of Anaesthetists of Great Britain and Ireland. In addition, he was appointed vice-provost to the University of Wales. Furthermore, he was elected President of the European Academy of Anaesthesiology and, in 1984, founded their journal, *The European Journal of Anaesthesiology*. He was appointed a Member of the Order of the British Empire (OBE) in 2000. His association with WFSA formally began when he joined the Education Committee in 1976. He was elected secretary in 1992 and President at the 11th World Congress in Sydney, Australia in 1996.

12th President

Thomas Christopher Kenneth Brown (1935). President 2000-2004

T.C.K. Brown, known as Kester, was born in Kenya on 9 December 1935. He graduated from St. Andrew's University in Scotland in 1960. He did his internship in London, Ontario. He then worked as a general practitioner for a while in Yellow Knife in the Northwest Territories, which involved giving anaesthetics after 2 weeks' training! He moved on to Vancouver for his formal anaesthetic training. He then spent 6 months at the Toronto Children's Hospital before emigrating to Melbourne, Australia. He soon became involved in educational work, organising the scientific programme for the ASA annual meeting for 25 years. This led to his appointment to the WFSA Educational Committee of which he became chairman in 1987. It was a short step to becoming chairman of the WFSA Executive Committee in 1992. In 1998, he was made a member of the Order of Australia (AM) for his national and international services to teaching and research in anaesthesia. He was elected President of WFSA at the 12th World Congress in Montreal Canada in 2000.

22 WFSA ARCHIVES: LEGACY OF ORGANIZED WORLD ANAESTHESIA. ORIGIN AND DEVELOPMENT

P. Sim, J. Robins, J. Rupreht

Origin

The World Federation of Societies of Anaesthesiologists (WFSA) is an international organisation founded in 1955 to coordinate world anaesthesiology. It promotes international cooperation among anaesthesia communities, exchanges and shares knowledge through education and research, and promotes world health through high-quality anaesthesia care worldwide, particularly in aid to third-world countries. Founded in Scheveningen, The Netherlands, WFSA is governed by an Executive Committee, which oversees a network of committees to execute its programmes and projects worldwide. Every 4 years this world body gathers in a designated city in the world at the General Assembly of the World Congress of Anaesthesiology.

The issues of WFSA records and papers

The WFSA leadership comes from every corner of the world. The quadrennial World Congress of Anaesthesiology is the culmination of projects and programmes on education, clinical and scientific research, international aid, and world organisational affairs. The records and documents emanated by leaders the world over are understandably voluminous. No formal mechanism had been devised for the retention of such records, or plans for their active collection, systematic organisation, and permanent preservation. Leaders of WFSA retained their personal records in scattered corners of the world, and the bulk of each administration was kept as personal papers with no directive for organisation or retention. Expedient adaptation of filing systems depended upon the leadership's executive style and habits. Such state of official WFSA documentation prevailed for 3 decades after its founding. The elected offices of the presidency and the secretariat continued to generate most papers and records.

By 1986, the WFSA Honorary Secretary John S.M. Zorab of Bristol (UK) recognised the importance of retaining its organisational records for posterity. Dr. Zorab was a pragmatic visionary. He began collecting what was available of the WFSA papers and planned a comprehensive systematic process for collecting all existing past and future records of this world organisation of anaesthesiology. Collecting the existing papers of the organisation became his first target. Securing the cooperation of the Association of Anaesthetists of Great Britain and Ireland (AAGBI), Dr. Zorab collected and organised the papers of the second WFSA President, Sir Geoffrey Organe, and deposited them at the headquarters office of the AAGBI at 9 Bedford Square in London. This marks the beginning of a conscientious effort to archive WFSA records. Soon after, Zorab heard from WFSA past President, John J. Bonica, who was ready to deliver his cartons of official Presidential papers to 9 Bedford Square. This was followed by an announcement from the incumbent President Carlos P. Parsloe of Sao Paulo, Brazil that he would follow suit and organise and deliver his papers to London.

Wood Library Museum of Anaesthesiology: official WFSA archive repository. Plan for a trans-Atlantic move of the WFSA archive

The stark reality of the space requirements and anticipated volume flow of documents from two WFSA Presidents to the archive concerned Dr. Zorab. He had witnessed first hand the space limitation at 9 Bedford Square and the ever-growing volume of papers passing through his office during his active years as a key WFSA officer. Dr. Zorab sought Dr. Bonica's advice on the possible transfer of the WFSA archive to the American Society of Anaesthesiologists, thinking that the Wood Library/Museum of Anaesthesiology (WLM) would be an ideal and logical home for WFSA official records. Dr. Bonica suggested that he contact the WLM directly.

In early 1990, Dr. Zorab initiated a unilateral cross-Atlantic proposal to invite the cooperation of the WLM as a repository of WFSA presidential papers. He projected that to accommodate the records of 9 past WFSA Presidents in 36 years, it would need a capacity of approximately 25 filing cabinet drawers. At its March 1990 meeting, the WLM board debated the Zorab proposal. Still using a facility built 3 decades ago, the WLM Board of Trustees was mindful of limited available space on premises, but noted the importance of this archive. The trustees were willing to rent temporary storage for such important international anaesthesia records until new permanent facilities became available in 1992. In accepting the organisational papers, the WLM normally required the donor organisation to pay for maintenance of its archive, such as cost of storage facilities and equipment, and expected the donor organisation to pay for shipping costs for the delivery of records. In this case, the WLM was willing to forego the customary requirements to accept, preserve, and maintain the records of this world leader organisation of anaesthesiology at no operating cost to the donor organisation. It only asked the donor organisation for a one-time donation of U.S. $ 100.00 per linear foot of files delivered to this designated WFSA archive repository. WFSA would arrange with its past leaders to forward their records independently from all corners of the world to the WLM. The records should be organised before shipping. The WLM would be responsible for the maintenance of these papers and records and make them accessible for future research. Dr. Zorab relayed this provisional WLM response to his Executive Committee, which met later in August 1990 in Warsaw, Poland. By September 1990, the WFSA Executive Committee accepted these conditions in principle, as it had to ascertain the actual cost for the transfer of records before a formal agreement could be drawn up.

2-Year hiatus on WFSA archive issue

Two years elapsed before the WFSA archive issue resurfaced. The WLM librarian reported on 21 September 1992 that the incumbent WFSA President Say Wan Lim planned to forward his presidential records to the WLM on the advice of the WFSA Executive Committee chair, Dr. Bernard V. Wetchler, that WFSA had agreed on terms set by the WLM, although no official documents were drafted for transfer of WFSA archival papers. Meanwhile, the WLM had received 12 cartons of files from Professor Bonica, which included all Bonica papers from 1955 through 1988, measuring 15 linear feet. Dr. Bonica had meticulously organised his files, making it a model for future papers to be transferred to the WLM. In addition, the WLM received 4 linear feet of WFSA records from its treasurer, Dr. Richard Ament. A total of 19 linear feet of files had been received in September 1992.

The WLM President Elliott V. Miller invited the WFSA President Say Wan Lim to attend the October 1992 WLM board of trustees meeting for a dialogue on the issue. Dr. Lim accepted the invitation, but could not make the meeting due to an unforeseen flight delay in Malaysia. The WLM trustees debated this issue, and without any hesitation re-affirmed its commitment to accept this important archive on the terms it had previously elaborated.

In April 1993, WLM finally became the official repository of WFSA archival records. The WFSA Executive Committee chair Bernard V. Wetchler informed the WLM that WFSA had approved this official designation. Again, there was no official communication from the WFSA to confirm. The WLM librarian followed through with a letter to Professor M.D. Vickers, Honorary Secretary of WFSA, to confirm this agreement. Along with his letter was an invoice for U.S. $ 1,900.00 according to the agreed charge for the 19 linear feet of archival files deposited at the WLM. Within a week, Professor Vickers responded with a cheque in payment to WLM, and informed the librarian that other presidential papers, i.e., those of Sir Geoffrey Organe, Carlos Parsloe, and John Zorab, were forthcoming.

Document and record collecting

Policies and procedures

Appointment of WFSA honorary archivist. In 1992 the WFSA Executive Committee appointed Joseph Rupreht, MD, PhD, of Rotterdam, The Netherlands, as honorary archivist to serve as a liaison officer between the donor organisation and the official archive repository. Dr. Rupreht would also supervise the administration of the WFSA archive records. He subsequently visited the WLM to discuss organisational matters, which included the use of archive material for exhibition at WFSA general assemblies. By 1995, WFSA officers agreed that the honorary archivist might claim expenses of up to U.S. $ 250.00 per annum. WFSA would also fund quadrennial visits of the honorary archivist to the WLM at, U.S. $ 500.00 per visit.

Document collection, retention and disposal. In consultation with the honorary archivist, Professor Vicker drafted a document, dated 2 January 1996, detailing the policies and procedure for WFSA document collection, retention, and disposal. This advised WFSA officers to retain all documents and records when they organised their files to be forwarded to the WLM. Records requiring confidential consideration would be reviewed by the Honorary Secretary and the honorary archivist of the Federation. Sensitive materials would hence be treated with confidence and be appropriately designated with restrictions on their usage.

Dr. Rupreht respected the necessity of observing closure of confidential documents, but he contended that all archival documents are historical evidence, which should be made available for research at some time. He also encouraged donors to submit their records and documents intact. Professor Vickers was more realistic on document confidentiality. He was concerned that indiscriminate collecting of documents for the archive without restriction would cause parties to be less candid and frank in their exchanges. However, should document-initiating parties be given the right to designate confidentiality, the document retention period would tend to be unnecessarily prolonged. Both the Honorary Secretary and the honorary archivist, however, had total confidence in the professionalism of the administrators at the WLM to honor confidentiality.

All things considered, it was suggested that an ad hoc Scrutiny Committee comprising the President, Honorary Secretary, and honorary archivist of the WFSA, ex officio, be charged with the task of determining confidentiality of documents on a case-by-case basis. Additionally, should there be request for study of confidential material on file, the committee would decide its availability according to the purpose and nature of the request and the sensitive nature of the files to be revealed at a specific time. The honorary archivist expressed hope that the Scrutiny Committee would be temporary, and the designation of confidential matters would eventually be vested upon the honorary archivist who, after all, should have the confidence of the WFSA administration upon his appointment. Dr. Rupreht further suggested that the policies and procedure document be made available to all WFSA officers when each assumes office. The purpose was to make them aware of their mission in retaining historical records and documents for future research. This would also hopefully make them fair in their designation of confidential materials for the archive.

Document and record collection priorities. The WFSA Honorary Secretary and honorary archivist, upon discussion, recommended the following categories for document retention and disposal.

Records and documents for mandatory retention
By WFSA secretary
1. Agenda and minutes of General Assemblies and Executive Committee meetings
2. Annual reports
3. Committee reports to the assembly
4. Minutes of Standing Committee meetings
5. Correspondence with all member societies

By WFSA treasurer
1. Audited accounts

By WFSA publications editors
1. All WFSA publications and *Anaesthesia Worldwide*

Prima facie case for retention
1. From initiators of correspondence copied to Executive Committee, officers, and committee chairs

Prima facie case for retention under embargo
1. All confidential documents designated by ad hoc Scrutiny Committee
2. Documents designated by originators as confidential

Records for short-term retention
1. Ballot papers kept for the period of time legally required for possible challenge

Prima facie case for destruction
1. Memoranda to and from the WFSA administrative officer
2. Correspondence non-essential to WFSA affairs

Incumbent officers were also advised to deliver their papers for archival deposition 6 months after leaving office. For reasons of confidentiality, embargoed papers may remain confidential for 5, 10, or 15 years, to be determined by the ad hoc Scrutiny Committee on a case-by-case basis. In no case should a confidential paper be embargoed for more than 16 years.

From record retention to organised professional archive: observation and after-thoughts

Above is an account of the development of a concept to retain organisational records of an international professional organisation into an official professional archive. It emanated from an idea in 1986 by an active leader of an established organisation who had served in many official capacities for an extended period of time. Having witnessed and contributed to the history of this world professional body, Dr. John Zorab saw the need for collecting, retaining, and organising the records of his organisation for posterity. He thought it was a simple process to collect and keep vital and relevant records for history in 1986. A few years later, he recognised the overwhelming volume of documents he had amassed, and projected the proliferating volume to increase exponentially. This increase of historical records from all parts of the world not only required an enormous amount of storage space, but demanded professional organisation to make retrieval of information possible. In 1990, he convinced his professional brethren to seek assistance and cooperation from an established institution supported by a member society.

World organised anaesthesia involved a world body of leaders in action. Decisions on issues would take time, and policies were formulated only slowly and informally. There was a lack of action on the archive issue for 2 years following the Zorab proposal to formalise an official repository for the WFSA archive. It was not until 1992 that the WFSA Executive Committee approved Dr. Zorab's recommendation to designate the WLM the official repository of the WFSA archive. No formal agreement was drafted or signed. An honorary archivist, who would be a liaison officer for WFSA, was appointed to direct and oversee the transfer of archival records from papers to permanent archive. It took much persuasion and persistence for the honorary archivist to convince the WFSA administration of the vital role of his office. It would require time and attention, as well as a minimum of international travel, like all other organisational personnel, in order for that office to be effective. The honorary archivist eventually secured modest funding for his annual expenses, and was given a travelling allowance to visit the WLM on archival business every 4 years. The scope of collection and retention of papers and records for WFSA has also expanded from the mere collecting of presidential papers. WFSA has moved in the right direction in collecting and managing its official archive. By the end of a decade since its inception, in 1996, a policy procedure for managing this international professional archive was drafted by the then WFSA Honorary Secretary.

Still pending is important unfinished business on the WFSA archive. As an established institution managing archive collections of organisations, institutions, and individuals, the Wood Library/Museum of Anaesthesiology operates in accordance with the best professional standards of the archives community. It has employed a full-time archivist, assigned adequate and environmentally ideal space to house its collection, and has assigned generous funding on the preservation and management of all archive records. To facilitate its work, and for the best interest of all, the WLM requires the donor parties who have entrusted their papers and records for safe keeping at the WLM to sign deeds of gifts. This would allow the WLM total operational freedom on their respective records according to initially established stipulations on access to their collections for research. We have yet to convince the WFSA administration of the necessity of this last step of confidence to bring this important archive collection to an important closure, as a way to assure its value for posterity. We are, however, very hopeful, judging from the development of this process described above, that the WLM will eventually gain the full and complete confidence of the donor organisation of the WFSA archive.

APPENDIX

STATUTES

SECTION 1: NAME AND OBJECTIVES

Art 1.01 NAME
The Organisation bears the name: World Federation of Societies of Anaesthesiologists.

Art 1.02 OBJECTIVES
The objectives of the Federation are exclusively educational, scientific and charitable in nature and are to make available the highest standards of anaesthesia and resuscitation to all peoples of the world and to disseminate the same amongst them and it shall, in pursuit of those aims, try:
a. to assist and encourage the formation of national Societies of Anaesthesiologists;
b. to promote education and the dissemination of scientific information;
c. to arrange at regular intervals a World Congress of Anaesthesiologists and sponsor Regional Congresses; to encourage meetings of special groups within the speciality and make provision for them to meet where appropriate at the above Congresses;
d. to recommend desirable standards for the training of anaesthesiologists;
e. to provide information regarding opportunities for postgraduate training and research;
f. to encourage research into all aspects of anaesthesiology
g. to encourage the establishment of safety measures including the standardisation of equipment;
h. to advise, upon request, national and international organisations;
i. to apply all other lawful means which may be conducive to the objects of the Federation.

Art 1.03 TAXATION STATUS IN USA
Within the meaning of Section 501(c) (3) of the United States Internal Revenue Code:
a. no part of the net earnings of the Federation shall inure to the benefit of any private stockholder or individual, except that reasonable compensation may be paid for services rendered and payments may be made in furtherance of the objects set forth in Article 1.02 hereof;
b. no substantial part of the activities of the Federation shall be the carrying on of propaganda, or otherwise attempting to influence legislation;
c. The Federation shall not participate in, or intervene in (including by the publishing or distribution of statements) any political campaign on behalf of any candidate for public office; and
d. the Federation shall not carry on any other activities not permitted to be carried on by an organisation exempt from United States income tax under Section 501(c) (3) of the United States Internal Revenue.

Art 1.04 FINANCIAL ARRANGEMENTS

If the Federation is treated as a "private foundation" within the meaning of Section 509 of the United States Internal Revenue Code:

a. the Federation shall distribute its income for each taxable year at such time and in such manner as not to become to the tax on undistributed income imposed by Section 4942 of the United States Internal Revenue Code;

b. the Federation shall not engage in any act of self-dealing as defined in Section 4941(d) of the United States Internal Revenue Code;

c. the Federation shall not retain any excess business holdings as defined in Section 4943(c) of the United States Internal Revenue Code;

d. the Federation shall not make any investments in such manner as to subject it to tax under Section 4944 of the United States Internal Revenue Code; and

e. the Federation shall not make any taxable expenditure as defined in Section 4945(d) of the United States Internal Revenue Code.

SECTION 2: MEMBERSHIP

Art 2.01 CATEGORIES OF MEMBERSHIP

a. Full membership
b. Associate membership
c. Corresponding membership

Art 2.02 FULL MEMBERSHIP

Full membership of the Federation shall be granted to National or Regional Societies by the General Assembly in accordance with the Statutes following the procedure determined by the Bylaws.

Annexe I to these Statutes lists the Member Societies at the date of adoption of these Statutes (2000) and their geographical grouping for the purposes of Article 4.0.2.

Art 2.03 ASSOCIATE MEMBERSHIP

Associate membership of the Federation may be granted to Societies which are unable, by virtue of Government action, to comply with their obligation to pay the annual subscription, as determined by the Bylaws.

Art 2.04 CORRESPONDING MEMBERSHIP

Corresponding membership of the Federation may be granted to groups of anaesthesiologists where there are fewer than ten anaesthesiologists in a country. (accepted 2000)

Art 2.05 LIMITATIONS

Only one National Society from each country shall be admitted to membership of the Federation unless the General Assembly on the advice of the Executive Committee, determine otherwise.

Art 2.06 RESIGNATION

In any year, prior to October 1st, a Member Society may give three months notice of termination of membership to the Secretary, provided that all arrears of subscription. if any, have been paid.

Art 2.07 SUSPENSION

If a Member Society fails to reply to enquiries or questionnaires from the Secretary or does not pay its dues for two consecutive years, the Executive Committee may suspend the membership of that Member Society.

Art 2.08 TRANSFER TO ASSOCIATE MEMBERSHIP

If a Member Society is unable to pay the annual subscription, the Executive Committee may transfer the Member Society to Associate Member status according to the procedure specified in the Bylaws.

Art 2.09 EXPULSION

The membership of any Member Society may be terminated by a resolution of the General Assembly according to the procedure specified in the Bylaws 1.09-1 to 1.09-5 if a change in the nature of the activities of a Member Society makes it inappropriate for continued membership.

Art 2.10

If a suspended Member Society fails to respond for a period of two years following its suspension, its membership will be regarded as lapsed.

Art 2.11 RIGHTS

Any Member Society which, for any reason, ceases to be a Member of the Federation shall forfeit all rights pertaining to membership.

SECTION 3: GENERAL ASSEMBLY

Art 3.01 MEETINGS

The General Assembly shall meet in ordinary session on the occasion of each World Congress. It shall meet in extraordinary session as circumstances may require.

Art 3.02 POWERS AND FUNCTIONS

The General Assembly is the supreme decision making body and shall be entitled to take account of all matters unless they are explicitly excluded or specifically delegated elsewhere by the Statutes.

Its functions shall be:

1. To determine the policy of the Federation.
2. To elect the Officers of the Federation and the members of the Executive Committee, in the manner prescribed in the Bylaws.
3. To determine the annual subscription, supervise the financial policy, receive, scrutinise and accept the audited accounts, and approve the budget.
4. To receive, approve and if necessary take such action as is deemed appropriate on the reports of the Executive Committee and other Committees.

Art 3.03 DELEGATES

The Federation shall be governed by a General Assembly composed of Delegates from the Full Member Societies, which meet in ordinary session at each World Congress.

Art 3.04 NUMBER OF DELEGATES

Full Member Societies shall be entitled to send Delegates to the General Assembly according to the number of members for which it has paid membership fees, on the following scale:

NUMBER OF MEMBERS	NUMBER OF DELEGATES
Less than 251	1
251-500	2
501-1000	3
1001-2000	4
2001-3000	5
each further 1000 or fraction thereof	1

Art 3.05 ALTERNATES

A Member Society may appoint Alternates for any or all of its Delegates.

Art 3.06 NOTIFICATION

Member Societies are recommended to confirm to the Secretary the name(s) of their Delegate(s) and Alternate(s) four weeks before the first session of the General Assembly and MUST do so at least 24 hours before the opening of the first session of the General Assembly or they may be excluded by the Executive Committee from participating.

Art 3.07 VOTING IN THE GENERAL ASSEMBLY

Unless otherwise determined, one Member of each delegation will cast the vote(s) of the Member Society: that delegate will cast as many votes as there are Delegates or Alternate Delegates of that Society actually seated at the meeting. The method of voting may be varied by the Rules of Procedure which will be adopted at each General Assembly.

Art 3.08 MAJORITY REQUIRED

Any resolution to amend the Statutes or to dissolve the Federation or to admit or to expel any Member Society requires an affirmative vote of two-thirds of the Delegates or Alternate Delegates present at that General Assembly, abstentions being null and void. All other resolutions shall be determined by a simple majority of the votes cast.

Art 3.09 ENTITLEMENT TO VOTE: EQUALITY OF VOTES

Only Delegates or Alternate Delegates of Full Member Societies who are not in arrears and have paid their dues for the current year are entitled to vote. If the vote is equally divided the Presiding Officer shall be entitled to cast a vote.

Art 3.10 AGENDA AND PROCEEDINGS

The Agenda of the General Assembly meetings shall be prepared by the Executive Committee and forwarded to the Member Societies with the notice calling the Assembly.

Art 3.11 OFFICERS AND VICE-PRESIDENTS

The Officers of the Federation shall be a President, a Secretary and a Treasurer and the Chairman of the Executive Committee, who shall be nominated and elected as prescribed in the Bylaws. The Federation will also have three or more Vice-Presidents who shall be nominated and elected as prescribed in the Bylaws.

Art 3.12 MINUTES

The proceedings of the General Assembly, which shall include the full wording of all Resolutions, shall be recorded in the Minutes, signed by the President and Secretary. The Secretary shall keep a copy available for inspection. A copy of the Minutes shall be forwarded to all Societies.

Art 3.13 AMENDMENT OF THE STATUTES

The General Assembly shall not be entitled to amend the Statutes or move the dissolution of the Federation unless the matter has been notified to all Member Societies not less than three months prior to the meeting or unless Delegates of more than two-thirds of Full Member Societies are present at the meeting.

Art 3.14 ADDITIONAL BUSINESS

The General Assembly shall deal with the items on the agenda and any such matters as it may decide to add thereto. However, any such added business must be referred to the Executive Committee for review and recommendation if it involves expenditure for which provision has not been made.

Art 3.15 EXTRAORDINARY MEETINGS OF THE GENERAL ASSEMBLY

Extraordinary meetings of the General Assembly may be convened either by the Executive Committee or at the request of not less than two-thirds of the Member Societies. In the latter case, if the meeting has not been convened within two years, those Member Societies requesting the meeting may convene a General Assembly unless a regular General Assembly convenes before the end of those two years. Such a meeting shall elect its own Presiding Officer.

SECTION 4: EXECUTIVE COMMITTEE

Art 4.01 FUNCTIONS
The Executive Committee shall carry out the resolutions of the General Assembly and take all measures within the limits of these resolutions, designed to further the aims of the Federation.

Art 4.02 COMPOSITION
The Executive Committee shall consist of the President, Secretary, Treasurer and 12 elected members and, (if appointed) Deputy Secretary and Deputy Treasurer together with the chairmen of the Standing Committees. Of the elected members, at least one must be from each of the following geographical groupings:
a. Africa and the Middle East
b. Asia
c. Australia, New Zealand and the Pacific Islands
d. Central and South America, Mexico and the Caribbean Islands e. Europe and Israel
e. The United States of America and Canada.

Art 4.03 LEGAL ACTIONS
The Chairman of the Executive Committee and the Secretary shall represent the Federation legally against any third parties.

Art 4.04 NOMINATION OF SECRETARY AND TREASURER
The Executive Committee shall make a nomination for the post of Secretary and communicate this nomination to all Member Societies at least four months prior to the General Assembly. The Executive Committee shall likewise make a nomination for the post of Treasurer. Counter nominations may be made by any three Member Societies and must be received by the Chairman of the Executive Committee at least one month before the meeting of the General Assembly.

Art 4.05 MEETINGS
The Executive Committee shall meet as and when the interests of the Federation so require.

SECTION 5: FINANCE

Art 5.01 FUNDS
The funds of the Federation will be derived from:
a. Subscriptions;
b. Subsidies, gifts and bequests;
c. Interest;
d. Surplus funds accruing from congresses sponsored by the Federation

Art 5.02 OFFICIAL YEAR: AUDIT
The official year coincides with the calendar year. The Treasurer shall prepare the accounts and budgets of the Federation as at December 31 each year and prepare the same for inspection by March 31 following.
In Alternate years, the Treasurer shall forward to the Executive Committee with the accounts, an Audit, certified by an accountant approved by the Executive Committee, covering the accounts for the two previous years.

SECTION 6: REPORTS

Art 6.01 ANNUAL REPORTS
The Secretary shall forward to all Member Societies an Annual Report of the Federation.

Art 6.02 ANNUAL ACCOUNTS
The Annual Accounts shall be sent to Member Societies with the Annual Report.

SECTION 7: DISSOLUTION

Art 7.01 DISSOLUTION
Upon any dissolution of the Federation, or any partial or entire liquidation of its property or assets, all of the Federation's property shall, after making provision for discharge of all of the Federation, be paid over and transferred to such one of more organisations of institutions which are exempt from United States income Tax under Section 501(c)(3) and described in Section 170(c) (2) of the United States Internal Revenue Code of 1954 as the General Assembly shall determine.

In the event of liquidation following a resolution to dissolve the Federation, liquidation shall be carried out by the person appointed by the General Assembly for that purpose, which shall decide upon his powers and, if relevant, his emoluments.

Failing the appointment of a liquidator, liquidation shall be carried out jointly by the Executive Committee then in office acting as a Panel of Liquidators. Such panels have powers without restrictions or limitations.

SECTION 8: BYLAWS AND TEXT

Art 8.01 BYLAWS
Any matters left in these Statutes to be regulated by Bylaws and such other matters for which no provisions have been made in these Statutes, shall be provided for in Bylaws. In any conflict of interpretation the Statutes shall take precedence.

Art 8.02 TEXT
The English text of the Statutes and of the Bylaws shall be considered as authoritative.

SECTION 9: MISCELLANEOUS

Art 9.01 UNITED STATES TAX LAWS
All references herein to identified sections of the United States Internal Revenue Code shall include the corresponding section(s) of any further United States Internal Revenue Laws.

Netherlands	Nederl. Ver. voor Anesthesiol.	883	3
Norway	Norsk Anestesiologisk Forening	525	3
Poland	Polish Soc. of Anaesth.	2000	4
Portugal	Soc. Portuguesa de Anestesiologia	600	3
Romania	Romanian Soc. of Anaesth.&Int. Care	250	1
Slovak Republic	Slovak Soc. of Anaesth.& Int. Care	251	2
Slovenia	Slovenian Soc. of Anaesthesiology	100	1
Spain	Spanish Soc. of Anaesth.	1000	3
Sweden	Swedish Soc. for Anaesth. And Int. Care	1420	4
Switzerland	Swiss Soc. of Anaesth.	490	2
Turkey	Turkish Soc of Anaesth	550	3
U. K.	Ass. of Anaesth. of Great Britain & Ireland	3864	6
Ukraine	Anaes. Assoc. of Ukraine	112	1
Uzbekistan	Uzbekistan Soc. Of Anaesthesiology & Int. Care	16	1
Yugoslavia	Ass. of Anaesth. of Yugoslavia	710	3

F	**Canada and the United States of America**		
Canada	Canadian Anaesthesiologists' Society	1481	4
U.S.A.	American Society of Anesthesiologists	23613	26

(s) = Suspended Status

Membership numbers are those submitted for 2000. Where no returns were received the last figure known was used.

BYLAWS

SECTION 1: MEMBERSHIP

1.01 ELIGIBILITY

a) National Societies Eligibility for membership in the Federation is a membership of at least ten anaesthesiologists.

b) Regional Societies Eligibility for membership in the Federation is a membership of at least ten anaesthesiologists practising in geographical adjacent areas where no National Society exists.

c) National group of anaesthesiologists < 10 Corresponding membership of the Federation may be granted to groups of anaesthesiologists where there are fewer than ten anaesthesiologists in a country.

1.02 APPLICATION

A Society desiring to become a Member of the Federation shall make application in writing to the Secretary of the Federation.

1.03 APPROVAL

The Executive Committee, after due enquiry and payment of dues, may grant provisional membership to that Society, until the next General Assembly. Societies being admitted to membership during the course of a year may be required to pay only a reduced membership subscription.

1.04 ENROLMENT

When a Member Society has been admitted, the name of the Society shall be entered into the official Register of the Federation and the Annexe to the Statutes.

1.05 LIMITATIONS

If a nation, because of prevailing political circumstances, is divided into two or more parts with separate Governments, the General Assembly, on the advice of the Executive Committee, may recognise more than one Society. Each Society will be representative of a part of the country, with the same requirements, obligations and duties, rights and privileges, as are accorded to other Member Societies, as provided for in the Bylaws.

1.06 RIGHTS AND PRIVILEGES

Full Member Societies which are not in arrears (1.08-1) enjoy all rights and privileges of the Federation. Full Member Societies which are in arrears shall not be permitted to vote.

Associate Member societies enjoy all rights and privileges except that they are not represented in the General Assembly.

Suspended Member Societies have no rights or privileges except that they will continue to receive all official communications addressed to Member Societies.

1.07 OBLIGATIONS AND DUTIES

Each Member Society shall:

a. do all in its power to promote the knowledge of, and an interest in, the objectives and work of the Federation;

b. keep the Secretary informed of any events and developments in its country of interest to the Federation;

c. make prompt reply to all enquiries and questionnaires from the Secretary, or within the time limit specified by the Secretary.

1.08 ANNUAL SUBSCRIPTIONS

Each Member Society shall pay an annual subscription. The subscription year is the current calendar year.

1.08-1 DUE DATES

Annual subscriptions are due by the 1st April each year. If the subscription has not been paid by the due date, the Member Society shall be deemed to be in arrears for that year.

1.08-2 AMOUNT

The amount of the subscription of Member Societies shall be determined by the General Assembly on the recommendation of the Executive Committee.

Member Societies are liable for the subscription due in the calendar year in which their notice terminates or in which they are expelled.

1.08-3 REFUNDS

Annual subscriptions which have been paid, other than those for provisional Societies (1.03) shall not be refunded.

1.08-4 ARREARS

If a Member Society fails to meet the full requirements of 1.08 or 1.08-1, it will be adjudged to be in arrears for that year.

1.09 EXPULSION

1.09-1 INVESTIGATION

If any cause for expulsion of a Member Society is alleged, the Chairman of the Executive Committee shall set up an ad hoc Enquiry Committee, composed of at least 5 members of the Executive Committee to investigate the cause or claim of cause and determine whether the matter shall be referred to the full Executive Committee for a hearing.

1.09-2 NOTICE

If the ad hoc Enquiry Committee determine that the matter shall be heard by the full Executive Committee, the Executive Committee shall submit the findings to the Member Society concerned for explanation or comment. It shall inform the Member Society of the right of appeal and that, in the event of such an appeal, a hearing will be given to the complainant (or his representative) and to a representative of the Member Society whose conduct or policy has been the subject of complaint.

1.09-3 HEARING

The Executive Committee shall give the complainant (and the Member Society involved), at least thirty days notice of the date, time and place of the meeting of the Executive Committee at which the matter is to be considered.

The proceedings of the meeting will not be invalidated by the absence of a representative of the Member Society provided due notice has been given.

1.09-4 REPORT

The Executive Committee shall make a written report to the General Assembly with a recommendation that either no action shall be taken or the facts are considered to justify expulsion and the Member Society be expelled from the Federation.

1.09-5 ACTION

The recommendations of the Executive Committee involving the expulsion of a Member Society shall be presented to the General Assembly for approval. A two-thirds vote of the Delegates or Alternate Delegates present at the General Assembly is required for expulsion, abstentions being null and void.

1.10 SUSPENSION

Suspension of a Member Society by the Executive Committee shall be until the next General Assembly but can be revoked at any time.

If a representative of a suspended Member Society is an Officer or Member of the Executive Committee, the Executive Committee may, at its discretion, declare the position vacant.

1.11 ASSOCIATE MEMBER SOCIETIES

Member Societies which are unable to meet a requirement of Bylaw 1.08-4 may, by a decision of the Executive Committee, be transferred to Associate Member status.

1.12 REINSTATEMENT TO FULL MEMBERSHIP

1.12-1 EXPELLED SOCIETIES

A Member Society which has been expelled from membership pursuant to the provisions of Article 2.08 of the Statutes may be reinstated following application to the Executive Committee in the same manner as provided for with original application for membership and by paying such arrears of subscription as the Executive Committee, at its discretion, may determine.

1.12-2 ASSOCIATE MEMBER SOCIETIES

An Associate Member Society may be transferred to full membership, following a recommendation by the Executive Committee, approved at the General Assembly.

1.12-3 SUSPENDED SOCIETIES

A Member Society which has been suspended may be reinstated following application to the Executive Committee and the payment of such arrears of subscription, up to a maximum of two years' subscription, as the Executive Committee, at its discretion, may determine.

SECTION 2: GENERAL ASSEMBLY

2.01 COMPOSITION

The General Assembly is composed of:
a. The President
b. Voting Delegates of Member Societies
c. Officers and Chairmen of Standing Committees. These may not vote unless they are also voting Delegates of a Member Society.
d. Representatives of international medical organisations representing interests relevant to anaesthesiology may be admitted an participate (without vote) in the General Assembly, by decision of the Executive Committee.

2.02 DELEGATES

The term Delegate, as used in these Bylaws, means a Delegate or Alternate Delegate seated in place of the Delegate, as the representative of his Member Society in the General Assembly.

2.02-1 REQUIREMENTS

Each Delegate shall be a physician anaesthesiologist in good standing in the Member Society that he represents.

2.02-2 REPRESENTATION

No Delegate shall be a Member of delegation of more than one Member Society.

2.02-3 OFFICE

No Delegate shall hold more than one elected office at one time.

2.02-4 SEATING

No Delegate shall be recognised in the General Assembly until his credentials have been certified by the Committee on Credentials.

2.02-5 SUBSTITUTION

A Delegation shall serve without substitution at all meetings of the General Assembly unless a substitution is consented to and an Alternate is so certified by the Committee on Credentials.

2.02-6 VOTING of DELEGATES

No one other than Delegates or Alternate Delegates may vote.

2.03 MEETINGS

The General Assembly shall meet during each World Congress and at such other times and places as may be determined by the Executive Committee. It may recess from time to time, as is necessary to complete its business.

2.04 RULES OF PROCEDURE

Rules of Procedure shall be prepared by the Executive Committee and adopted by the General Assembly, as the first item of business, to regulate the conduct of the meeting. A motion to adopt, amend, suspend or re-apply the Rules of Procedure requires an affirmative vote by a simple majority of the votes cast.

2.05 PRESIDING OFFICER

The President elected at the preceding General Assembly or, in his absence, the Chairman of the Executive Committee, shall serve as the Presiding Officer.

2.06 QUORUM

Fifty per cent of the voting Delegates, certified by the Credentials Committee of the General Assembly, shall constitute a quorum. (14-04-96)

2.07 VOTING

Voting shall be by a show of hands unless, before the vote is taken, ten Delegates present a request that the vote be by secret ballot.

2.07-1 VOTING FOR OFFICERS

Voting for election of Officers and Members of the Executive Committee shall be by secret ballot unless the number of nominated candidates is the same as the number of vacancies, in which case the vote may be taken by a show of hands.

2.07-2 ELECTION OF OFFICERS

A majority of votes cast shall be necessary to elect. If on any ballot no nominee shall receive a majority of the votes cast, the candidate receiving the smallest number of votes shall be eliminated and the balloting shall proceed in that manner until a majority is obtained.

2.08 ELECTION OF NOMINATIONS COMMITTEE

The General Assembly will select eight Member Societies from which the Nominations Committee will be constituted according to the procedure laid down in Bylaw 4.06-2.

2.09 EXPENSES

The expenses of Delegates attending meetings of the General Assembly shall not be a charge upon the funds of the Federation.

2.10 EXTRAORDINARY MEETINGS

Extraordinary Meetings of the General Assembly may be convened as governed by Art 3.15 of the Statutes. If convened by the Executive Committee, written notice of the time and place of the meeting shall be mailed to each Member Society at least six months in advance.

2.11 OFFICERS AND CHAIRMEN OF STANDING COMMITTEES

All Officers (Art 3.11) and Chairmen of Standing Committees (Bylaw 4.01) shall be, or have been, Delegates to the General Assembly.

2.11-1 ELECTION

All Officers shall be elected by the General Assembly at a meeting held during the regular World Congress in the manner provided in Bylaws 2.07-1 and 2.07-2

2.11-2 TERMS OF OFFICE AND DUTIES

2.11-2.1 PRESIDENT

The term of the office of the President extends from the close of the General Assembly at which he was elected, until the installation of his successor at the end of the next regular General Assembly. No Delegate may be elected to serve as President for more than one term.

The President
- shall preside over the sessions of the General Assembly;
- he/she shall attempt in all ways possible to contribute to the welfare of the people through the medical specialty of anaesthesiology, furthering the aims of the Federation to the fullest extent and perform such other services of leadership as are customary;
- he shall be an ex-officio Member, without vote, of all Committees of the Federation
- and shall perform such other duties as are provided in the Bylaws.

2.11-2.2 VICE PRESIDENT

The term of office of Vice-President extends from the close of the General Assembly at which election takes place until the close of the next regular General Assembly. No one may be elected to, or serve as, Vice-President for more than one term.
- A Vice-President shall, when so requested by him, assist the President in the performances of his duties, and shall, when so requested, represent the President at meetings and functions of the Federation and allied organisations.

2.11-2.3 SECRETARY

The term of office of the Secretary extends from the close of the General Assembly at which he/she was elected until the close of the next regular General Assembly. No Delegate may be elected to serve for more than two terms as Secretary. The Secretary shall:
a. serve as the Secretary of the General Assembly and as Secretary of the Executive Committee;
b. execute all official documents when an official signature is required, provided that the Executive Committee may authorise any other officer to execute official documents when necessary or appropriate;
c. supervise the safekeeping of all records in the Secretariat other than those pertaining to financial matters;
d. maintain a Register of Member Societies
e. notify all Member Societies of all meetings, regional and international of the Federation;
f. forward to all Member Societies an Annual Report of the Federation;
g. perform such other duties as provided in the Bylaws.

2.11-2.4 TREASURER

The term of office of the Treasurer extends from the close of the General Assembly at which he/she was elected until the close of the next regular General Assembly. No Delegate may be elected to serve for more than two terms as Treasurer. The Treasurer shall:
a. act as the official custodian of all funds of the Federation, except as otherwise specifically provided in the Bylaws;
b. be responsible for a detailed accounting of all receipts and disbursements and the safekeeping of the financial records and securities of the Federation as detailed in guidelines prepared for this purpose;
c. submit a written report at each meeting of the Executive Committee and General Assembly concerning the financial transactions of the Federation, the funds in his care and his actions as Treasurer;
d. recommend a per diem allowance applicable for the following two years for approval by the Executive Committee, and
e. perform such other duties as provided in the Bylaws.

2.11-2.5 DEPUTY SECRETARY

On recommendation of the Secretary, the Executive Committee may appoint a Deputy Secretary for the same term of office as the Secretary.
This position shall not be an officer.
The Deputy Secretary will be a Member of the Executive Committee without vote unless also an elected Member of the Committee.
The Secretary shall inform him/her regularly of all affairs of his office, so that he/she would be able to take over the duties of the Secretary at any moment of his term if so required.

2.11-2.6 DEPUTY TREASURER

On the recommendation of the Treasurer, the Executive Committee may appoint a Deputy Treasurer for the same term of office as the Treasurer.
This position shall not be that of an officer.

The Deputy Treasurer will be a Member of the Executive Committee without vote unless also an elected Member of the Committee.

The Treasurer shall inform him/her regularly of all financial matters of the Federation, so that he/she would be able to take over the duties of the Treasurer at any moment of his term, if so required.

2.11-3 VACANCIES

If for any reason the incumbent in any elected or appointed office of the Federation becomes unable or unwilling to perform the functions of his/her office or is removed from office, such office shall be declared vacant. Vacancies in office shall be filled in the following manner:

2.11-3.1 PRESIDENT

The Chairman of the Executive Committee shall immediately undertake his statutory duties and will assume the title of Acting President.

The office of President shall remain vacant until the next General Assembly.

2.11-3.2 VICE-PRESIDENT

Vacancies shall remain unfilled until the next regular General Assembly.

2.11-3.3 SECRETARY AND TREASURER

The Executive Committee shall request the Deputy Secretary or Deputy Treasurer to take over the office for the rest of the term. If no appointment of Deputy Secretary or Deputy Treasurer has been made, the Executive Committee shall appoint a Secretary or Treasurer to fill the vacancy.

SECTION 3: EXECUTIVE COMMITTEE

3.01 COMPOSITION

The composition of the Executive Committee is laid down in Art 4.02 of the Statutes. The President has no vote except as provided in Bylaw 3.15. The Deputy Secretary and the Deputy Treasurer have no vote unless they are also elected members of the Committee.

3.02 ELECTION

Members of the Executive Committee shall be elected by the General Assembly, as provided in Sections 2.07-1, 2.07-2 and 4.06-2-3.

3.03 ELIGIBILITY

Members must be a Delegate of a Member Society at the General Assembly at which they are elected.

3.04 TERM OF OFFICE

Members shall be elected for a term of eight years. Retiring Members are not eligible for immediate re-election.

3.05 DUTIES

a. It shall carry out the resolutions of the General Assembly and take all measures designed to further the purposes of the Federation.
b. It shall prepare the Agenda of the General Assembly and forward the same to the Member Societies with notice of the Assembly.
c. It shall nominate candidates for the posts of Secretary and Treasurer, having regard to the provisions of Bylaw 3.07.
d. Prior to the General Assembly, it shall consider the proposed budget prepared by the Finance Committee and Treasurer's report of anticipated income and expenditure and shall prepare a recommended budget to present to the General Assembly.
e. It shall review the report of the Finance Committee regarding the amount and manner of payment of the annual subscriptions, and present recommendations to the General Assembly for appropriate action.

    f.   It shall choose the members and Chairman of all Standing Committees having regard to the provision of Bylaw 4.01.

    g.   It shall elect a Chairman according to the procedure laid down in Bylaw 3.15. Following the election of Chairman it shall elect a Vice-Chairman in a similar manner.

    h.   It shall approve the repository of the Federation's funds.

    i.   It shall perform such other duties as are prescribed in the Bylaws.

3.06 POWERS

In addition to these duties, the Executive Committee:

    a.   may invite, at its discretion, other organisations to send observers to the General Assembly;

    b.   may appoint a Deputy Secretary and Deputy Treasurer, who must have been a Delegate of a Member Society;

    c.   may appoint Special Committees to further expedite and carry on activities resulting from implementation of Federation purposes and aims;

    d.   may co-opt additional members to serve until the next General Assembly. Co-opted members are not entitled to vote;

    e.   may amend the Bylaws according to the procedure of Bylaw 7.01.

3.07 NOMINATION OF SECRETARY AND TREASURER

The Executive Committee shall nominate a candidate for the office of Secretary and another candidate for the office of Treasurer as laid down in Art 4.04 of the Statutes and having regard to the provisions of Bylaws 2.11-1 and 2.11-3.3.

3.08 MEETINGS

The Executive Committee shall meet whenever the interests of the Federation so require, at the time and place established by the Chairman or his deputy, and it may recess from time to time, as necessary to complete its business.

3.09 PRESIDING OFFICER

The Chairman, or in his absence the Vice-Chairman, shall preside over meetings of the Executive Committee.

3.10 QUORUM

No business shall be transacted unless at least 10 voting members are present.

3.11 VOTING

Unless otherwise provided in the Bylaws, a simple majority shall be sufficient to carry a resolution. In the event of an equality of votes the Chairman may cast a further vote.

3.12 BUSINESS BY CORRESPONDENCE

The Chairman of the Executive Committee shall have the power to decide what Committee business may be conducted by correspondence. He/she may request the members of the Executive Committee to cast their vote on such business in writing, by telegram, cablegram, e-mail or facsimile, all with confirmation of receipt.

3.13 MINUTES

The Secretary shall keep the Minutes of the proceedings of each meeting of the Committee. The Minutes shall be circulated to the members of the Committee within three months of the meeting and be confirmed by the Committee at its next meeting.

3.14 SPECIAL MEETINGS

Upon receiving a request signed by not less than 8 members of the Committee and specifying the business for which a Special Meeting is needed, the Chairman shall call a Special Meeting.

3.14-1 TIME AND PLACE OF SPECIAL MEETING
The time and place at which a Special Meeting shall be held, and its purpose shall be specified in the official notice calling the meeting.

3.14-2 BUSINESS
No business shall be transacted at a Special Meeting other than that for which the meeting was called.

3.15 ELECTION OF CHAIRMAN AND VICE-CHAIRMAN
It shall elect its Chairman by secret ballot in the following manner:
The Secretary shall provide each voting Member of the Committee with a list of all the members of the Committee. Each voting Member shall mark thereon his choice for Chairman. Any candidate who receives a majority of the votes is elected. If no candidate achieves a majority, the procedure will be repeated; the candidate or candidates with the least number of votes, and all those with no votes being ineligible. The process will be repeated until one candidate polls a majority of votes.
In the event that there is an even number of members present and the final two candidates poll an equal number of votes, the matter will be resolved by reference to their respective number of votes on the most recent ballot at which there was not an equality of votes. In the event that two candidates have polled an equal number of votes at every ballot, the President shall have a casting vote.

3.15.1 VICE-CHAIRMAN
The Vice-Chairman shall be elected in a similar manner from amongst those members who have served on the Committee during the previous four years. The Vice-Chairman will serve until the next (interim) meeting of the Executive Committee.

3.15.2 VICE CHAIRMAN AT INTERIM MEETING
At an Interim meeting of the Executive Committee, a Vice Chairman shall be elected from amongst those members elected at the previous General Assembly, using the election procedure of 3.15-.1.

3.16 CASUAL VACANCIES
When a casual vacancy arises from any cause, the Executive Committee itself shall appoint a successor to fill the vacancy until the next General Assembly. In so doing, as far as possible, the geographical representation of the Executive Committee shall be preserved.
Such appointees shall be eligible for a further full term of office, provided that they fulfil the requirements of Bylaw 3.03.

SECTION 4: OTHER COMMITTEES

4.0 TYPES OF OTHER COMMITTEES
The Federation has three types of other Committees:
Standing Committees, Ad Hoc Committees and Special Committees.

4.01 STANDING COMMITTEES
a.   Committee on Finance
b.   Committee on Statutes and Bylaws
c.   Committee on Education
d.   Committee on Publications

4.01-1 MEMBERSHIP OF STANDING COMMITTEES
They are composed of Delegates to the General Assembly chosen by the Executive Committee and ratified by the General Assembly, subject to Bylaw 2.11. The members of the committee on Publications need not be Delegates or former Delegates.

4.01-2 TERM OF OFFICE
Each Committee shall continue from the General Assembly at which it is appointed until the next regular General Assembly. No Delegate shall normally serve on the same Standing Committee for more than two consecutive four year terms.

4.02 FINANCE COMMITTEE

Composition:

A Chairman and four other Delegates from five Member Societies, two of whom shall be elected from amongst the elected members of the Executive Committee), plus the Secretary, Treasurer and Deputy Treasurer (if any).

Duties:

a. establish the formula for the manner of payment of the annual subscription of the Member Societies of the Federation;
b. propose to the Executive Committee the amount of annual subscription required;
c. prepare a budget of anticipated income and expenditure to apply to the succeeding fiscal years until the next General Assembly;
d. report their recommendations to the Executive Committee;
e. perform such other functions as are provided in the Bylaws.

4.03 STATUTES AND BYLAWS COMMITTEE

Composition:

A Chairman and five other Delegates from each of the regions of WFSA as stated in Art 4.02 of the Statutes. At least two of whom, were Members of the previous Committee.

Duties:

Recommend to the Executive Committee amendments to the Statutes and Bylaws which it considers will facilitate the work of the Federation.

4.04 EDUCATION COMMITTEE

Composition:

A Chairman and eight other Delegates from nine Member Societies.

Duties:

a. to initiate and carry out the aims of the Federation with regard to education;
b. training and the dissemination of scientific information.

4.05 PUBLICATIONS COMMITTEE

Composition:

A Chairman and five other members. Membership of this committee should have regard to the world-wide interests of the Federation and its publications.

The Chairman of the Education or his nominee and the Editor of the WFSA Newsletter shall be members of the Publications Committee, ex officio.

Duties:

To review and disseminate existing WFSA publications; to liaise with the Education Committee; to further the aims of the Federation by encouraging appropriate publications; to arrange for the preparation and distribution of a WFSA Newsletter.

The Editor of the WFSA Newsletter shall be appointed by the Executive Committee.

4.06 AD HOC COMMITTEES

The Ad Hoc Committees of the Federation are:
1. Credentials Committee
2. Nominations Committee
3. World Congress Venue Committee

4.06-1 CREDENTIALS COMMITTEE

Composition:

Chairman and six Delegates of as many Member Societies from the WFSA regions.

Prior to the first session of the General Assembly, the Executive Committee will appoint the Chairman and one Delegate from each Region.

Duties:

a. Report on the eligibility of each Delegate (as defined under 2.02) attending the General Assembly;
b. Certify credentials and authorise seating of Delegates to the General Assembly;
c. Determine and announce the official quorum for all sessions of the General Assembly.

4.06-2 NOMINATIONS COMMITTEE

4.06-2-1 Composition:

A Chairman, appointed by the Executive Committee, and ten Delegates of as many Member Societies of whom at least one shall be from each of the regions in Art 4.02 of the Statutes. A member society elected to the Nominations Committee must be in good standing with the Federation (and not in arrears).

4.06-2-2 Nomination and Election:

The Executive Committee shall nominate sixteen Full Member Societies at least one year prior to the next World Congress. A postal ballot shall then be conducted of all Full Member Societies to elect ten of these sixteen Societies. "Registered" mail shall be used.

Prior to the World Congress, the Executive Committee shall appoint a Chairman of the Nominations Committee. The Executive Committee shall, at its first meeting, choose one delegate from each of the ten elected Member Societies, who shall constitute the Nominations Committee.

The Executive Committee shall be empowered to fill any vacancy.

4.06-2-3 NOMINATIONS

The Nominations Committee, having regard to Bylaws 2.11-1, 3.03 and 3.04 shall propose:

a. the name of a candidate for election as **President**;
b. the names of three or more candidates for election as **Vice-President**;
c. the names of as many Delegates as there are vacancies for election to the **Executive Committee**.

Other nominations for membership of the Executive Committee may be made in advance, in writing, by any three Member Societies, such nominations to reach the Secretary at least 48 hours before the second session of the General Assembly.

4.06-3 WORLD CONGRESS VENUE COMMITTEE

4.06-3-1 Composition:

A Chairman appointed by the Executive Committee and eight Delegates of as many Member Societies of whom at least one shall be from each of the regions in Art 4.02 of the Statutes.

4.06-3-2 Duties:

To select the host Society and the venue of future World Congresses.

4.07 OTHER AD HOC COMMITTEES

Other Ad Hoc Committees may be appointed by the General Assembly as the necessity arises.

4.08 SPECIAL COMMITTEES

The Special Committees of the Federation are those appointed by the Executive Committee for four years for specific purposes.

4.08-1 MEMBERSHIP SPECIAL COMMITTEE

Membership is not restricted to Delegates. Special Committees have power of co-option. International medical organisations which have been granted formal liaisons with the Federation may nominate a member to any relevant Special Committee.

4.08-2 TERM OF OFFICE

No Member shall serve on the same Special Committee for more than two consecutive four year terms.

SECTION 5: FUNDS AND EXPENDITURE

5.01 FUNDS

Funds of the Federation are derived from the following sources:

a. Annual subscriptions paid by Member Societies, the scale of which shall be related to the number of members in the Member Society, in amount established as provided in the Bylaws;

b. Subsidies, Gifts and Bequests bestowed on the Federation and accepted by the Executive Committee;

c. Interest on Capital;

d. Surplus Funds arising from congresses held under the auspices of Federation.

5.02 EXPENDITURES

The Funds of the Federation may be expended by the Executive Committee within the limits of the budget approved by the General Assembly and subject to any limitations provided for in the Statutes and Bylaws.

5.03 PAYMENT

Cheques issued by the Federation must bear the signature of one of the following three officers of the Federation:

a. The President

b. The Secretary

c. The Treasurer

provided, however, that the Executive Committee may authorise the establishment of special bank accounts and authorise the issuance of cheques on such accounts by such persons as the Committee may determine.

5.04 AUDIT

Prior to March 1st in Alternate years, the Treasurer shall forward to the Executive Committee an Audit, certified by an accountant approved by the Executive Committee, listing income received, the amounts receivable, the allocation of and disbursement made of Federation's Funds during the preceding two years.

SECTION 6: SECRETARIAT OF THE FEDERATION

6.01 LOCATION

The Federation shall have its principal office in the United Kingdom, at 8th Floor, Imperial House, 15-19 Kingsway, London WC2B 6TH United Kingdom, or at such other address as the Executive Committee may from time to time determine.

The Executive Committee shall from time to time establish the mailing address of the Federation, which shall normally be the same address or that of the Secretary.

The accounts of the Federation shall be kept at the office of the Treasurer.

6.02 EXPENSES OF SECRETARIAT

The expenses of the Secretariat and the editorial expenses shall be defrayed out of the general funds of the Federation.

SECTION 7: THE BYLAWS: AMENDMENT AND INTERPRETATION

7.01 AMENDMENT

The Bylaws may be amended by the Executive Committee. Proposals to amend the Bylaws must be notified in writing by the Chairman to all members of the committee and require an affirmative vote by ten voting members.

7.01-1 NOTIFICATION AND RATIFICATION

Amendments must be notified to each Member Society as soon as possible. They must be included on the agenda of the next General Assembly as the first item of business following the adoption of the Rules of Procedure and must be formally approved by a simple majority of those voting, abstentions being null and void.

7.01-2 ALTERATIONS TO AMENDMENTS

The General Assembly may, by a simple majority, alter the form of an amendment in any manner not exceeding the original intent.

7.02 GENDER

Throughout these Bylaws, words importing the masculine gender shall be read as also importing the feminine gender.

7.03 LANGUAGE

The English text of the Bylaws shall be considered as authoritative.

7.04 STATUS

These Bylaws are to be interpreted as complying with the Statutes and nothing in the Bylaws can override any provision of the Statutes.

RULES OF PROCEDURE

GENERAL ASSEMBLY

1.00 PURPOSE

1.1 These Rules of Procedure shall govern all deliberations of the General Assembly and of Committees of the WFSA where appropriate.

2.00 MEETINGS OF THE GENERAL ASSEMBLY

2.1 The General Assembly, shall meet as required in Art 3.01 and Bylaw 2.03, provided, however, that there shall be a minimum of two meetings at each World Congress separated by at least twenty-four hours.

2.2 Any person registered for the Congress may be admitted as an observer to the General Assemblies within the limits of space.

2.3 Delegates of Member Societies with a single vote may have the assistance of an adviser within the limits of space but such advisers may be required to withdraw whilst ballots are conducted.

2.4 A nominated representative of an Associate Member Society may address the General Assembly at the discretion of the President.

2.5 Smoking is not permitted during the General Assembly.

3.00 CREDENTIALS COMMITTEE

3.1 DUTIES

The duties of the Credentials Committee are laid down in Bylaw 4.06-1

3.2 APPEALS

An appeal from any ruling of the Credentials Committee may be entered by any Member Society and such appeal must be entered immediately following the report of the Credentials Committee to the General Assembly. A majority vote shall decide the issue of appeal.

3.3 CREDENTIALS OFFICER
The Chairman of the Credentials Committee shall:
a. Ensure that only certified Official Delegates or Alternate Delegates are seated.
b. Assist the President to preserve order.
c. He shall act under the direction of the President.

3.4 REGISTRATION OF MEMBERS
The Credential Committee shall:
a. Determine whether a quorum is present:
b. Maintain a running tally of the total number of voting members present.

4.0 REFERENCE COMMITTEE ON STATUTES AND BYLAWS

4.1 COMPOSITION:
The Reference Committee shall consist of not less than five members. It shall include the Chairman of the Committee on Statutes and Bylaws and any members of that Committee attending the Congress, the Secretary of the WFSA and the Chairman and one other Member of the Executive Committee nominated by the Executive Committee.

4.2 DUTIES
a. All motions to amend the Statutes or Bylaws other than those already approved by the Executive Committee and ratified by the General Assembly, shall be referred to the Reference Committee for its consideration.
b. Such meetings shall be held at the time and place as shall have been announced before or at the first meeting of the General Assembly. Only one Delegate specified from each Member Society may participate but other Delegates may attend as observers within the limitations of space.
c. The Reference Committee shall report its recommendation to the second General Assembly.

5.0 ADDITIONAL REFERENCE COMMITTEES
5.1 The Chairman of the Executive Committee shall recommend to the President any additional Reference Committee which needs to be appointed, designating the duties and composition of such Committees.
5.2 All Member Societies have a right to appoint one Delegate to appear before a Reference Committee.
5.3 The Reference Committee Chairman, the President or the Chairman of the Executive Committee may request the presence and testimony of non-Delegates when necessary.

6.0 ORDER OF BUSINESS

6.1 FIRST MEETING OF THE GENERAL ASSEMBLY
Order of Business. The order of business shall include:
a. Report of the Credentials Committee and Roll Call
b. Adoption of the Rules of Procedure
c. Admission of new Member Societies
d. Motions to adopt changes in Bylaws
e. Receipt of Minutes of the last session of the General Assembly
f. Matters arising from the Minutes not already on the agenda
g. Consideration of suspended Member Societies
h. Expulsion of Member Societies
i. Report of the Chairman of the Executive Committee
j. Report of the Secretary
k. Report of the Treasurer
j. Announcement of Reference Committee hearings
l. Election of Societies to form Nomination Committee
m. Election of World Congress Venue Committee
n. Report of World Congress Organising Committee(s)
o. Any other business
p. Recess of first meeting

6.2 SECOND MEETING OF THE GENERAL ASSEMBLY

Order of Business. The order of business shall include:

a.   Report of the Credentials Committee and Roll Call
b.   Receipt of Minutes of the last session of the General Assembly
c.   Matter arising from the Minutes not already on the agenda
d.   Report(s) of Reference Standing Committee(s)
e.   Reports of Standing Committees
f.   Reports of Special Committees
g.   Reports of Ad Hoc Committee (other than listed)
h.   Election of Standing Committees
i.   Election of Secretary
j.   Election of Treasurer
k.   Report of Nominations Committee
l.   Installation of President and adjournment

6.2-2 REPORTS OF REFERENCE COMMITTEE

The General Assembly shall receive the full report of any Reference Committee on the items of business that were referred to it at the first General Assembly.

6.2-3 ACTION

Each item of business so reported upon shall be subject to full debate, amendment or other action which the General Assembly desire to take upon it, except that any item may not be amended to any degree that materially alters the original intent.

6.2-4 NEW BUSINESS

No new items of business may be introduced from the floor at the second General Assembly unless it was introduced at the first meeting and, if thought advisable, referred to a Reference Committee except as provided for in Section 4 or 5 of these Rules of Procedure.

6.2-5 FAILURE TO REPORT

If a Reference Committee fails to report to the second General Assembly upon any item that was referred to it at the first General Assembly, such item may be placed before the General Assembly by the President and shall be so placed upon the request of any delegate.

7.00 RESOLUTIONS AND MOTIONS

7.1   All resolutions shall be submitted in writing.
7.2   All resolutions must be made by an Officer or a Delegate except:
   7.2-1 Reference Committee Chairman may make motions pertaining to any matter which has been referred to or considered by their Committee.
   7.2-2 Standing or other Committee Chairman may make motions pertaining to any matter relevant to the report of their respective committee.
7.3   The President may, at his discretion, direct that complicated motions or amendments to resolutions be submitted in writing.

8.00 DEBATE

8.1   Delegates may discuss any matter which is before the General Assembly.
8.2   Committee Chairmen may discuss any report of their Committee.
8.3   The Chairman of the Executive Committee shall be granted the floor without regard to the ordinary limitations on debate provided, however,
   a.   that no other Member be deprived of his parliamentary rights;
   b.   that he shall be bound by the usual rules of parliamentary decorum,
   c.   that he shall be subject to any special rules to limit debate which are in effect at the time.

9.00 VOTING

9.1   The method of voting shall be by the Member Societies as determined in the Statutes and Bylaws except that individual voting by Delegates may be permitted on any question when agreed by a simple majority of the Delegates present and voting.
9.2   When the Presiding Officer is in doubt as to the outcome of a vote, he shall call for another vote indicating the exact number of votes on each side.

10.00 APPEALS, CHALLENGES AND CLAIMS OF ILLEGALITY

    10.1   Decisions of the Chair must be challenged immediately and before other business has intervened.

    10.2   All other appeals, challenges of claims of illegality must be raised at the same session at which the action under question occurred.

11.00 PARLIAMENTARY AUTHORITY

    11.1   These Rules of Procedure shall be the primary authority in all deliberations of the General Assembly.

    11.2   No provision of these Rules of Procedure shall be effective if such provision is in violation of the Statutes or Bylaws of the Federation.

    11.3   "Roberts' Rules of Order-Newly Revised" shall be the Parliamentary Authority in matters not covered by the Statutes, Bylaws and Rules of Procedure.

    11.4   Any matter remaining unresolved shall be decided by the General Assembly by a simple majority vote.

12.00 SUSPENSION OF THE RULES OF PROCEDURE

    12.1   The General Assembly may, by a simple majority vote, amend or temporarily suspend the Rules of Procedure, abstentions being null and void.

    12.2   The General Assembly may, by unanimous consent, grant any motion, action or request not consistent with these Rules of Procedure and/or parliamentary procedure.

    12.3   No amendment to, nor suspension of, the Rules of Procedure and no motion, action or request shall be valid if such suspension, motion, action or request is in violation of the Statutes of Bylaws of WFSA.

Douglas R. BACON

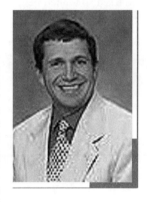

Douglas R. Bacon, MD, MA received a Bachelor of Science in Medicinal Chemistry and a Bachelor of Arts in History from the State University of New York at (SUNY) Buffalo, and completed medical school at SUNY Stony Brook. His anaesthesiology residency was completed at the affiliated hospitals of SUNY Buffalo. After completing his medical training, Dr. Bacon completed his Master of Arts in History at SUNY Buffalo. Doug has published extensively on the history of anaesthesiology in the United States with a special interest in the history of organisations devoted to the specialty. He was an editor of the *History of Anesthesia*, a compilation of essays from the 5th International Symposium on the History of Anaesthesia held in Santiago de Compestela, Spain in 2001. He currently serves as a consultant anaesthesiologist at the Mayo Clinic and is Professor of Anaesthesiology and History of Medicine at the Mayo Clinic College of Medicine in Rochester, Minnesota, USA. He is a member of the organising committee for the 6th International Symposium on the History of Anaesthesiology to be held in Cambridge, England, in September 2005 and serves on the editorial boards of the *Journal of Clinical Anesthesia*, *Regional Anesthesia and Pain Medicine*, and *The Bulletin of Anesthesia History*. Dr. Bacon is the current American Society of Anesthesiologists *Newsletter* editor.

T.C. Kester BROWN

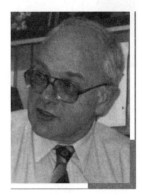

T.C. Kester Brown has been involved in teaching and training anaesthesiologists for over 30 years. He had already organised the annual meeting programme for the Australian Society of Anaesthesists for 12 years when he was elected to the WFSA Education and Scientific Affairs Committee in Manila in 1984. He was asked to take over the chairmanship in 1987 and continued until the World Congress in The Hague. He was elected to the Executive Committee in 1992, becoming deputy chairman and then chairman from 1996 to 2000. At the World Congress in Montreal he became president. He chaired the scientific programme committee for the 1996 World Congress in Sydney at which invited speakers from 56 countries participated.

He has travelled all over the world teaching and promoting the World Federation. He has also trained people from many countries in his department at the Royal Children's Hospital in Melbourne during his 26 years as director. He has written books, chapters, many scientific papers, mainly on paediatric anaesthesia, and produced several films and videos for teaching.

Martin CHOBLI

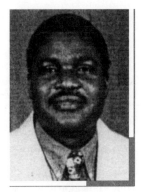

Born: 01-01-1948, Benin

Secondary studies: Benin 1961-1968
University Medical Studies: Clermont-Ferrand (France) 1969-1975
Specialty in Anaesthesia and Intensive Medicine: 1975-1978
(French National Diploma of Anaesthesia)
Diploma of Disaster Medicine, Bordeaux (France) 1986

Scientific societies
Associate Member of French Society of Anaesthesia (SFAR)
Member of WFSA, Member of WFSA Education Committee, Member of WFSA African Regional Section's board
Member of International Society for the Study of Pain (IASP)
Member and Past President of Society of Anaesthesia of African French-Speaking Countries (SARANF)

Posts
University
Professor, Head of Department of Anaesthesia and Intensive Medicine since 1986
Lecturer 1981-1986

Hospital
Head of First Aid Ambulance Service (SAMU BENIN) since 1998
Head of Emergency Medicine Unit since 1998
Head of Anaesthesia and Intensive Care Unit 1982-1998

Elena A. DAMIR

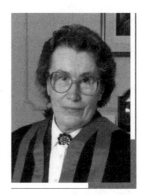

Date of birth: 13 June 1928
Nationality: Russian
Knowledge of languages: Fluent in English and German
Education: 1946-1952 1ˢᵗ Moscow Medical Institute (School)

Training

1952-1954: General Surgery: Ordinatura, Clinic of Surgery,
2ⁿᵈ Moscow Medical Institute (School) based in 1ˢᵗ Moscow
Clinical Hospital
1954-1957: Thoracic and Heart Surgery: Aspirantura in the
same clinic. Qualification Surgeon
January 1958 to January 1959 Anaesthesiology, WHO
course in Copenhagen. Qualification Anaesthesiologist

Work

1959-1960: Dozent, Clinic of Thoracic Surgery and Anaesthesiology of Central Institute
of Postgraduate Training of Physicians
1960-1998: Professor and Chairlady, Clinic of Anaesthesiology and Reanimatology
(Resuscitation) of Russian Medical Academy of Post-diploma Training of Physicians;
Department of Anaesthesiology, Botkin Hospital, Moscow
1999 to present: vice-chairman of above

Scientific societies

1958-1989: All-Union Society of Anaesthesiologists and Reanimatologists, executive
committee member (international contacts)
1990-1998: President of All-Russian Society of Anaesthesiologists and Reanimatologists
1980-1988: WFSA, member of committee on resuscitation
1988-1996: WFSA, member of Executive Committee
1996-2000: WFSA, vice-president

Honours

1988: Honorary Scientist of Russian Republic
1980-1992: Honorary member of Societies of Anaesthesiology of Bulgaria, DDR, Hungary, Poland, Romania
1998: Fellow by election, FRCA
2002: Honorary member of the Society of Anaesthesiology of Germany

Publications

1967: Textbook *Practice of Anaesthesiology*, 5 books on different topics in anaesthesiology
1969: Doctor of Sciences Thesis
135 publications in medical journals

Michael B. DOBSON

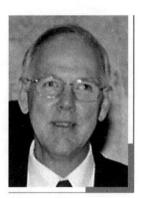

Consultant Anaesthetist Nuffield Department of Anaesthetics, Oxford Radcliffe Hospital, OX3 9DU, UK
Honorary Senior Clinical Lecturer, University of Oxford, Oxford, UK
Tel.: +44-1865-778513, Mobile +44-79-73737380,
e-mail: michael.dobson@nda.ox.ac.uk
Age 56 years

Qualifications
M.B., Ch.B. (Edinburgh), 1970
M.R.C.P.(UK) 1974
F.F.A.R.C.S. (Eng.) 1976 (now F.R.C.A)

Clinical interests
Anaesthesia in developing countries
Obstetric and vascular anaesthesia

Academic and professional interests
Education in Anaesthesia, including development of electronic and distance learning materials
WHO Expert Panel Member-Blood Safety, and District Hospital Services
Liaison officer between WHO and WFSA
Regional anaesthetic assessor for the UK Confidential Enquiry into Maternal Deaths

Publications
Anaesthesia at the District Hospital (book, WHO, sole author)
Surgical Care at the District Hospital (book, WHO, clinical editor)
Various publications on oxygen concentrators, appropriate technology, draw-over anaesthesia etc.

Memberships
Fellow of the Royal Society of Medicine
Honorary member of the Australian Society of Anaesthetists
Academician member, European Academy of Anaesthesiology

Roger **ELTRINGHAM**

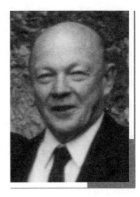

Roger Eltringham is a graduate of St. Andrews University, Scotland. He is a consultant anaesthetist in Gloucester, England.

He became a member of the Education Committee in 1988 when he took responsibility for organising refresher courses in English-speaking countries in Africa. He was very successful and was a major contributor to the great expansion of the activities of the Education Committee during the next 8 years. He has also been involved in several courses in Russia. In 1996 he transferred to the Publications Committee as chairman. He brought together World Anaesthesia and WFSA in the production of *Update in Anaesthesia*, edited by Iain Wilson and also, for 4 years, the newsletters. He has promoted and organised book and journal distribution to needy departments.

He has also taken an interest in equipment for the less-affluent world. He has been involved in the development and promotion of the Glostavent.

Roger Eltringham has been one of the most-active contributors to the World Federation during the past 16 years.

Antonino GULLO

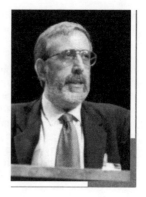

Training and specialties
Anaesthesia and Resuscitation, Paediatrics, Clinical Toxicology, Cardiology

Associated Professor
From 1989, Anaesthesiology, Trieste University School of Medicine

Full Professor
From 1990, Intensive Care, Trieste University School of Medicine

Director
From 1990, School of Anaesthesiology and Resuscitation
From 1993, Section of Anaesthesia, Intensive Care, and Pain Therapy
From 2002, Department of Perioperative Medicine, Intensive Care, and Emergency, Trieste University School of Medicine

Teaching
Trieste University School of Medicine: Intensive Care, Anaesthesiology and Emergency Medicine
Specialty schools: Anaesthesia and Resuscitation, Obstetrics and Gynaecology, Vascular Surgery, Emergency Surgery and First Aid, Urology, Otorhinolaryngology, Ortopaedics and Traumatology, General Surgery, Thorax Surgery, Gastroenterology

Promotion of
From 1987, Course on Anaesthesia, Pain, Intensive Care, and Emergency Medicine (APICE)
From 1991, Post-graduate Course of Anaesthesiology under the aegis of Foundation for European Education in Anaesthesiology (FEEA)

Publications
460 publications; over 100 of them are reviewed on MedLine, on aspects of perioperative and critical care medicine
As author and editor of several volumes and monographs on topics concerning anaesthesia and intensive care, cardiopulmonary resuscitation, trauma, and education.
From 1998 he has been the editor of the Collection of Anestesia e Medicina Critica and "Topics in Anaesthesia and Critical Care Medicine" (edited by Springer Verlag Italia)

Involvement with scientific committees and organisations
Participation in several national and international congresses. In 1997 he participated as a representative at the World Congress on Critical Care in Ottawa. He is one of the founder members of the European Society of Anaesthesiology.

Cultural involvement
He promotes advances in critical care in Eastern European countries (Poland, Romania, Croatia, Slovenia, Serbia-Erzegovina, Macedonia, Bulgaria, and Russia), as well as in his own country

Main interests and activities

Teaching and training, continuous search for collaboration with national and international experts.

In 1986 he organised the first edition of APICE (Anaesthesia, Pain, Intensive Care and Emergency Medicine), which in 1996 became a School of Critical Care. It is an international symposium on critical care and is of increasing importance due to the presence of more than 200 invited speakers who contribute to every edition (75% of them are foreigners). In November 2003 the APICE International Symposium was the 18th. OFA (Organ Failure Academy), founded in 1992, it gives the possibility for top experts in sepsis and organ dysfunction to meet.

ETAIC (Education and Training in Anaesthesiology and Intensive Care), association created in collaboration with the Ljubljana Clinical Centre (Slovenia) in order to promote the improvement of standards of specialized training.

Most-recent assignments

Co-operation with Institute of Critical Care Medicine, Palm Spring, USA. During the last World Congress of Intensive and Critical Care Medicine (Sydney, October 2001) he was elected as member of the WFSICCM board, as Italian representative of this prestigious society together with other 14 colleagues from different countries of the five continents. Since May 2002 he has been member of the ESICM council, being one of the two ESICM representatives elected for Italy. He is president of the World Congress of Societies of Intensive and Critical Care Medicine, 2009, Florence, Italy

Cedric H. HOSKINS

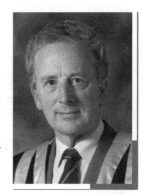

Born at Cheviot in the South Island of New Zealand on 25 May 1929

Early education in the South Island and completed at Mount Albert Grammar School in Auckland where he was a prefect. University education at the Auckland University and at the Otago University in Dunedin, to graduate MB ChB in 1954. Following internships and 2 years of general medical practice returned to Auckland to commence postgraduate training in anaesthesia.

Married to Doreen, a registered nurse, in 1955. They have four daughters and 12 grandchildren.

In April 1963 sailed to England with his wife and children to complete anaesthetic specialist training at some of the leading postgraduate centres in London. Admitted to the Diploma of Fellow, Faculty of Anaesthetists, Royal College of Surgeons, England in July 1964. Before returning to New Zealand spent 3 months as a senior anaesthetist at the Sundsvall Hospital in Sweden.

Back in Auckland in mid 1965 as a specialist anaesthetist with the Auckland Area Health Board and later as a specialist anaesthetist in private practice. Was a member of the board of trustees for the Lavington Trust Hospital (1975-1981). Developed an interest in the then new concept of day stay surgery including the design and function of such units, being a Director of the Auckland Surgical Centre from 1986. Was a contributor to *Anaesthesia For Day Stay Surgery* Healy TEJ (ed) 1990. Elected to the Diploma of Fellow of the Faculty of Anaesthetist, Royal Australasian College of Surgeons in June 1970 and a founding Fellow of the Australian and New Zealand College of Anaesthetists in March 1992. Retired from anaesthetic practice early in 1999. Was Secretary of the New Zealand Society of Anaesthetists 1968-1969 and President 1977-1979. As president attended the 5th Asian and Australasian Congress of Anaesthesiologists in New Delhi where New Zealand was elected to host the next AACA. With his wife, he was a member of the organising committee for the 6th AACA held in Auckland in 1962. Elected to the New Zealand Committee of the Faculty of Anaesthetists, Royal Australasian College of Surgeons in 1980, serving for 12 years, 2 as chairman. The visit to New Delhi for the 5th AACA in 1978 began an 18-year association with the WFSA. Firstly as secretary and chairman of the board of the AARS, 1978-1986. Was a member of the Executive Committee of the WFSA, 1984-1992 and vice president of the WFSA, 1992-1996.

As a teenager began a life long love for the sea. Sailed 4-m sailboats while at school. When back in Auckland in the 1960s and 1970s, enjoyed 5- to 6-m powerboats with the family. Back to sail with a 9-m keel yacht for family cruising and racing on the magnificent coast around Auckland. Built his own 10.6-m keel yacht, which was launched and sailed from 1996. During this time involved in yacht club and race management, being Rear Commodore of the Royal Akarana Yacht Club, 1986-1990. Was part of the on the water Race Committee for the Louis Vuitton Cups 1999-2000 and 2002-2003, and for the America's Cups 2000 and 2003 with the Royal New Zealand Yacht Squadron. In 1998 returned to power boating with the purchase of a 10-m launch. As skipper of this launch is actively involved with the Auckland Volunteer Coast Guard Service in search and rescue.

Maarten MAUVE

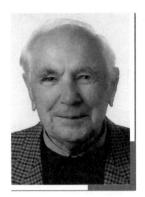

Born: 18th of May, 1912
Place of birth: The Hague

Education and Profession:
1939-19478: General practitioner
from 1947 onwards: Trainee Anaesthesia Amsterdam University Hospital (Professor D.M.E. Vermeulen-Cranch)
1948: Co-founder of the Netherlands' Society of Anaesthetists of which president 1951-1956
1951-1964: Anaesthetist of a general hospital and a paediatric hospital, both Amsterdam
1953-1955: Honorary Secretary of the World Congress of
Anaesthesiologists, September 5th-10th in Scheveningen (The Netherlands) at which congress the WFSA was established.
1964-1971: Anaesthesiologist Amsterdam University Hospital
1971-1982: Professor Anaesthesiology University of Utrecht
1992: Honorary President of the 10th WFSA World Congress, The Hague.
Author of "Episodes from the History of the Establishment of the World Federation of Anaesthesiologists".

Otto MAYRHOFER-KRAMMEL

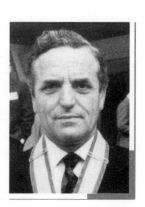

Born 2 November 1920, Vienna, Austria. Father Karl M.
(born 1894), Engineer

Education
Medical School, University of Vienna 1939-1944, Graduation MD, 8 December 1944, University of Vienna

Career
Career 1945 9 months internal medicine, 1945-1946
12 months pathology, 1946-1947 12 months surgery
From September 1947 to April 1948 basic training in anaes-
thesia on a WHO stipend in the UK. London (teacher Dr.
Bernard G.B. Lucas) and Glasgow (teacher Dr. Tony Pinkerton)
From May 1948 Head of Anaesthesia Service, Department of Surgery 2, University Hos-
pital, Vienna
First Monograph published 1949 *Intratracheale Narkose*, Maudrich, Vienna
From July 1949 to October 1950 resident training at Department of Anesthesiology,
Columbia, Presbyterian Medical Center, New York City (teachers Virginia Apgar and
Manny Papper)
November 1950 Diploma Fellow of the American College of Anesthesiology
1951 Return to Vienna
Introduction of succinyl choline into clinical practice, based on own experiments (BMJ
1952, p1332)
1952 Head Division of Anaesthesia in the Department of Surgery
1955 Associate Professor
1961 Full Professor and Chairman Department of Anaesthesiology, University of Vienna
1976-1978 Vice-Dean Medical Faculty, University of Vienna
October 1991 to present Emeritus Professor

Professional achievements
1951 Founder President Austrian Society of Anaesthesiology
1952 Co-founder (with Rudolf Frey and Werner Hugin) of the first German Journal *Der
Anaesthsis*
1955 co-editor and author of *Lehrbuch der Anaesthesiologie*, Springer, Heidelberg (four
Editions up to 1986)
More than 200 publications, covering aspects of anaesthesia and intensive care medicine

Functions within the WFSA
1955 Official Delegate of the Austrian Society at Founding Congress in Scheveningen
1955-1964 Member of Executive Committee
1964-1972 Secretary
1972-1976 President
1976-1980 Chairman of Membership Committee

Honours
Honorary MD/Diplomas of Universities of Szeged (Hungary), Reims (France), and Poz-
nan (Poland)
Honorary Member Anaesthesia Societies of Austria, Australia, Bolivia, Chile, Cuba,
Ecuador, Germany, Great Britain and Ireland, Hungary, Peru, Poland, Romania, Rus-
sia, Spain, West Africa, Yugoslavia, and of the European Academy of Anaesthesiology
Full Member by election of the Austrian Academy of Science and of the German Acad-
emy of Natural Scientists-Leopoldina (Halle)

Anneke E.E. MEURSING

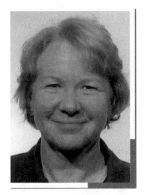

Education and medical career
1964-1971 Medical School State University Leiden, The Netherlands
1971-1973 Doctor of Tropical Medicine and Hygiene, Amsterdam
1974-1976 District Medical Officer, Uganda (MEMISA), Nkozi and Rubaga Hospital
1976-1977 Internal Medicine, Leiden, The Netherlands
1977-1981 Anaesthesia Education, State University Leiden
1981 Junior Consultant Anaesthesia, State University Leiden
1982-1985 Consultant Anaesthetist, Sophia Children's Hospital, Erasmus University Rotterdam
1985 PhD Thesis Tracheal length in the very small infant, Erasmus University Rotterdam
1985-1986 Consultant, Royal Children's Hospital, Melbourne, Australia
1985-1999 Director of Paediatric Anaesthesia, Rotterdam
1989-1999 Director of Paediatric Anaesthesia, The Hague (in addition to Rotterdam)
1995 Locum, Royal Children's Hospital, Melbourne, Australia
1999-2002 Associate Professor of Anaesthesia, College of Medicine, Blantyre, University of Malawi to help set up a physician training programme in anaesthesia
2002 to present Senior Consultant Anaesthesia, Erasmus University Medical Centre, Rotterdam, The Netherlands

Scientific work
Paediatric Anaesthesia >80 invited lectures worldwide, 14 chapters in books, >50 abstracts, >35 publications. Member of the Editorial Board of *Paediatric Anaesthesia*. Theses in Finland and The Netherlands
Safety in Anaesthesia Chairman, National Mortality Study, The Netherlands resulting in one thesis with honours (Dr. S.Arbous), three papers published and three papers submitted

Committee work
1982-1990 Founding member and President, Dutch Society Paediatric Anaesthesia
1983-1991 Honorary Secretary of Dutch Anaesthesia Association (NVA)
1986-1990 Overseas member of Executive Committee Association of Paediatric Anaesthetists of Great Britain and Ireland
1986-1992 Honorary Secretary, 10th World Congress of Anaesthesiologists, The Hague
1986-1999 Founding Member and Secretary (1986-1997) and later President-elect (1997-1999) of Federation of European Associations of Paediatric Anaesthesia
1992-1996 Member of Executive Committee, World Federation of Societies of Anaesthesiologists (WFSA)
1996-2004 Secretary General, WFSA

Emmanuel PAPPER†

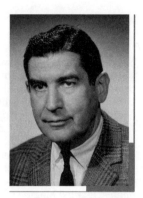

Emmanuel Papper, MD, PhD, was born on 12 July 1915 in the Harlem section of New York City and grew up in the greater New York City area. He graduated second in his class from Columbia University during the heart of the Great Depression. Manny attended New York University School of Medicine and trained in anaesthesiology under Emery A. Rovenstine at the NYU/Bellevue programme. A decorated veteran of World War II, Dr. Papper served with distinction in the European Theatre of Operations, as one of a handful of board-certified anaesthesiologists. Returning from the war, Manny came back to New York City, Bellevue Hospital, and Dr. Rovenstine. Over the next few years, Dr. Papper would leave Bellevue and become Professor and Chairman at Columbia University. He was President of the American Society of Anesthesiologists in 1968, and a director of the American Board of Anesthesiology. He left Columbia and went to the University of Miami as one of the first anaesthesiologists to be dean of a school of medicine. Manny was one of the driving forces behind National Institutes of Health funding for anaesthesiology research in the 1960s, which permitted the tremendous growth of research within the specialty. Dr. Papper was also one of the founding members of the Association of University Anesthesiologists, an organisation devoted to academic anaesthesiology in the United States and which will celebrated its 50th anniversary this May. Dr. Papper died on 2 December 2002 at the age of 87 years.

Nagin PARBHOO

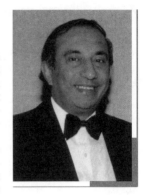

Nagin Parbhoo was born in Wynberg Village (now known as Little Chelsea), Cape Town on 3 May 1942. A recipient of a Cape Town Municipal Bursary, he matriculated from Livingstone High School and then commenced studies at Grant Medical College, University of Bombay, as a holder of a Government of India Scholarship for Medical Studies.

On his return to South Africa, he worked in Port Elizabeth, first in the Livingstone Hospital and later as a general practitioner with a special interest in anaesthetics, an interest that led him to specialise and obtain the FFA (SA) in 1983 and become a full-time specialist on the staff of Groote Schuur Hospital (of Professor Chris Barnard fame), University of Cape Town. Since 1987 he has been in private practice while retaining his connection with Groote Schuur Hospital as a part-time senior lecturer until 1995.

Nagin has been actively involved in the affairs of the South African Society of Anaesthesiologists. In 1987 he was invited to be their Honorary Archivist and in this capacity he has written the society's history in a publication *Five Decades-The SA Society of Anaesthetists 1943-1993*.

Since 1982 he has been keenly involved in historical aspects of anaesthesia and contributed much time and effort to collection of old anaesthetic equipment. The Department of Anaesthesia, University of Cape Town honoured him in March 2000 by naming the collection 'The Nagin Parbhoo Museum of Anaesthesia'.

Nagin was the honorary editor of *Pipeline*, the newsletter of the SA Society of Anaesthesiologists from 1993 to 2001. In December 2002, he was awarded the doctorate MD (UCT) for his thesis on *The Department of Anaesthesia, UCT 1920-2000. A History*.

Carlos Pereira PARSLOE

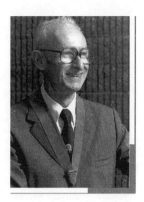

Born in Santos, State of São Paulo, Brasil on 28 November 1919

Education
Graduated from High School in Santos,1935
Medical School, "Faculdade Nacional de Medicina da Universidade do Brasil", Rio de Janeiro, Brasil, Graduation 1943
Internship, Illinois Masonic Hospital in Chicago, 1946
Residency in Anaesthesiology with Professor Ralph Waters, State of Wisconsin General Hospital, University of Wisconsin, Madison, Wisconsin, 1946-1948

Clinical practice
"Santa Casa da Misericórdia Hospital", Santos, from December 1948 to March 1952
Hospital Samaritano, São Paulo, Brasil, 1955 to 2003
Secretary, First Board of Directors, Department of Anaesthesia, Associação Paulista de Medicina (State of São Paulo Medical Association)

Academic association
1952-1954 and 1963, Research Associate, Department of Anaesthesiology, University of Wisconsin Medical School, Madison, Wisconsin, Chairman, Professor O.S. Orth.
Visiting Professor, Department of Anaesthesiology, Medical College of Ohio, Toledo, Ohio, chairman, Professor Lucien E. Morris, 1974

Professional organisations
Brasilian Society of Anaesthesiology, Board of Directors, Member and Chairman, International Affairs Committee for a number of years, Member, Committee for Specialist Title for several years
Editorial Board, *Brasilian Journal of Anesthesiology* (Revista Brasileira de Anestesiologia) for several years
President, State of São Paulo Society of Anaesthesiologists, 1973
Honorary Member, Brasilian Society of Anesthesiology and from the following State Societies of Anesthesiology: Paraná, Rio Grande do Sul, Pernambuco, and Minas Gerais
Benemerit Member, State of São Paulo Society of Anesthesiology
Benemerit Physician, Sociedade Hospital Samaritano, São Paulo
Board of Editors, *Survey of Anesthesiology*, for several years
Confederation of Latin American Societies of Anesthesiology (CLASA) Prize, 1981

Honorary Fellowships
Royal College of Anaesthetists (FRCA), 1986
Australian and New Zealand College of Anaesthetists (ANZCA), 1989
Honorary Member, The Association of Anaesthetists of Great Britain and Ireland (AAGBI), 1989

WFSA activities
Chairman, Scientific Committee, Brasilian Society of Anesthesiology Organising Committee for the Third World Congress of Anaesthesiology, São Paulo, Brasil, 1960-1964
Committee on Education and Scientific Affairs, 1964-1972
Executive Committee, 1972-1980
Vice-President, 1980-1984
President, 1984-1988
Honorary President, 10th World Congress of Anaesthesiologists, the Hague, Holland, 1992

Judith A. ROBINS

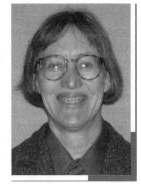

Judith A. Robins earned a Master's degree in history and a Master's degree in Librarianship from the University of Denver, Denver, Colorado, 1984. She has worked as an archivist for Bowling Green State University (Bowling Green, Ohio), Thomas Jefferson University (Philadelphia, Pennsylvania), and the Center for Judaic Studies (Philadelphia, Pennsylvania.) She has also worked as a freelance knowledge assets manager. She has held the position of Collections Supervisor at the Wood Library-Museum of Anesthesiology from 1999 to the present, with responsibility for archives, manuscripts, ephemera and artifacts.

Michael ROSEN

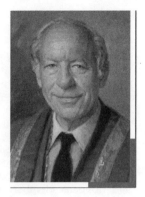

Professor Michael Rosen was born (17-10-27) in Dundee and educated there, graduating at St. Andrews University (1949). After army service in Egypt and Cyprus, he trained at Newcastle with Professor E.A. Pask and in Cardiff with Professor W.W. Mushin. In 1960 he held a Fellowship at Cleveland with Dr. R.A. Hingson. Appointed a consultant anaesthetist in Cardiff in 1961, a study of the use of suction in clinical medicine led to Chairmanship of British Standard Committee for Hospital Vacuum Services and for Dental Services, which are still in existence. He specialised mainly in obstetric anaesthesia and postoperative pain management with over 150 publications and 13 books, including *Central Venous Cannulation* (1981), *Obstetric Anaesthesia and Analgesia* (1982), *Patient-Controlled Analgesia* (1985), *Difficult and Tracheal Intubation* (1985), and *Consciousness Awareness and Pain in General Anaesthetics* (1987).

In 1983 he was elected as Honorary Professor in Anaesthetics, Wales. During the period 1986-1988 he was President of the Association of Anaesthetists of Great Britain and Ireland, and in 1988-1991 President of the College of Anaesthetists (Founding President of the Royal College). In 1989 he was appointed Commander of the British Empire. He is an Honorary Member of French, Australian, Japanese, Malaysian, College and University Anaesthetists Association (USA). He is a Fellow of the Royal College of Surgeons of England, of the Royal College of Obstetrics and Gynaecologists, and Honorary Doctor of Laws (Dundee University).

Joseph RUPREHT

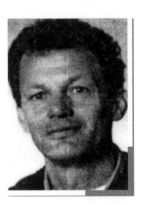

Born: 18th of December, 1946
Place of birth: Slovenia

Education and Profession
Classical gymnasium Celje
Medical studies, Ljubljana
1971-1972: Military service; former JNA.
1973-1977: Anaesthesia residency at Rotterdam.
1982: Organized the 1st International Symposium on the
History of Anaesthesia; Rotterdam.
1993: Honorary Member of Slovenian Society of Anaesthesiologists.
1995: Honorary Extraordinary Professor of Anaesthesia in Ljubljana, Slovenia
1998-2002: Reconstruction of cultivated landscape; 5 km pear tree lane at Wijk en
Aalburg.

Interests
- Lifelong interest in dendrology and landscaping.
- Lifelong service to the academic Anaesthesiology at Rotterdam.
- Served as the first Honorary Archivist of the World Federation of Societies of Anaes-
thesiologists.

Philippe André SCHERPEREEL

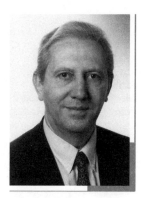

Professor of Anaesthesiology, Chairman of the Department of Anaesthesia and Intensive Care, Lille University Hospital, France

Personal data
Date of birth: 12 August 1940
Place of birth: Roubaix, 59100, France
Citizenship: France
Marital status: Married, three children

Medical education
1958-1965 Lille School of Medicine

Postgraduate training
1965-1970 Interne Lille University Hospital, Cardiology, Pneumology, Nephrology, Endocrinology

Qualifications
MD Thesis 18 June 1970, Lille, France
Registered Medical Council, no. 4950
Specialist qualification in anaesthesiology and intensive care 1975

Professional appointments
1968-1971 Research Assistant, Biochemistry Laboratory
1970-1973 Assistant Professor, Intensive Care Medicine, Calmette Hospital, Lille University Hospital, France
1974-1975 Assistant Professor, Anaesthesiology, Pitié Salpetrière Hospital, Paris, France
1975-1977 Professor, Anaesthesiology and Intensive Care, Lille, University Hospital, France
1978 to present Professor Anaesthesiology and Intensive Care, Chairman Department of Anaesthesiology and Intensive Care, Lille University Hospital, France

Certificates
1968 General Biochemistry, Lille Medical School
1969 Molecular Biochemistry, Lille Medical School
1969 Master of Human Biology, Lille Medical School
1970 Diploma of Research in Human Biology, Lille Medical School

Educational appointments
1971 to present Anaesthesia and Intensive Care (D.E.S.A.R.)
1978 to present National Diploma of Emergency Medicine (CMU) and Disaster Medicine (CMC), Director
1986 to present Evaluation and Treatment of Pain, Lille Medical School

Research
1968-1971 Biochemistry of lipids-CNRS, INSERM
1988 presented Research in medical informatics, European Union programmes (AIM, TANIT)
1993 presented Research in Applied Physiology (CIVIS), Vasoreactivity and tissue oxygenation

Expertise
1985-1995 National Committee of Homologation
1985 to present Expert Clinician
1992 to present Expert in the Court of Justice

Affiliations
French Society of Anaesthesia and Intensive Care (SFAR)
French College of Anaesthesiology
Fellow of the Royal College of Anaesthesiology (FRCA)
Honorary Member of the German Society of Anaesthesiology
French-speaking African (SARANF) Society
Algerian Society
Romanian Society
Italian Society
Polish Society
Member of the Spanish (SEDAR) Society
Member of the International Society of Pain Clinicians (ISCP)
Member of the International Association for Study of Pain (IASP)
Doctor Honoris Causa of the Stradins University of Riga (Latvia)

Committee work
1990-1992 President of the Scientific Committee (SFAR)
1992-1994 President of the French Society of Anaesthesia and Intensive Care (SFAR)
1994-1998 President of the French College of Anaesthesiologists
1993-1997 President of the European Board of Anaesthesiology and of the Section Anaesthesiology of the UEMS
1985-2000 Vice-President of the Foundation for European Education in Anaesthesiology (FEEA)
2000 to present President of the Foundation for European Education in Anaesthesiology (FEEA)
1990-2000 Member of the Senate and of the Executive Committee of the European Academy of Anaesthesiologists (EAA)
1988-2000 Member of the Committee on Publications of the World Federation of Societies of Anaesthesiologists (WFSA)
1996-2000 Member of the Executive Committee (Educational Matters) of the European Academy of Anaesthesiologists (EAA)
1997 to present Member of the National Committee of the Universities (CNU section 48-1)
2000 to present Member of the Executive Committee of the WFSA
2002 President Elect of the Confederation of the European National Societies of Anaesthesiologists (CENSA)
2004 President of the XIII World Congress of Anaesthesiologists (WCA 2004)

Publications
Member of several editorial boards/scientific committees
Participation, examination of MD theses, 560
Communications at meetings, 210
General reviews, 175
Original papers, 146
Editions of books 10

Koki SHIMOJI

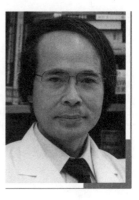

Personal data
Citizenship Status: Japan
Born: Okinawa, Japan (21 November 1935)
Married: Yoko Sano
Children: Yuko (1973), Kaoru (1974)

Education, training, and academic appointments
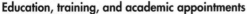
1954-1960: Kumamoto University School of Medicine (MD)
1961-1965: Kyoto University Faculty of Medicine, Graduate School (Dr med Sci)
1965-1966: Instructor, Department of Anaesthesiology, Kyoto University School of Medicine
1966-1967: Mayo Graduate School of Medicine
1968-1973: Associate Professor, Department of Anaesthesiology, Tokyo Medical and Dental University School of Medicine
1973-1974: Associate Professor, Department of Anaesthesiology, Kumamoto University School of Medicine
1974-2001: Professor and Chairman, Department of Anaesthesiology, Niigata University School of Medicine, Director of Intensive Care Unit, University Hospital
1975-2001: Visiting Professor, Yamagata and Yamaguchi University School of Medicine
1981-2001: Visiting Professor, Kyoto University Faculty of Medicine
1988: President, Japan Society of Cerebral Blood Flow and Metabolism
1993-2001: WFSA Pain Committee Member (1998-2001 Chairman)
1994 to present: Member of AUA
1996: President, Jpn Soc EEG and EMG
1997: President, JSA (Jpn Soc of Anesthesiologists)
1997 to present: FRCA
1999 to present: Education Committee Member, JASP
2001 to present: Professor Emeritus, Niigata University
2001: Visiting professor University of London
2001 to present: Visiting professor, Ansted University
2002 to present: Professor, Institute of Neurosciences, Ube Frontier University

Patrick SIM

Patrick Sim, MLS, received his undergraduate degree in history from Truman State University in Kirksville, Missouri, and his Master of Library Science degree from the State University of New York at Albany. He has been Librarian of the Wood Library-Museum of Anesthesiology since 1971.

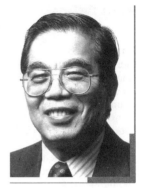

Michael D. VICKERS

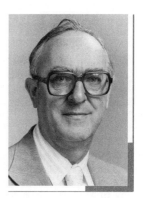

Career in WFSA
Member Scientific Affairs Committee 1976/80
Chairman, Statutes and Bylaws Committee 1980/84
Vice chairman, Executive Committee 1984/88
Chairman, Executive Committee 1988/92
Honorary Secretary 1992/96
President 1996/00

Other Appointments
Professor of Anaesthetics and Intensive Care UWCM,
Cardiff 1976-96
Vice Provost, University of Wales College of Medicine
1992/95
Chairman, North Glamorgan NHS Trust 1996-2000
Hospital & Medical Director, King Khalid Hospital Jeddah 1985-6
President, Association of Anaesthetists of Gt. Britain & Ireland 1982-4
President, European Academy of Anaesthesiology 1988 -91
President, National Association of Theatre Nurses 1976-9

Editorships
European Journal of Anaesthesiology
1984-94
Today's Anaesthetist
1994-2001

Books (Joint author or editor)
Medicine for Anaesthetists, 1ˢᵗ-4ᵗʰ eds (Latest 1999)
Drugs in Anaesthetic Practice, 3ʳᵈ-8ᵗʰ eds (Latest 1999)
Principles of Measurement, 1ˢᵗ-3ʳᵈ eds (Latest 1991)
Anaesthesia: Basic Principles of Education and Training (1994)
Patient Controlled Analgesia (1985)
Ethical Issues in Anaesthesia (1994)
OSCEs for Anaesthetists (1995)

David John WILKINSON

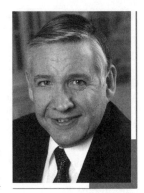

Consultant Anaesthetist, Boyle Department of Anaesthesia, St Bartholomew's Hospital, London EC1A 7BE

Qualifications LRCP. MRCS, MBBS, DRCOG, FRCA, Hon. FCARCSI

1994 to present
Worshipful Society of Apothecaries of London Lecturer in the History of Medicine to St. Bartholomew's Hospital Honorary Member of the Faculty of History and Philosophy of Medicine and Pharmacy, Worshipful Society of Apothecaries of London

2003 to present
Vice President, Association of Anaesthetists of Great Britain and Ireland

2002 to present
President, Confederation of European National Societies of Anaesthesiologists (CENSA)
Academician, European Academy of Anaesthesiology

2000 to present.
Member, Executive Committee, World Federation of Societies of Anaesthesiologists
Chairman, World Federation of Societies of Anaesthesiologists (WFSA) Statutes and Bylaws Committee

1982-1995
Curator of Charles King Collection of Historical Anaesthetic Apparatus, Association of Anaesthetists of Great Britain and Ireland

1994-2001
Honorary Archivist, Association of Anaesthetists of Great Britain and Ireland

1986-1996
Medical Director, Day Surgery Centre, St. Bartholomew's Hospital, London

1996-1998
Honorary Secretary, Association of Anaesthetists of Great Britain and Ireland

1998-2003
Honorary Treasurer, Association of Anaesthetists of Great Britain and Ireland (AAGBI)

1997-2000
Chairman, Department of Anaesthesia, St. Bartholomew's Hospital, London

Author of multiple chapters, papers and presentations on day-stay surgery and history of anaesthesia
Lewis Wright Memorial Lecturer 2003
Visiting Professor to Mayo Clinic, Rochester, Minnesota, USA October 2002
Editor of *Proceedings of the History of Anaesthesia Society* (1986-1993)

John Stanley Mornington ZORAB

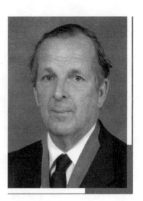

Born: 16-01-1929

Education
Armed Services: Royal Corps of Signals Regiment
Undergraduate: Guy's Hospital (University of London)
1949-1956
Qualification: LRCP (Lon), MRCS (Eng) 1956
DA 1958
FFARCS 1962

Current post
Consultant Anaesthetist Emeritus, Frenchay Hospital, Bristol 1996

Past appointments
World Federation of Societies of Anaesthesiologists
Secretary 1980-1988
President 1988-1992
European Academy of Anaesthesiology
Chairman of Examination Committee 1978-1999

Other
WFSA Newsletter (Editor) 1980-1988
EAA Newsletter (Editor) 1997-2002
Current Opinion in Anaesthesiology (Section Editor) 1999-2002

Abbreviations

AACA, Asian and Australasian Congress of Anaesthesiology
AAGBI, Association of Anaesthesists of Great Britain and Ireland
AARS, Asian/Australasian Regional Section
ABA, American Board of Anesthesiology
ABS, American Board of Surgery
AEF, Anaesthesia Educational Foundation
AMA, American Medical Association
AOSRA, Asian and Oceanic Society of Regional Anesthesia
ARS, African Regional Section
ASA, American Society of Anaesthesiologists
ASRA, American Society of Regional Anesthesia
AUA, Association of University Anaesthetists
CENSA, Confederation of European National Societies of Anaesthesiologists
CESA, Committee on Education and Scientific Affairs
CIOMS, Council for International Organisation of Medical Sciences
CLASA, Confederación Latinoamericana de Sociedades de Anestesiologia
DfID, Department of International Development (UK)
EAA, European Academy of Anaesthesiologists
ECA, European Congress of Anaesthesiology
EDA, European Diploma in Anaesthesiology
EEC, Economic European Community
ERS, European Regional Section
ESA, European Society of Anaesthesiology
ESRA, European Society of Regional Anesthesia
FAR, Federation of Anaesthesiologists and Reanimatologists
FEEA, Foundation for European Education of Anaesthesiology
FUINANAC, Fundación para la Investigatión en Anesthesologia A-C
IARS, International Anesthesia Research Society
IASP, International Society for the Study of Pain
ISA, International Symposium of Anaesthesiology
JMH, Japanese Ministry of Health and Welfare
JSA, Japanese Society of Anaesthesiologists
LASRA, Latin-American Society of Regional Anesthesia
MASA, Medical Association of South Africa
NARS, National Anesthesia Research Society
NGO, Non-Governmental Organization

NYSSA, New York State Society of Anaesthesiologists
OBE, Order of the British Empire
PAHO, Pan-American Health Organisation
PRC, People's Republic of China
PTC, Primary Trauma Care
SAA, Society of Arab Anaesthesiologists
SARANF, Society of Anaesthesia and Intensive Care of Sub-Saharan Africa
SASA, South African Society of Anaesthetists
SFAR, French Society of Anaesthesia and Resuscitation
SIAARTI, Società Italiana di Anestesia, Analgesia, Rianimazione e Terapia Intensiva
UEMS, European Union of Medical Specialists
UNESCO, United Nations Educational, Scientific and Cultural Organisation
UNHDR, United Nations Human Development Report
VETS, Voluntary Educational Teams
WASA, West African Society of Anaesthesiologists
WCA, World Congress of Anaesthesiologists
WFSA, World Federation of Societies of Anaesthesiologists
WHO, World Health Organisation
WMA, World Medical Association

Name index

Publication index

EDITORS' NOTE

*W*e wish to express our gratitude to all the Contributors and to all those who helped in collecting the material for this book: without their invaluable cooperation, the publication of this volume would not have been possible.

We are aware that some photographs appear more than once throughout the book: we considered the possibility of deleting some of them, but we eventually decided to respect the authors' original manuscripts.

The collection of these documents has taken a long time and requested much effort, and though we tried to include the most important stages of WFSA history, it is possible that some information is incomplete or not included. We would therefore like to apologize for any errors or omissions that we have unintentionally made.

Trieste and Rotterdam, March 2004 **A. Gullo**
J. Rupreht